Textbook of
Preclinical Conservative Dentistry

Textbook of
Preclinical Conservative Dentistry

Third Edition

Editors

Nisha Garg
MDS (Conservative Dentistry and Endodontics)
Professor
Department of Conservative Dentistry and Endodontics
Bhojia Dental College and Hospital
Baddi, Himachal Pradesh, India

Amit Garg
MDS (Oral and Maxillofacial Surgery)
Dean Academics
Professor and Head
Department of Oral and Maxillofacial Surgery
BRS Dental College and Hospital
Panchkula, Haryana, India

Foreword
Mahesh Verma

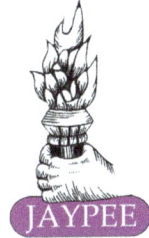

JAYPEE BROTHERS MEDICAL PUBLISHERS

The Health Sciences Publisher

New Delhi | London

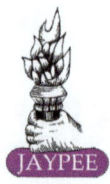

Jaypee Brothers Medical Publishers (P) Ltd

Headquarters
Jaypee Brothers Medical Publishers (P) Ltd
EMCA House, 23/23-B
Ansari Road, Daryaganj
New Delhi 110002, India
Landline: +91-11-23272143, +91-11-23272703
+91-11-23282021, +91-11-23245672
Email: jaypee@jaypeebrothers.com

Corporate Office
Jaypee Brothers Medical Publishers (P) Ltd
4838/24, Ansari Road, Daryaganj
New Delhi 110 002, India
Phone: +91-11-43574357
Fax: +91-11-43574314
Email: jaypee@jaypeebrothers.com

Overseas Office
J.P. Medical Ltd
83 Victoria Street, London
SW1H 0HW (UK)
Phone: +44 20 3170 8910
Fax: +44 (0)20 3008 6180
Email: info@jpmedpub.com

Website: www.jaypeebrothers.com
Website: www.jaypeedigital.com

© 2022, Jaypee Brothers Medical Publishers

The views and opinions expressed in this book are solely those of the original contributor(s)/author(s) and do not necessarily represent those of editor(s) of the book.

All rights reserved. No part of this publication may be reproduced, stored or transmitted in any form or by any means, electronic, mechanical, photocopying, recording or otherwise, without the prior permission in writing of the publishers.

All brand names and product names used in this book are trade names, service marks, trademarks or registered trademarks of their respective owners. The publisher is not associated with any product or vendor mentioned in this book.

Medical knowledge and practice change constantly. This book is designed to provide accurate, authoritative information about the subject matter in question. However, readers are advised to check the most current information available on procedures included and check information from the manufacturer of each product to be administered, to verify the recommended dose, formula, method and duration of administration, adverse effects and contraindications. It is the responsibility of the practitioner to take all appropriate safety precautions. Neither the publisher nor the author(s)/editor(s) assume any liability for any injury and/or damage to persons or property arising from or related to use of material in this book.

This book is sold on the understanding that the publisher is not engaged in providing professional medical services. If such advice or services are required, the services of a competent medical professional should be sought.

Every effort has been made where necessary to contact holders of copyright to obtain permission to reproduce copyright material. If any have been inadvertently overlooked, the publisher will be pleased to make the necessary arrangements at the first opportunity.

Inquiries for bulk sales may be solicited at: jaypee@jaypeebrothers.com

Textbook of Preclinical Conservative Dentistry

First Edition: 2013
Second Edition: 2017
Third Edition: *2022*

ISBN: 978-93-5465-485-5

Dedicated to

Prisha
and
Vedant

Contributors

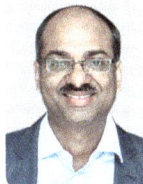

Amit Garg MDS
Dean Academics
Professor and Head
Department of Oral and
Maxillofacial Surgery
BRS Dental College and Hospital
Panchkula, Haryana, India

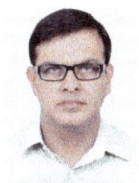

JS Mann MDS
Professor
Department of Conservative
Dentistry and Endodontics
Government Dental College and Hospital
Patiala, Punjab, India

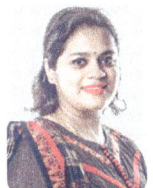

Lora Mishra MDS
Professor
Department of Conservative
Dentistry and Endodontics
Faculty of Institute of Dental Sciences
Siksha 'O' Anusandhan
Bhubaneswar, Odisha, India

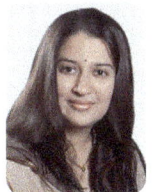

Mahima Tilakchand MDS
Professor
Department of Conservative
Dentistry and Endodontics
SDM College of Dental Sciences
Dharwad, Karnataka, India

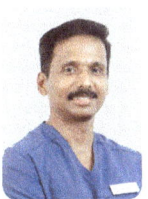

Mohan Bhuvaneswaran MDS
Director
Vignesh Dental Hospital
Chennai, Tamil Nadu, India

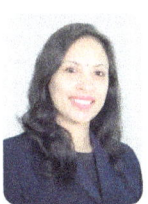

Nisha Garg MDS
Professor
Department of Conservative
Dentistry and Endodontics
Bhojia Dental College and Hospital
Baddi, Himachal Pradesh, India

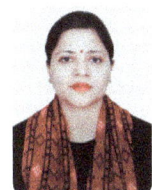

Neetu Jindal MDS
Professor and Head
Department of Conservative
Dentistry and Endodontics
Surendera Dental College and
Research Institute
Sri Ganganagar, Rajasthan, India

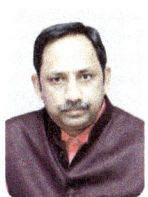

P Karunakar MDS
Principal
Professor and Head
Department of Conservative
Dentistry and Endodontics
Panineeya Institute of Dental Sciences and
Research Center
Hyderabad, Telangana, India

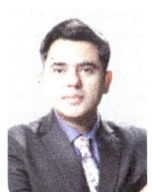

Prashant Bhasin MDS
Professor and Head
Department of Conservative
Dentistry and Endodontics
Sudha Rastogi Dental College and Hospital
Faridabad, Haryana, India

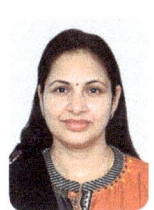

Renu Aggarwal MDS
Professor
Department of Conservative
Dentistry and Endodontics
Surendera Dental College and Research
Institute
Sri Ganganagar, Rajasthan, India

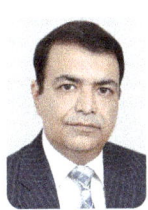

Sanjay Miglani MDS FISDR PHD
Professor and Head
Department of Conservative
Dentistry and Endodontics
Faculty of Dentistry Jamia Millia Islamia
New Delhi, India

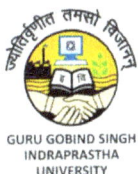

Prof. (Dr.) Mahesh Verma
प्रो. (डॉ.) महेश वर्मा

MDS, MBA, PhD, FDSRCS (Eng),
FDSRCS (Edin) FDS RCPSG (Glas)

Padma Shri Awardee
Dr. B. C. Roy Awardee
National Science & Technology Awardee

Vice Chancellor

Foreword

In the recent years there is clearly upsurge of advancement in the basic and clinical sciences especially in the field of Conservative Dentistry and Endodontics which has brought in numerous innovations and improvements in the practice of Dentistry. It has also become a mainstay and major chunk of dental practice for every practitioner today. Acquainting hands-on skills and correlating it with anatomy, use of materials, handling instruments in Preclinical Conservative Dentistry goes a long way in providing strong foundation for every dental student. Besides, before a dental student is exposed to clinical setup, he should also be familiar with basic etiquettes and operatory management for not only successful outcome but greater patient satisfaction. The Editors of the book Dr Nisha Garg and Dr Amit Garg has very painstakingly compiled all these information in the *"Textbook of Preclinical Conservative Dentistry"*. The publishing of third edition of the book in a short span is a testimony of its useful acceptance and popularity amongst students widely.

A dedicated efforts has been put in by the contributing authors in systematically sectioning the book into 12 chapters covering varied range of topics from fundamental to acquiring skills in preparations and material management. Most of the contributors are senior faculty and domain experts having brought collective excellence which is the hallmark of the textbook. The contributors have covered these topics in a simple language, illustrations diagrams and interpretation of real photographs to make it user friendly and attractive.

The text would be extremely useful in preparing the students with sequence of procedures carried out in practice making learning very easy. The undergraduate students would find the updated contents in the present edition very easy to assimilate preparing them well for clinical practice.

I congratulate all the contributors and wish many more editions of the publications.

Prof (Dr) Mahesh Verma

Preface to the Third Edition

Coming with the 3rd edition of the *Textbook of Preclinical Conservative Dentistry*, we would like to express our appreciation in a kind manner for the previous editions that were accepted by dental students across the country. We begin with thanking God, who gave us the power to believe in our passion and pursue our dreams. We wouldn't have achieved this without having faith in you, Almighty.

The scope of the 3rd edition is basically simple yet comprehensive which serves as an introductory for dental students. This book covers basic tooth anatomy, cutting instruments, principles of tooth preparation, dental materials and their manipulation so as to have fundamental knowledge before handling patients in clinics.

Emphasis is laid upon the language, which is simple, understandable and exclusively designed for beginners in conservative dentistry. The line diagrams are an expressive interpretation of tooth preparation procedures, which are worked upon and simplified to render a more comparable form to real photographs.

In an attempt to improve the book for better clarification of the subject, many eminent personalities were invited to edit and put down the important chapters in the form of text and photographs. We are grateful to Dr P Karunakar, Dr Lora Mishra, Dr Mahima Tilakchand, Dr Mohan Bhuvaneswaran, Dr Prashant Bhasin, Dr Sanjay Miglani for providing us photographs related to preclinical and clinical work for better understanding of the subject.

We fall short of words for Dr JS Mann, Dr Neetu Jindal, Dr Renu Aggarwal for critically evaluating the chapters and bringing them in their best form.

We offer our humble gratitude and sincere thanks to Mr Vikram Bhojia (Secretary, Bhojia Trust) for providing a healthy and encouraging environment for our work.

We would like to express our thanks to our colleagues for their 'ready to help' attitude, constant guidance and positive criticism which helped in the improvement of the book.

We are grateful to Hu-Friedy, GC Fuji, Coltene Whaledent and Dentsply for using their images in our book.

We hope that all these modifications will be appreciated and it yields a book that is valuable for preclinical dentistry.

We thank Shri Jitendar P Vij (Group Chairman), Mr Ankit Vij (Managing Director), Mr MS Mani (Group President), Dr Madhu Choudhary (Publishing Head–Education), Ms Pooja Bhandari (Production Head), Dr Astha Sawhney (Development Editor), Mr Rajesh Sharma (Production Coordinator), Ms Seema Dogra (Cover Visualizer), Mr Binay Kumar (Proofreader), Mr Deep Kumar (Typesetter), Md Sohail (Graphic Designer) and their team members, for showing personal interest and trying to give their level best to create the book as it is now.

We shall be grateful to our readers if they critically analyze the text and send us useful suggestions to improve the quality of the book for next edition.

More info:
https://www.youtube.com/channel/UCFAshHeRKl170TMg6wvcSPw
Instagram account: nisha.garg.311
"Nisha Garg dental academy" app available on play store/app store.
For any query, WhatsApp at 9876160546

Nisha Garg
Amit Garg

Preface to the First Edition

Operative dentistry is one of the oldest branches of dental sciences forming the central part of dentistry as practiced in primary care. It occupies the use of majority of dentist's working life and is a key component of restorative dentistry. The subject and clinical practice of conservative dentistry continues to evolve rapidly as a result of improved understanding of etiology, prevention and management of common dental diseases. The advances and developments within the last two decades have drastically changed the scope of this subject. But before taking professional training, gathering basic knowledge along with operating skill is mandatory.

The main objective of this book is to provide students with the knowledge required while they are developing necessary clinical skills and attitude in their undergraduate training in conservative dentistry and endodontics. We have tried to cover wide topics like morphology of teeth, cariology, different techniques, instruments and materials available for restorations of teeth along with the basics of endodontics.

So we can say that after going through this book, the student should be able to:
- Sit properly while operating and be able to organize their operating environment efficiently
- Understand the morphology of teeth and differentiate one tooth from another
- Chart teeth
- Understand basics of cariology, its prevention and conservative management
- Tell indications and contraindications of different dental materials
- Apply modern pulp protective regimens
- Select suitable restorative materials for restoration of teeth
- Understand the basics of endodontic treatment like what are the indications of endodontic treatment, basic instruments, access preparation, biomechanical preparation and obturation of root canal system.

Nisha Garg
Amit Garg

Contents

1. **Introduction to Preclinical Conservative Dentistry** 1
   - Need for preclinical conservative dentistry 1
   - Causes of loss of tooth substance 1
   - Objectives of operative dentistry 1
   - Objectives of preclinical conservative dentistry 3
   - Armamentarium 3
   - Preclinical tooth preparations 3
   - Shortcomings of preclinical practice 4
   - Scope of operative dentistry 4

2. **Tooth Nomenclature, Morphology, Anatomy and Physiology** 6
   - The crown and root 6
   - Elevations present on a crown 7
   - Depressions present on teeth 8
   - Other important terms 9
   - Nomenclature of teeth 9
   - Histological structures of teeth 12
   - Enamel 12
   - Functions of enamel 13
   - Dentin 13
   - Dental pulp 14
   - Periradicular tissue 15
   - Functions of teeth 15
   - Physiology form of the teeth 16
   - Conclusion 18
   - Morphology of individual teeth 18

3. **Carious and Non-carious Lesions of Teeth** 26
   - Etiology of dental caries 26
   - Classification of dental caries 27
   - Histopathology of dental caries 29
   - Diagnosis of dental caries 30
   - Recent methods of caries detection 30
   - Caries risk assessment 30
   - Prevention of dental caries 30
   - Noncarious lesions of teeth 31
   - Attrition 31
   - Abrasion 31
   - Erosion 32
   - Abfraction 32
   - Localized nonhereditary enamel hypoplasia 33
   - Localized nonhereditary enamel hypocalcification 33
   - Localized nonhereditary dentin hypoplasia 33
   - Localized nonhereditary dentin hypocalcification 34

4. **Dental Materials** 36
   - Classification of dental materials 36
   - Properties of dental materials to be considered 36
   - Dental cements 36
   - Zinc oxide-eugenol cement 37
   - Ethoxybenzoic acid reinforced cement 37
   - Polymer reinforced zinc oxide-eugenol cement 37
   - Zinc phosphate cement 38
   - Zinc silicophosphate cements 39
   - Calcium hydroxide 39
   - Zinc polycarboxylate cement/zinc polyacrylate cement 40
   - Glass ionomer cements 41
   - Composition 41
   - Setting reaction of glass ionomer cement 42
   - Dental amalgam 44
   - Clinical considerations 47
   - Steps to reduce mercury exposure in the dental clinic 48
   - Adhesive dentistry 48
   - Definitions 48
   - Enamel bonding 48
   - Dentin bonding 49
   - Evolution of dentin-bonding agents 49
   - Composites 50
   - Classification of composites 52
   - Cast metal alloys 53
   - Components of cast gold alloys 53
   - Classification of cast gold alloys 53
   - Waxes 54

5. **Instruments Used in Operative Dentistry** ... 58
   - Materials used for manufacturing cutting instruments 58
   - Classification 58
   - Nomenclature by GV Black 58
   - Parts of hand cutting instruments 59
   - Instrument formula 59
   - Different instrument designs 60
   - Description of various instruments 61
   - Hand cutting instruments 62
   - Restorative instruments 64
   - Instrument grasps 66
   - Finger rests 67
   - Methods of use of instruments 68
   - Rotary cutting instruments 68
   - Handpieces 68
   - Dental burs 68
   - Diamond abrasive instruments 70

- Matricing   71
- Matrix   71
- Classification   71
- Tofflemire universal matrix band retainer (designed by Dr BR tofflemire)   72
- Separation of teeth   73

6. Chair Position and Dental Operatory 80
- Operating stool   80
- Considerations for dentists while treating patients   80
- Dental chair positions   81
- Antisepsis in clinics   81
- Definitions   82
- Universal precautions   82
- Sterilization of dental handpiece   82
- COVID-19 and dentistry   82

7. Principles of Tooth Preparation 89
- Terminology   89
- Number of line and point angles in different tooth preparations   90
- GV Black's classification of tooth preparation   91
- Stages of cavity preparation   92
- Initial cavity preparation stage   92
- Final stages of tooth preparation   95

8. Tooth Preparation for Amalgam Restorations 106
- Class I cavity preparation for silver amalgam   106
- Class II cavity preparation for amalgam restoration   109
- Reverse curve   111
- Class III cavity preparation for amalgam restoration   112
- Class V cavity preparation   113

9. Tooth Preparation for Direct Composite Resin and Glass Ionomer Cements 117
- General principles for tooth preparation for composite restorations   117
- Steps of composite restoration on teeth   117
- Repair of composite restorations   121
- Tooth preparation for glass ionomer restoration   121
- Steps for placement of glass ionomer cement (GIC)   123

10. Cast Metal Restorations 126
- Steps of inlay preparation   126
- Cavity preparation for class II gold inlays   126
- Wax pattern fabrication   128
- Spruing the wax pattern   128
- Washing of wax pattern   129
- Investing the wax pattern   129
- Burnout of wax pattern/wax elimination and heating   130
- Casting machines   131
- Melting the alloy   131
- Trying in the casting   133
- Cementation of the casting   133

11. Basics of Endodontics 136
- Etiology of pulpal diseases   137
- Progression of pulpal pathologies   137
- Endodontic instruments   137
- Access cavity preparation   139
- Access cavity of anterior teeth   139
- Access cavity preparation for premolars   139
- Working length determination   140
- Significance of working length   141
- Irrigation of root canal system   142
- Cleaning and shaping   142
- Basic principles of canal instrumentation   142
- Techniques of root canal preparation   143

12. Examination Spotters 145
- Instruments   145
- Materials   154

Glossary *161*
Index *167*

Introduction to Preclinical Conservative Dentistry

Chapter Outline

- Need for preclinical conservative dentistry
- Causes of loss of tooth substance
- Objectives of operative dentistry
- Objectives of preclinical conservative dentistry
- Armamentarium
- Preclinical tooth preparations
- Shortcomings of preclinical practice
- Scope of operative dentistry

DEFINITIONS

Sturdevant—"**Operative dentistry** is defined as art and science of diagnosis, treatment planning and prognosis of defects of the teeth that do not require full coverage restorations for correction. Such treatment should result in the restoration of proper form, function and esthetics while maintaining the physiologic integrity of the teeth in harmonious relationship with the adjacent hard and soft tissues, all of which should enhance the general health and welfare of the patient".

Mosby's dental dictionary—"**Operative dentistry** deals with the functional and esthetic restoration of the hard tissues of individual teeth".

It plays an important role in enhancing dental health and now branched into dental specialties. But before practicing operative dentistry, one should understand the concept of tooth preparation because operative dentistry deals with diagnosis, prevention, interception and restoration of the defects of natural teeth.

Preclinical operative dentistry is a branch of operative dentistry where practical training is given for tooth preparation and restoration of teeth with various materials on dummy models in simulated oral environment.

NEED FOR PRECLINICAL CONSERVATIVE DENTISTRY

As we know oral cavity is a small area which consist of lips, cheeks, palate and a mobile tongue. To do tooth preparation in this area, a great skill is required. So, in order to have proper understanding of anatomical and dimensional considerations, it is always recommended to do tooth preparations on artificial acrylic teeth called typhodont teeth. Typhodont teeth are screwed on to the phantom head. By doing tooth preparation in dummy models, a person is able to juxtapose his acquired skill in clinical patient easily. Repeated tooth preparations in extracted natural teeth increase the skill and efficiency of the person. Moreover, this training increases the confidence and psychomotor skills for handling tissues.

Basic purpose of preclinical conservative dentistry is to make the students to gain expertise for restorative procedures before handling the patient. This develops confidence in the student before they manage the patient.

CAUSES OF LOSS OF TOOTH SUBSTANCE

- Dental caries (**Fig. 1.1**)
- Noncarious loss of tooth structure; attrition (**Figs. 1.2A and B**), abrasion (**Fig. 1.3**) and erosion (**Fig. 1.4**)
- Traumatized or fractured teeth (**Fig. 1.5**)
- Esthetic improvement (**Fig. 1.6**)
- Replacement or repair of restoration (**Fig. 1.7**)
- Developmental defects (**Fig. 1.8**).

OBJECTIVES OF OPERATIVE DENTISTRY

Following are the objectives of operative dentistry:

Diagnosis

Diagnosis is determination of nature of disease, injury or other defect by examination, test and investigation.

Prevention

It includes the procedures done for prevention before the manifestation of any sign and symptom of the disease.

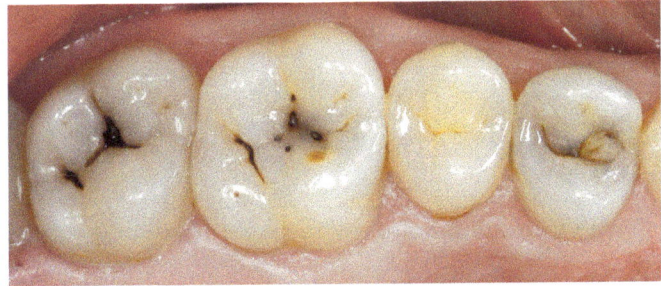

FIGURE 1.1: Clinical picture showing pit and fissure caries in premolar.

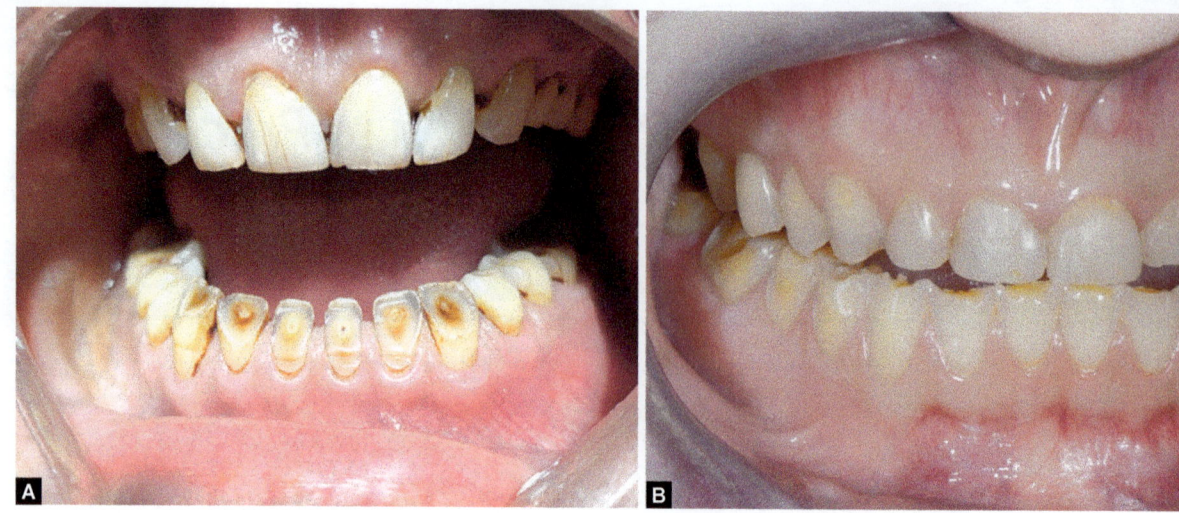

FIGURES 1.2A AND B: Clinical picture showing generalized attrition of mandibular anterior teeth.

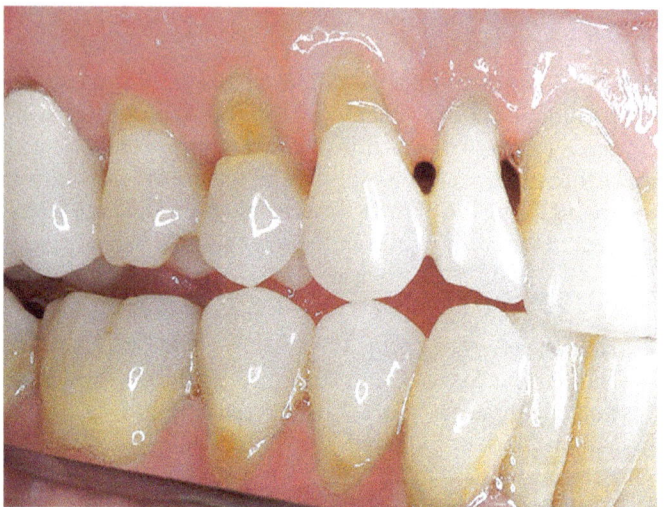

FIGURE 1.3: Clinical picture showing generalized abrasion of teeth.

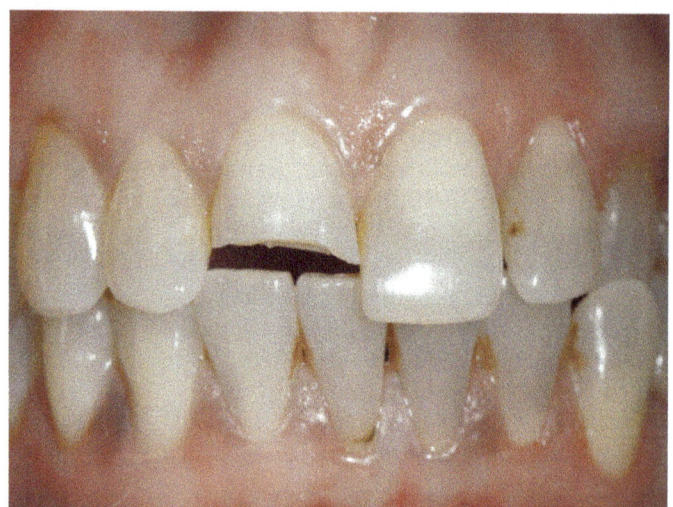

FIGURE 1.5: Clinical picture showing fractured central incisor which can be corrected by esthetic treatment.

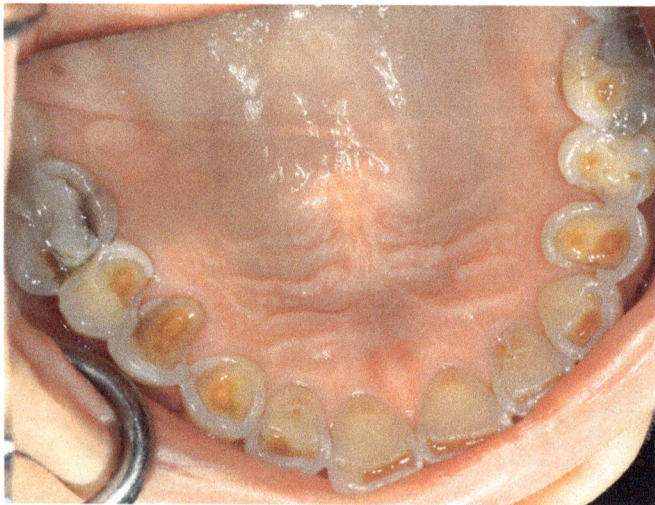

FIGURE 1.4: Clinical picture showing generalized erosion of maxillary anterior teeth.

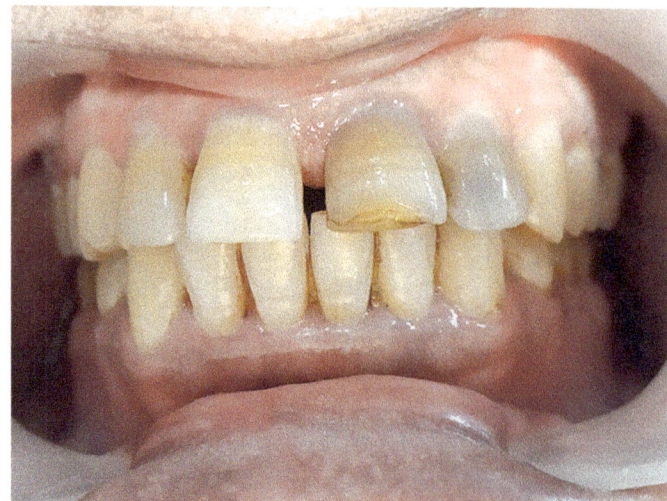

FIGURE 1.6: Clinical picture showing spacing between teeth which can be corrected by restorative procedures.

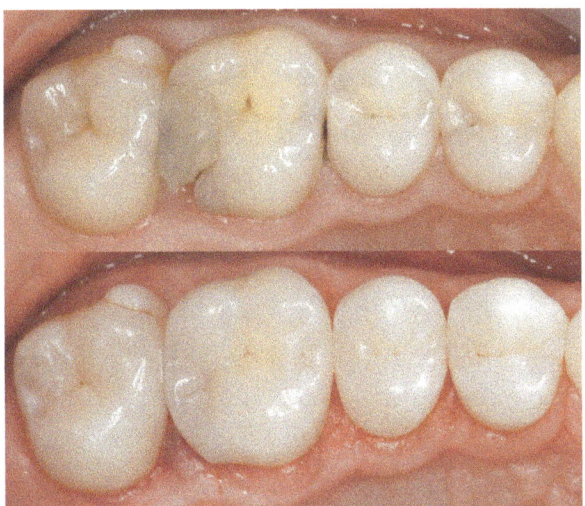

FIGURE 1.7: Clinical picture showing fractured composite restoration requiring replacement.

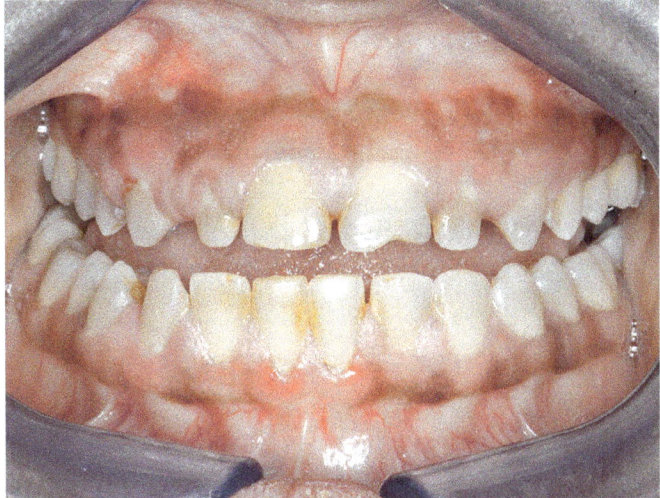

FIGURE 1.8: Clinical picture showing intrinsic discoloration of teeth which can be corrected by esthetic restorations.

Interception

It includes the procedures undertaken to prevent the disease from developing into a more serious or full extent.

Preservation

Preservation of the vitality and periodontal support of remaining tooth structure is obtained by preventive and interceptive procedures.

Restoration

It includes restoring form, function, phonetics and esthetics.

Maintenance

After restoration is done, it must be maintained for providing service for longer duration.

OBJECTIVES OF PRECLINICAL CONSERVATIVE DENTISTRY

- To have knowledge about anatomy of teeth
- To gain expertise for restorative procedures before handling the patient in simulated clinical conditions
- To gain expertise for restorative procedures before handling the patient by performing restorative procedures in simulated clinical conditions
- To gain expertise for manipulation of different dental materials
- To have knowledge of different instruments used in restorative dentistry
- To understand the fundamentals of tooth preparation.

ARMAMENTARIUM

Armamentarium (instruments) used in preclinical conservative dentistry should be arranged as following **(Fig. 1.9)**:

- **Exploring instruments:** Mouth mirror, straight probe, explorer and tweezers
- **Excavating instrument:** Spoon excavator
- **Cutting instruments:** Chisel, hatchet, gingival marginal trimmer and hoes
- **Mixing instruments:** Cement mixing spatula, mortar and pestle
- **Restoring instrument:** Plastic filling instrument, amalgam carrier, teflon-coated instruments
- **Condensers:** Round and parallelogram condenser
- **Carvers:** Diamond shaped (Frahm's), Hollenback's carver
- **Ball burnishers:** Egg shaped, ball shaped, beaver tail shaped, apple shaped, conical, bullet shaped, fish tail or hourglass shaped
- **Others:** Glass slab, Ivory no. 1 and 8 retainers and bands, Tofflemire retainer and bands, wedges, dappen dish
- Contrangle micromotor handpiece, round, straight, tapered, inverted cone diamond points.

PRECLINICAL TOOTH PREPARATIONS

Tooth Preparations on Plaster Models

Before going for tooth preparation on typhodonts or extracted teeth, it is advisable to practice on plaster models. These plaster models are prepared by pouring plaster of Paris in readymade tooth moulds. Students practice class I to V tooth preparations on these models. Working on plaster models have many advantages. Students can understand concept of tooth preparation better on bigger models. Outline form, line and point angles, convergence of walls, and carving can be understood in a better way on plaster models **(Figs. 1.10A to C)**. By these, student can easily replicate tooth preparations on typhodonts and extracted teeth.

Tooth Preparations on Typhodonts

Before going for tooth preparation in patient's mouth, it is always advisable to practice all types of tooth preparations on typhodonts and extracted teeth. Typhodonts are artificial acrylic teeth mounted on maxillary and mandibular arches which can be fixed to human-shaped rubber faces to simulate the oral cavities. Typhodonts can also be mounted separately on plaster moulds or blocks **(Fig. 1.10D)**. Typhodonts are advantageous because of their easy

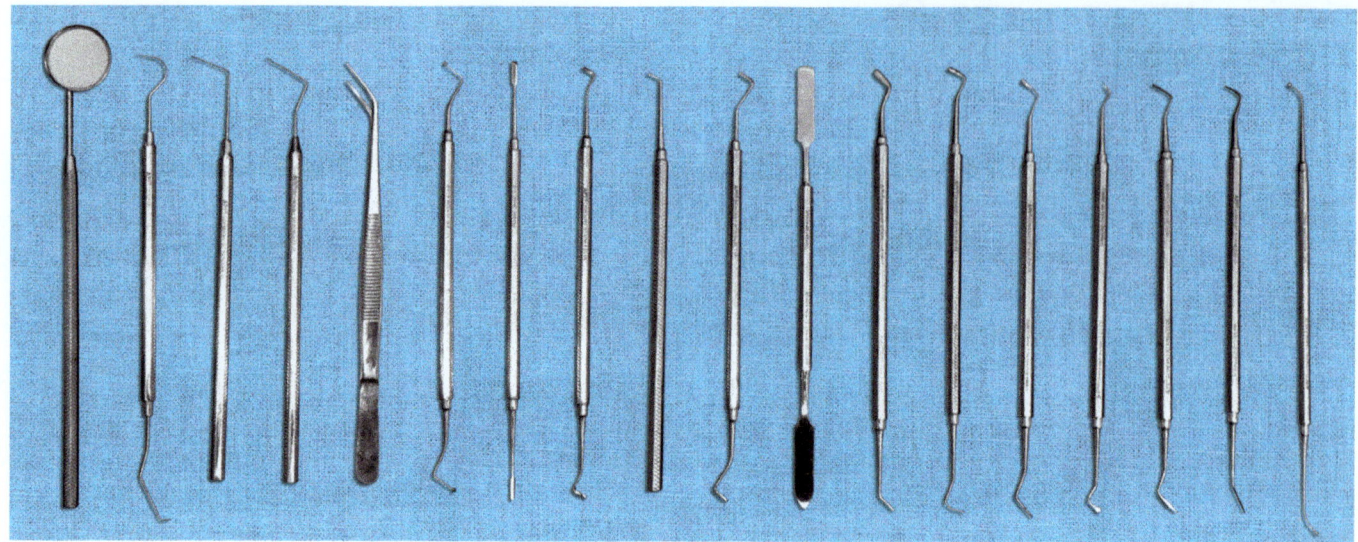

FIGURE 1.9: Photograph showing armamentarium required for restorative procedures.

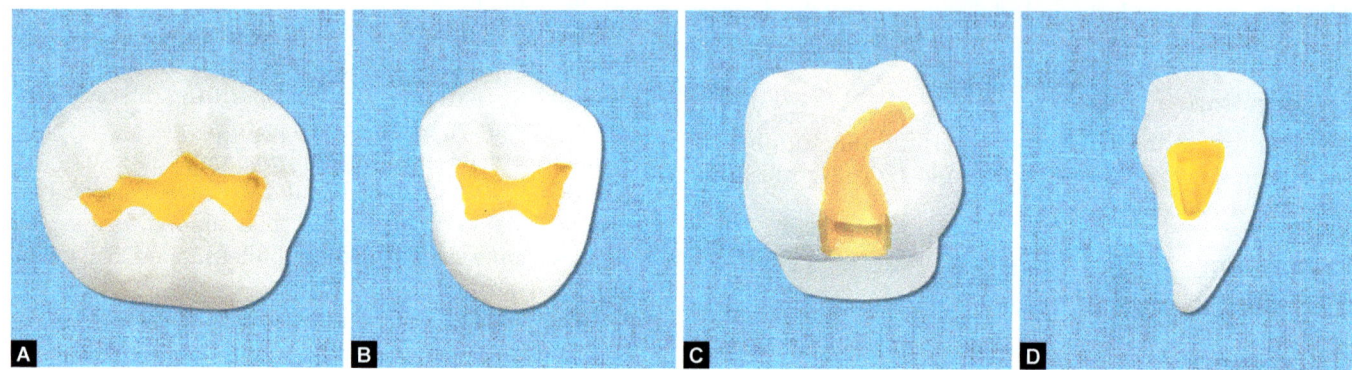

FIGURES 1.10A TO D: Photograph showing Class I and II and III tooth preparations on plaster model.

accessibility, availability in anatomical forms. But these have disadvantages like:
- There is no separation between enamel and dentin
- Because of their softness they get cut very fast.

Tooth Preparations on Extracted Teeth

After performing tooth preparations on plaster models and typhodonts, students are advised to practice on extracted natural teeth. These teeth should be mounted in plaster blocks or phantom jaws. These teeth have advantages over typhodonts because being natural, these show differentiation of enamel and dentin. But these teeth carry risk of contamination and they are not easily available.

SHORTCOMINGS OF PRECLINICAL PRACTICE

- Knowledge of saliva control and isolation cannot be experienced in preclinical work
- One cannot be familiar with tongue interference which is common while working on mandibular arch
- Retraction of soft tissues is completely different in patients
- Patient anxiety and apprehension cannot be experienced with mannequins.

SCOPE OF OPERATIVE DENTISTRY

- To have knowledge of dental anatomy and histology
- To understand the effect of the operative procedures on the treatment of other disciplines
- To know condition of the affected tooth and other teeth
- To examine not only the affected tooth but also oral and systemic health of the patient
- Provide optimal treatment plan to restore the tooth to return to health and function and increase the overall well-being of the patient
- Thorough knowledge of dental materials which can be used to restore the affected areas
- To understand the biological basis and function of various tooth tissues
- To maintain the pulp vitality and prevent occurrence of pulpal pathology.

VIVA QUESTIONS

Q.1 What is preclinical operative dentistry?

Ans. Preclinical operative dentistry is a branch of operative dentistry where practical training is given for tooth preparation and restoration of teeth with various materials on dummy models in simulated oral environment.

Q.2 Define operative dentistry?

Ans. According to Sturdevent, "operative dentistry is defined as science and art of dentistry which deals with diagnosis, treatment and prognosis of defects of the teeth which do not require full coverage restorations for correction". Such corrections and restorations result in the restoration of proper tooth form, function and esthetics while maintaining the physiological integrity of the teeth in harmonious relationship with the adjacent hard and soft tissues.

Q.3 Why is subject preclinical operative dentistry important?

Ans. Since, oral cavity is a small area which consist of lips, cheeks, palate, and a mobile tongue. To do tooth preparation in this area, a great skill is required. Repeated tooth preparation in extracted natural teeth increases the skill and efficiency of the person.

Q.4 Why should one practice on dummy models before doing patients?

Ans. By doing tooth preparation in dummy models, a person is able to juxtapose his acquired skill in clinical patient easily. Moreover, this training increases the confidence and psychomotor skills for handling tissues.

Q.5 What are different causes of loss of tooth structure?

Ans.
- Caries
- Noncarious loss of the tooth structure
- Malformed, traumatized, or fractured teeth
- Esthetic improvement
- Replacement or repair of restoration
- Developmental defects.

Chapter 2

Tooth Nomenclature, Morphology, Anatomy and Physiology

Chapter Outline

- The crown and root
- Elevations present on a crown
- Depressions present on teeth
- Other important terms
- Nomenclature of teeth
- Histological structures of teeth
- Enamel
- Functions of enamel
- Dentin
- Dental pulp
- Periradicular tissue
- Functions of teeth
- Physiology form of the teeth
- Morphology of individual teeth

In humans, teeth are present in jaws. There are two jaws, the term **mandibular** refers to the lower jaw, or mandible, the term **maxillary** refers to the upper jaw, or maxilla.

THE CROWN AND ROOT (FIGS. 2.1A AND B)

- **Crown:** Crown is covered with enamel
- **Root:** Root is covered with cementum
- **Cemento-enamel junction (CEJ):** The crown and root join at the cemento-enamel junction (CEJ). This junction is also called as the cervical line.

For purposes of description, the crowns and roots of teeth have been divided into thirds and these thirds are named according to their location.

Crown can be divided into thirds in three directions **(Fig. 2.2)**:
1. **Occluso-cervically:** Crown is divided into an incisal or occlusal third, a middle third, and a cervical third
2. **Mesiodistally:** Mesial, middle, and distal thirds
3. **Buccolingually:** Buccal, middle, and lingual thirds.

Root can be divided into thirds as cervical, middle third, and apical third.

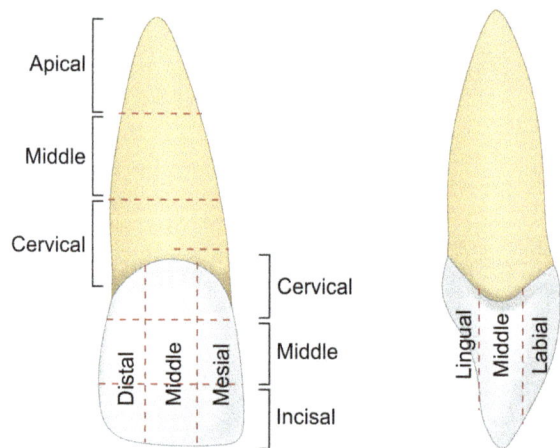

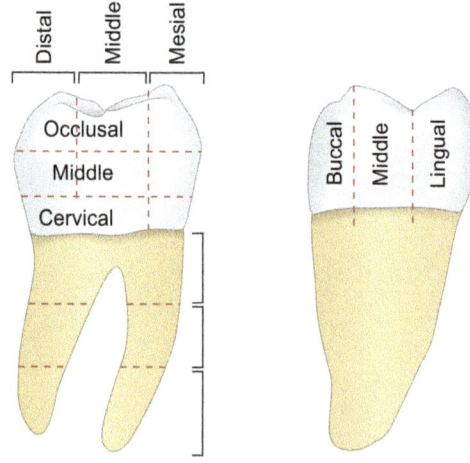

FIGURE 2.2: Division of crown and root in their respective thirds.

FIGURES 2.1A AND B: Schematic representation showing crown, root and CEJ.

Tooth Nomenclature, Morphology, Anatomy and Physiology

ELEVATIONS PRESENT ON A CROWN

Lobe (Fig. 2.3A)
A lobe is one of the primary sections of formation in the development of the crown. Cusps and mamelons are representative of lobes.

Mamelons (Fig. 2.3B)
These are small rounded projections on incisal surfaces of newly erupted incisors.

Cingulum (Fig. 2.3C)
It is the lingual lobe of an anterior tooth. It makes up the bulk of the cervical third of the lingual surface.

Cusp (Fig. 2.3D)
A cusp is an elevation on the crown portion of a tooth making up a divisional part of the occlusal surface.

Ridge (Fig. 2.3E)
Ridge is any linear elevation on the surface of a tooth and is named according to its location.

Marginal ridges: These are those rounded borders of the enamel that form the mesial and distal margins of the occlusal surfaces of premolars and molars and the mesial and distal margins of the lingual surfaces of the incisors and canines.

Triangular ridges: Triangular ridges descend from the tips of the cusps of molars and premolars toward the central part of the occlusal surfaces. They are so named because the slopes of each side of the ridge are inclined to resemble two sides of a triangle. They are named after the cusps to which they belong, e.g., the triangular ridge of the buccal cusp of the maxillary first premolar.

Transverse ridge: A transverse ridge is the union of two triangular ridges crossing transversely the surface of a posterior tooth.

Oblique ridge: The oblique ridge is a ridge crossing obliquely the occlusal surfaces of maxillary molars and formed by the union of the triangular ridge of the distobuccal cusp and the distal cusp ridge of the mesiolingual cusp.

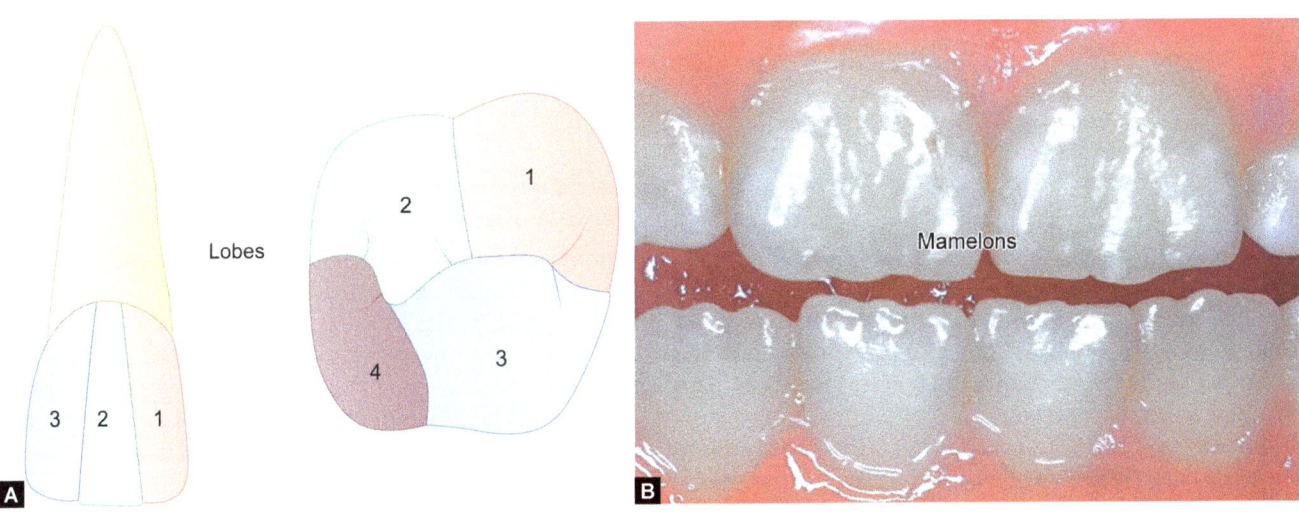

FIGURES 2.3A AND B: (A) Lobes; (B) Mamelons.

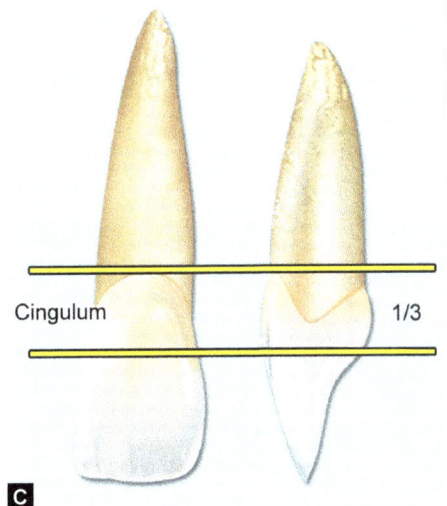
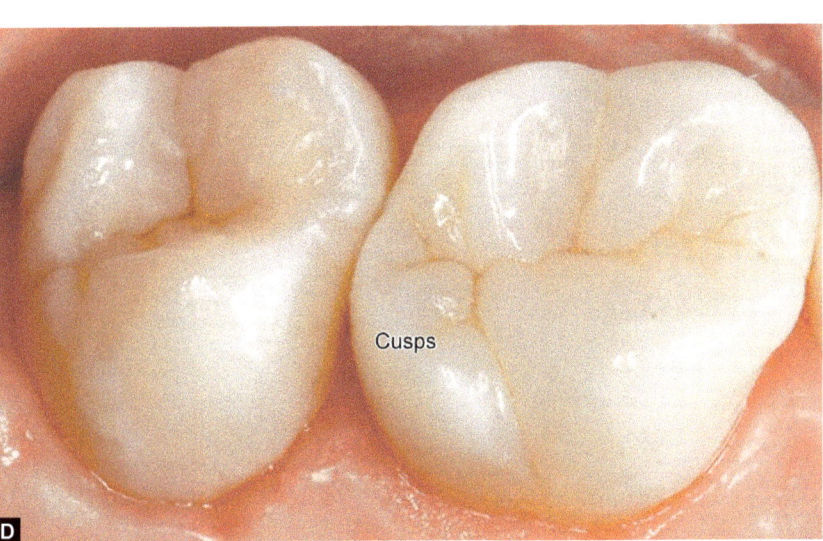

FIGURES 2.3C AND D: (C) Cingulum; (D) Cusps.

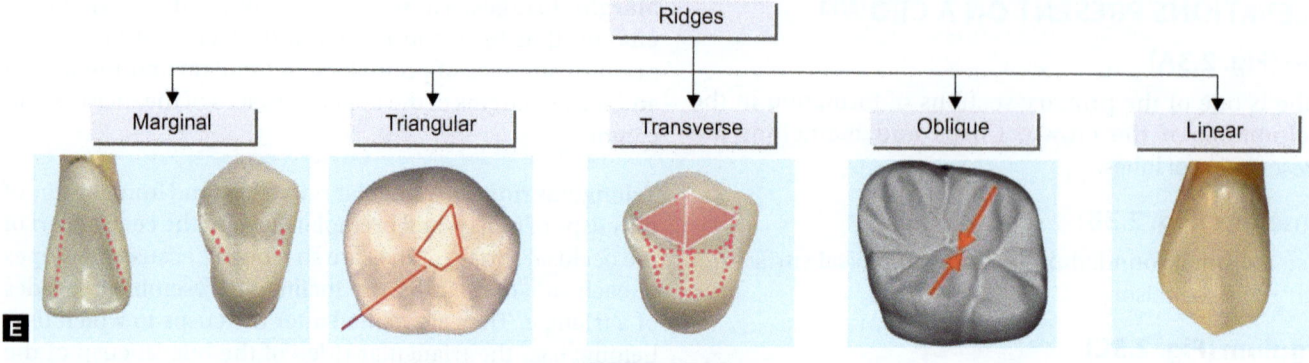

FIGURE 2.3E: Ridges.

DEPRESSIONS PRESENT ON TEETH (FIG. 2.4)

Pit: It is a sharp pin point depression on the surface of enamel.

Fossa: It is an irregular depression on the surface of tooth.

Central fossae: Central fossae are formed by the convergence of ridges terminating at a central point in the bottom of the depression where there is a junction of grooves.

Triangular fossae: These are found on molars and premolars on the occlusal surfaces mesial or distal to marginal ridges.

Sulcus: Sulcus is a long depression or valley on the surface of a tooth between ridges and cusps.

Groove: It is a shallow linear depression on the surface of a tooth.

Developmental groove: A developmental groove is a shallow groove between the primary parts of the crown or root.

Supplemental groove: A supplemental groove is a shallow linear depression on the surface of a tooth and does not mark the junction of primary parts.

Buccal and lingual grooves are developmental grooves found on the pits are small pinpoint depressions located at the junction of developmental grooves or at terminals of those grooves. For instance, central pit is a term used to describe a landmark in the central fossa of molars where developmental grooves join.

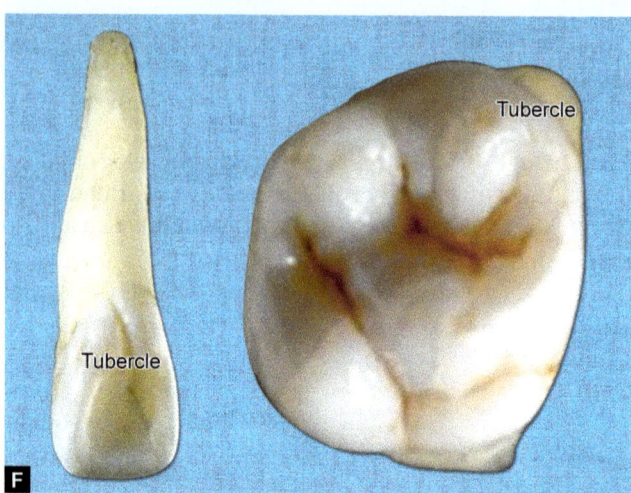

FIGURE 2.3F: Tubercle.

Tubercle (Fig. 2.3F)

A tubercle is a smaller elevation on some portion of the crown produced by an extra formation of enamel. It is commonly present as rounded projection on lingual surface of maxillary first molar and anterior teeth.

Tubercle differs from cusp in that it is formed of enamel only while cusp is formed of pulp horn which is covered by dentin and enamel.

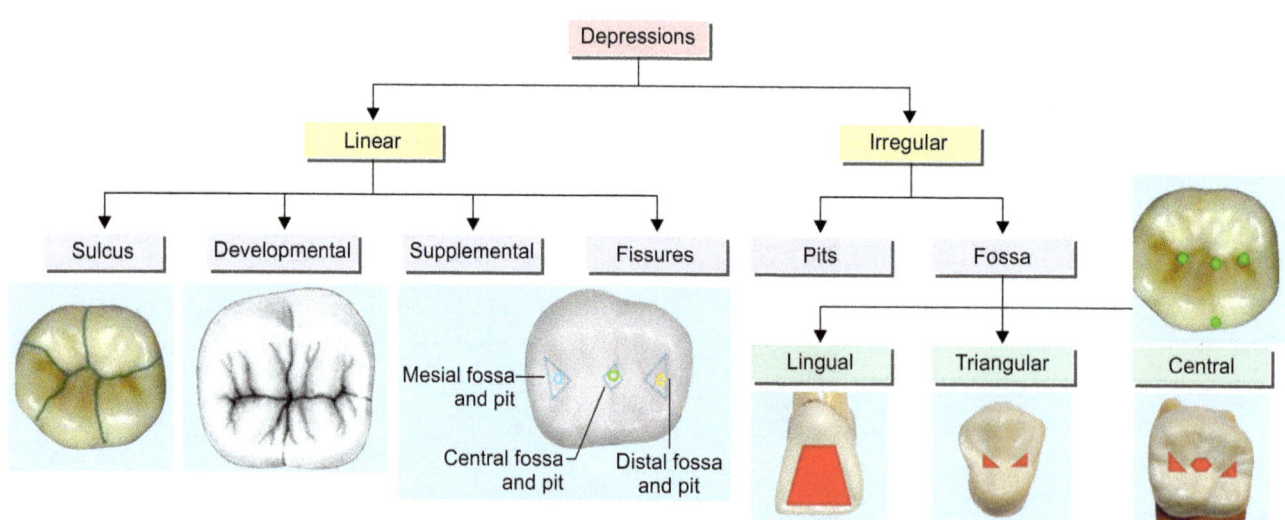

FIGURE 2.4: Schematic representation showing different types of depressions present on the crown surface.

Tooth Nomenclature, Morphology, Anatomy and Physiology

OTHER IMPORTANT TERMS (FIGS. 2.5 TO 2.8)

- **Facial:** The surface of tooth which faces towards the cheeks or lips is called facial surface.
- **Labial:** The surface of tooth which faces towards the lips is labial surface.
- **Buccal:** The surface of tooth which faces towards the cheeks is buccal surface.
- **Palatal/Lingual:** The surface of tooth that faces towards palate or tongue is palatal or lingual surface.
- **Midline:** It is an imaginary line dividing upper and lower arches in two equal halves.
- **Mesial:** The surface that is closest to the midline is mesial surface.
- **Distal:** The surface that is away from the midline is the distal surface.
- **Proximal:** Tooth surfaces that are next to each other are termed as proximal surfaces, (i.e., distal of central incisor and mesial of lateral incisor).
- **Incisal:** The biting edge of an anterior tooth is incisal surface.
- **Occlusal:** The chewing surface of posterior teeth is occlusal surface.

NOMENCLATURE OF TEETH

Though various nomenclature tooth nomenclature. The three most common systems used are the "FDI World Dental Federation" notation, the "Universal" system and the "Zsigmondy-Palmer" system.

Zsigmondy-Palmer System/Angular/Grid System

This is the oldest method of tooth notation introduced by Zsigmondy in 1861. Also known as angular or grid system.

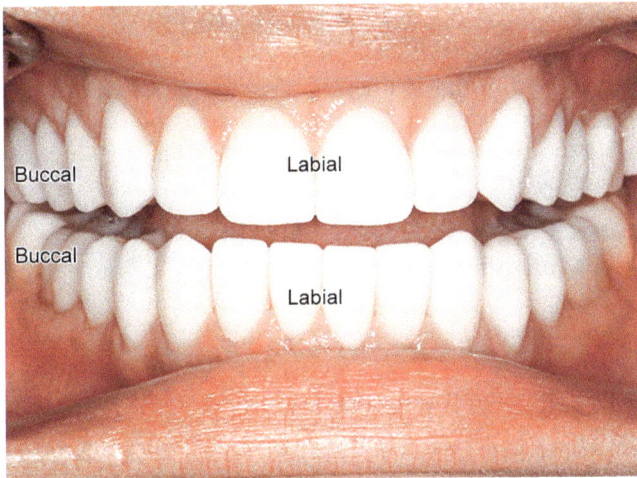

FIGURE 2.5: Labial and buccal surfaces of teeth.

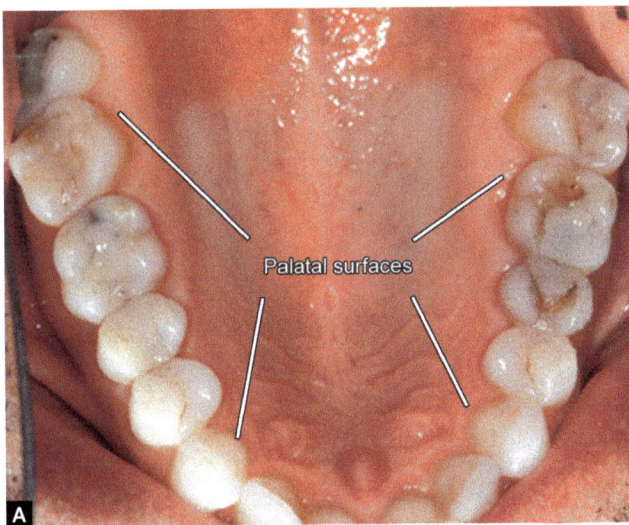

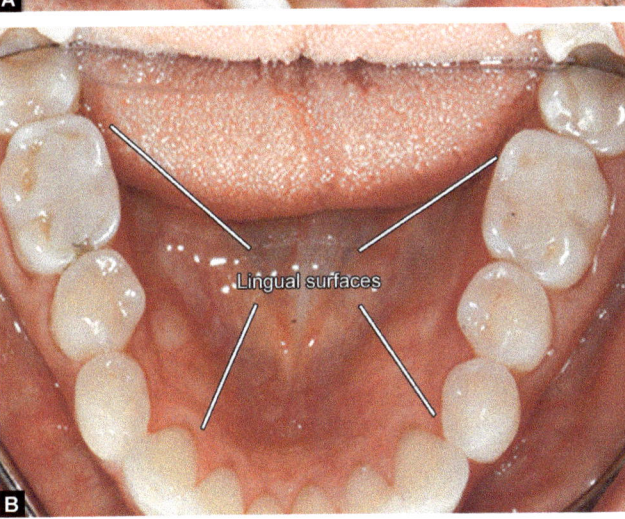

FIGURES 2.6A AND B: Palatal and lingual surfaces.

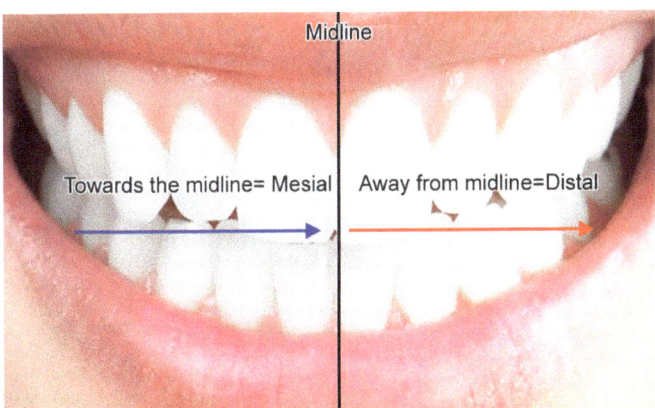

FIGURE 2.7: Mesial and distal surfaces of teeth.

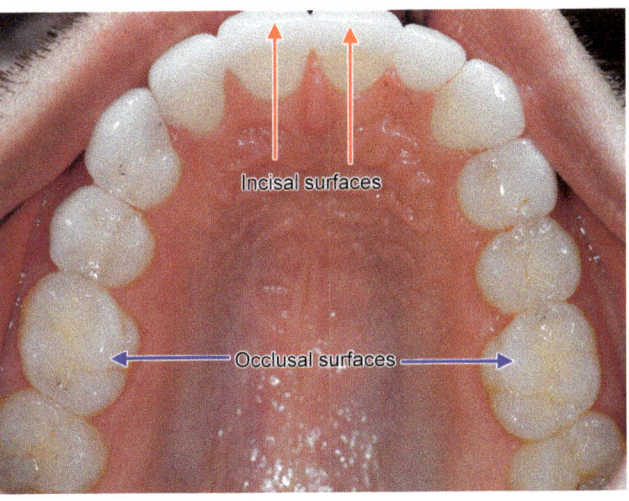

FIGURE 2.8: Incisal and occlusal surfaces.

Permanent Teeth (Figs. 2.9 A and B)

Permanent teeth are numbered 1–8, where 1 is central incisor, 4 is first premolar and 8 is third molar.

Each quadrant has unique L-shaped symbol to designate the quadrant to which tooth belongs. For example, for maxillary right, maxillary left, mandibular right and mandibular left symbols are respectively.

Primary Teeth (Figs. 2.10A and B)

Primary teeth are designated as A, B, C, D, E where A is central incisor and E is second molar.

Advantages	Disadvantages
■ Simple and easy to use ■ Less chances of confusion between primary and permanent tooth as there is different notation, e.g., permanent teeth are described by numbers while primary teeth by alphabets	■ Difficulty in communication ■ Confusion between upper and lower quadrants

Universal (National) System/ADA System

This system was introduced by the American Dental Association in 1968. It is most popular in the United States. Universal numbering system uses a unique letter or number for each tooth.

Permanent Teeth (Figs. 2.11A and B)

Numbering starts from maxillary right posterior tooth where tooth number 1 is the patient's upper right third molar and follows around the upper arch to the upper left third molar, tooth 16, descending to the lower left third molar, tooth 17, and following around the lower arch to the lower right third molar, tooth 32.

- If a third molar is missing, the first number will be 2 instead of 1, acknowledging the missing tooth.
- If teeth have been extracted or missing, they are also numbered.

Primary Teeth (Figs. 2.12A and B)

- But this method was modified where primary teeth are by English upper case letters A through T instead of numbers 1 to 20, with A being upper right second primary molar and T being the lower right second primary molar.

Advantage	Disadvantage
Unique letter or number for each tooth avoiding confusions	Difficult to remember each letter or number of tooth

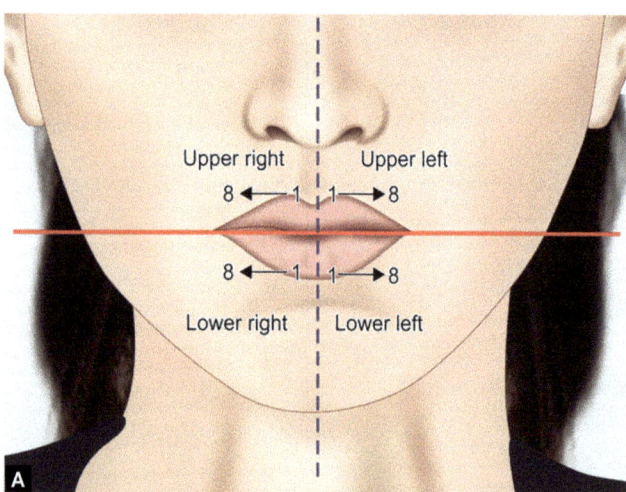

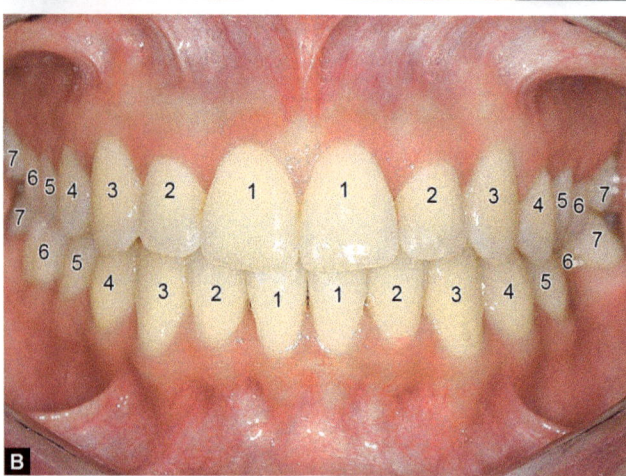

FIGURES 2.9A AND B: Zsigmondy-palmer tooth notation system for permanent dentition.

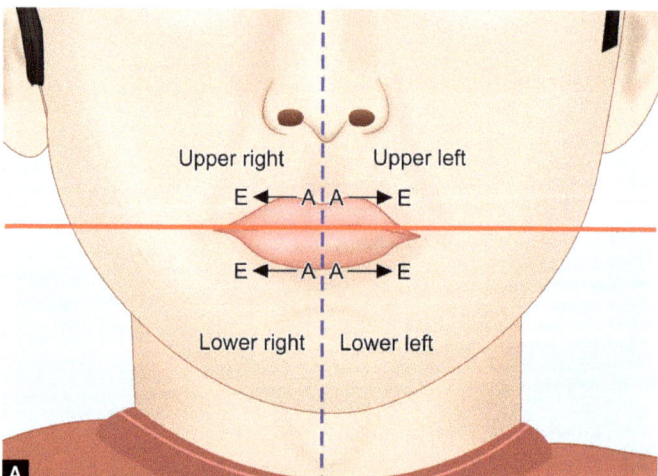

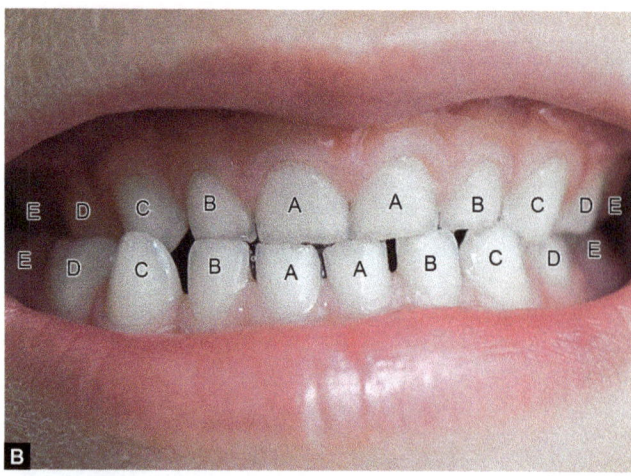

FIGURES 2.10A AND B: Zsigmondy-palmer tooth notation system for primary dentition.

Federation Dentaire Internationale (FDI) System

- This two-digit system was first introduced in 1971 and subsequently adopted by the American Dental Association (1996). FDI system is known as a "Two-Digit" system because it uses two digits; the first number represents a tooth's quadrant, and the second number represents the number of the tooth from the midline of the face
- Both digits should be pronounced separately in communication. For example, the lower left permanent second molar is "37"; it is not termed as "thirty-seven", but "three seven".

Permanent Teeth (Figs. 2.13A and B)

- In FDI notation, teeth are numbered as 1, 2,....8 where
  - 1—central incisor
  - 2—lateral incisor
  - 3—canine
  - 4 and 5—1st and 2nd premolars respectively
  - 6, 7, and 8—1st, 2nd, and 3rd molars.
- Quadrants are designated 1 to 4
  - 1—upper right
  - 2—upper left
  - 3—lower left
  - 4—lower right.
- This results in tooth identification a two-digit combination of the quadrant and tooth, e.g. the upper right canine is "13" (one three) and the upper left canine is "23" (two three).

Deciduous Teeth (Figs. 2.14A and B)

- In the deciduous dentition the numbering is correspondingly similar except that the quadrants are designated 5, 6, 7, and 8
- Teeth are numbered from number 1 to 5, 1 being central incisor and 5 is second molar.

Advantages	Disadvantages
Simple to understand, learn and pronounce	May be confused with universal tooth numbering system
Each tooth has specific number	
Easy for charting	

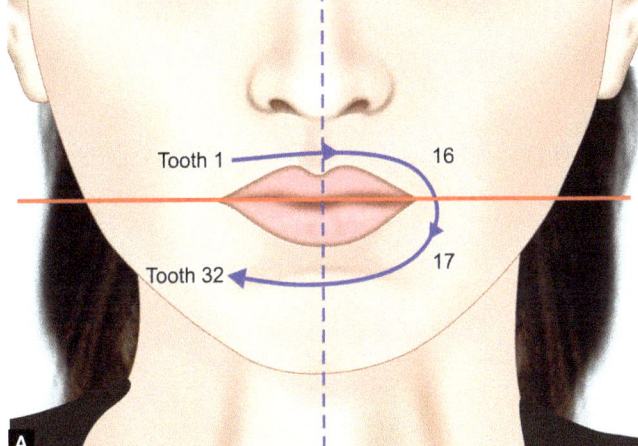

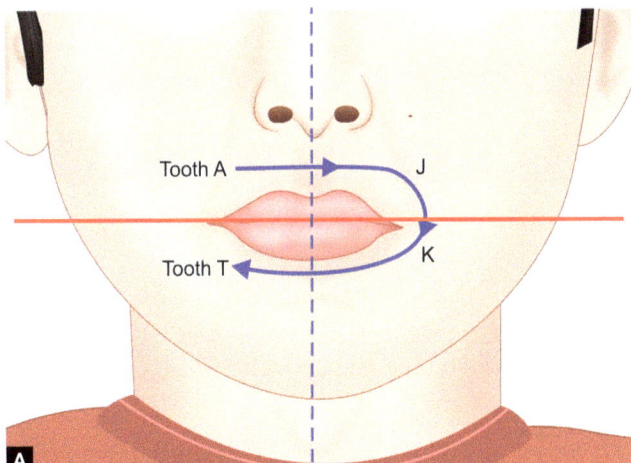

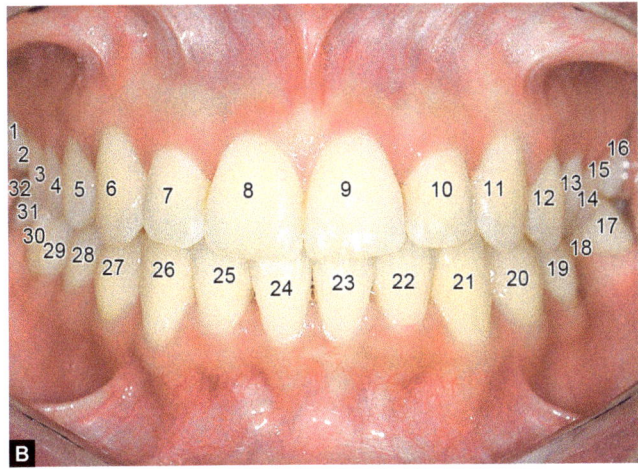

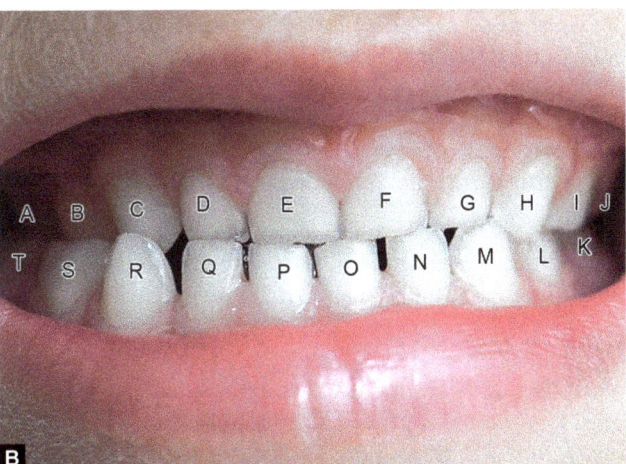

FIGURES 2.11A AND B: Universal tooth notation system for permanent dentition.

FIGURES 2.12A AND B: Universal tooth notation system for primary dentition.

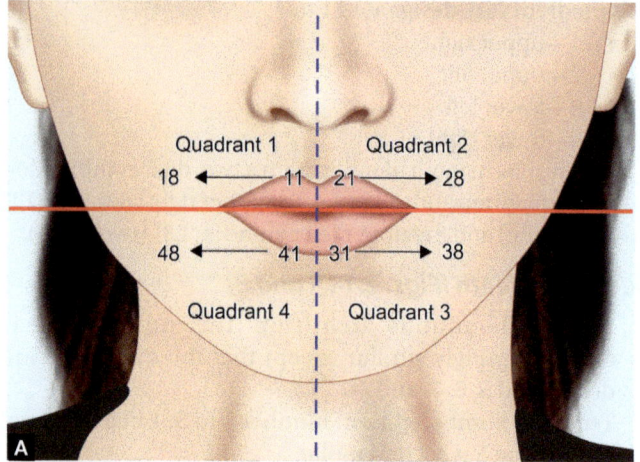
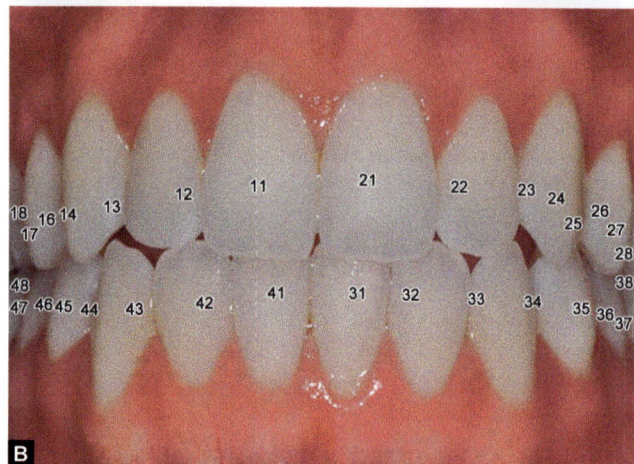

FIGURES 2.13A AND B: FDI tooth notation system for permanent dentition.

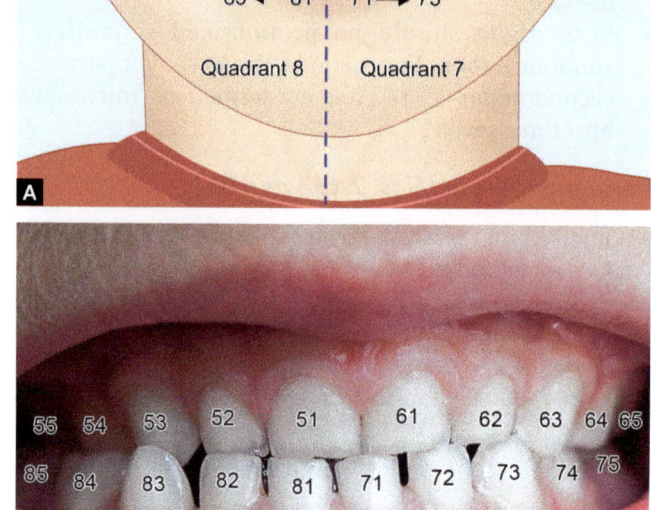

FIGURES 2.14A AND B: FDI tooth notation system for primary dentition.

HISTOLOGICAL STRUCTURES OF TEETH

Tooth is composed of three hard mineralized tissues (enamel, dentin, and cementum), and one soft tissue (pulp).

ENAMEL

Tooth enamel is the hardest and highly mineralized tissue which covers crown of the tooth. It is responsible for esthetics, texture, and translucency of tooth.

Composition

- **Inorganic contents (by volume):** Hydroxyapatite—96%
- **Organic contents (by volume):** Organic content and water 4%.

Significance: Poorly mineralized enamel appears whiter and more mineralized enamel appears more translucent.

Structure (Fig. 2.15)

Enamel is mainly composed of enamel rods/prisms covered by rod sheath and joined by interrod substance. Their number ranges from 5 to 12 million. Each rod is keyhole or paddle-shaped having head and tail, head is directed occlusally and tail toward cervical area.

Significance: Cervical enamel rods of deciduous teeth are inclined incisally or occlusally, while in permanent teeth

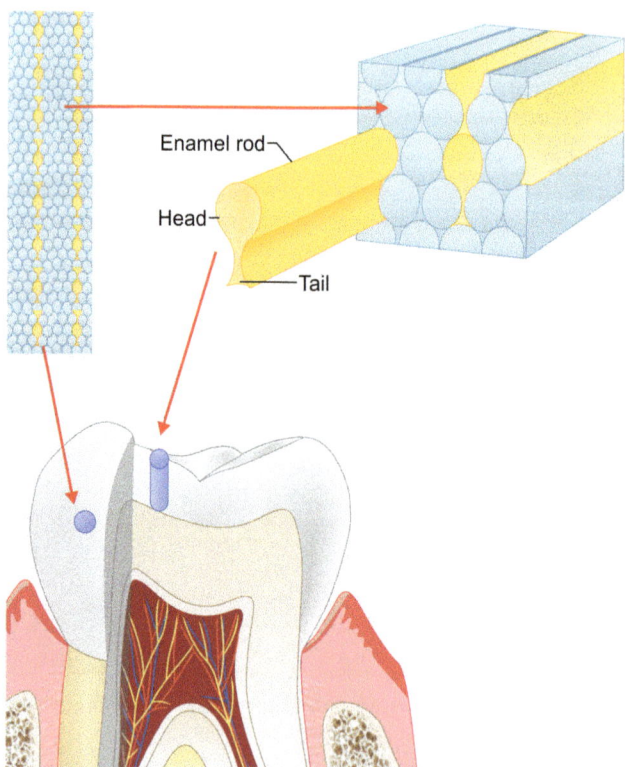

FIGURE 2.15: Schematic representation showing enamel rods.

these are inclined apically **(Fig. 2.16)**. Therefore to avoid unsupported enamel rods at gingival floor, cavosurface bevel (15 to 20°) at gingival margin is given by using gingival margin trimmer (GMT).

Thickness
Average thickness of enamel at incisal edges is 2 mm and at cusp tip of molars, it ranges from 2.3 to 3.0 mm. Thickness decreases gradually from cusps or incisal edges to cervical area and terminates at cemento-enamel junction (CEJ) as knife edge.

Color (Figs. 2.17A and B)
Enamel is translucent in nature. Color of tooth mainly depends on:
- Thickness of enamel; young anterior teeth appear translucent gray or bluish near incisal edges
- Shade of underlying dentin
- Anomalies occurring during developmental and mineralization stage, antibiotic usage and fluorosis, etc. affect the color of teeth.

Hardness
Enamel is the hardest substance in human body.

Significance: Because of more compressive strength of dentin than enamel, dentin acts as a cushion for enamel when masticatory forces are applied on it.

FUNCTIONS OF ENAMEL
- Hardest structure of tooth which supports masticatory forces
- Mainly responsible for esthetics, surface texture and translucency of tooth
- Protects the underlying dentin and pulp.

> **Box 2.1: Clinical significance**
> - **Color:** Color of the enamel varies because of age, ingestion of tetracycline or fluoride during the formative stages, extrinsic stains and developmental defects of teeth
> - **Attrition:** It is mechanical wear of enamel on occlusal and proximal surfaces
> - **Acid etching:** Acid etching forms micro- and macro tags in enamel which improves bonding between resin and enamel
> - **Permeability:** Enamel is semipermeable, that is why various fluids, pigments, ions, demineralization, remineralization, fluoride intake, and vital bleaching are possible.

DENTIN
Dentin is the most voluminous mineralized connective tissue of tooth. It is covered by enamel in crown portion and cementum in root part.

Composition
Dentin contains 64% inorganic hydroxyapatite crystals and 36% organic content (collagen) and water.

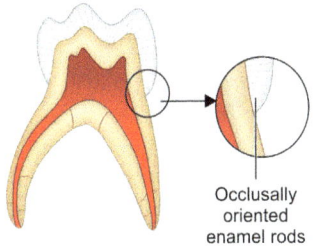
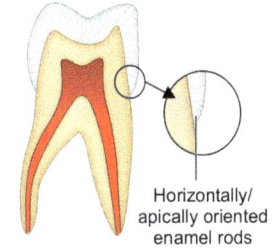

FIGURE 2.16: Schematic representation of direction of enamel rods in permanent and primary teeth.

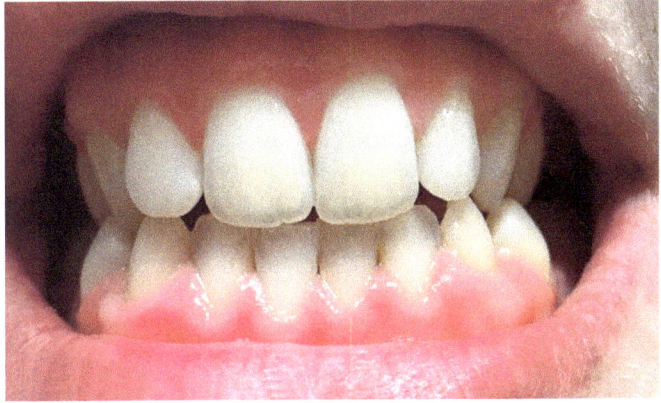

FIGURE 2.17A: Translucent gray or bluish color of enamel at the incisal edges.

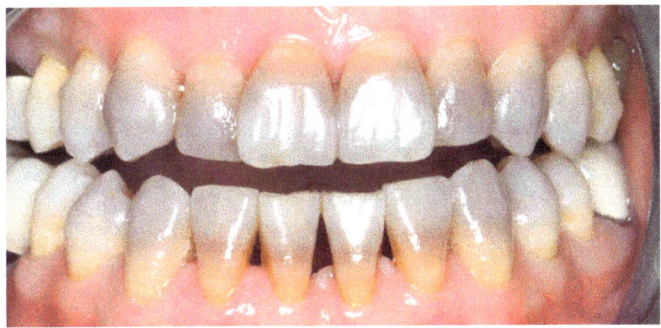

FIGURE 2.17B: Tetracyclin stains of teeth.

Color
Dentin is slightly darker than enamel. It is yellow white in young teeth and gets darker with age due to constant exposure to oral fluids, irritants and deposition of secondary or tertiary dentin.

Thickness
Dentin thickness (3 to 3.5 mm) is more on cusp tip and less in cervical area of tooth. Its thickness increases with age due to deposition of secondary and tertiary dentin.

Hardness
Hardness of dentin is one-fifth of enamel. Hardness of dentin increases with age due to its mineralization. **Table 2.1** shows differentiating features between enamel and dentin.

TABLE 2.1: Differences between enamel and dentin.

	Enamel	Dentin
Color	Whitish blue or white gray	Yellowish white or slightly darker than enamel
Sound	Sharp, high-pitched sound on moving fine explorer tip	Dull low-pitched sound on moving fine explorer tip
Hardness	Hardest structure of tooth	Softer than enamel
Reflectance	More shiny surface and reflective to light than dentin	Dull and reflects less light than enamel

Structure

Dentinal Tubules (Fig. 2.18)

Dentin is made up of dentinal tubules which follow a gentle "S"-shaped curve in crown and become straighter in incisal edges, cusps and root areas. Number of dentinal tubules increases from 15,000–20,000/mm^2 at DEJ to 45,000–65,000/mm^2 toward pulp.

Secondary Dentin (Fig. 2.19)

Secondary dentin is formed after completion of root formation. In this, the direction of tubules is more asymmetrical and complicated as compared to primary dentin.

Tertiary Dentin

Also known as reactive dentin, reparative dentin and irritation dentin. Tertiary dentin is formed in response to external stimuli like dental caries, attrition and trauma.

Table 2.2 is showing differences between primary, secondary and tertiary dentin.

Sclerotic Dentin

It occurs due to aging or chronic and mild irritation (such as slowly advancing caries) which causes a change in the composition of the primary dentin. Here, deposition of apatite crystals and collagen occurs in dentinal tubules. Due to filling of dentinal tubules with hydroxyapatite crystals, refractive indices of intertubular and peritubular dentin are equalized, giving transparent appearance to dentin. Sclerotic dentin is harder, denser, less sensitive, less permeable, and more protective of pulp against irritations when compared to primary dentin.

Functions of Dentin

- Provides color and elastic foundation for the enamel
- Offers protection of pulp
- Form bulk of the tooth
- Provides strength and durability of the crown.

DENTAL PULP (FIG. 2.20)

Dental pulp is soft tissue of mesenchymal origin located in the center of the tooth and shapes itself to miniature form of tooth. This space is called pulp cavity which is divided into pulp chamber and root canal.

Pulp Chamber

It is part of pulp cavity present in crown portion. The roof of pulp chamber consists of dentin covering the pulp chamber occlusally.

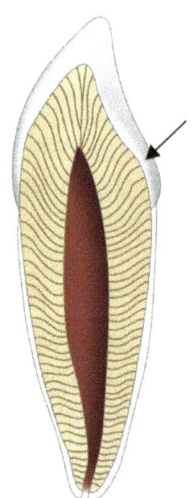

FIGURE 2.18: Schematic representation of dentinal tubules.

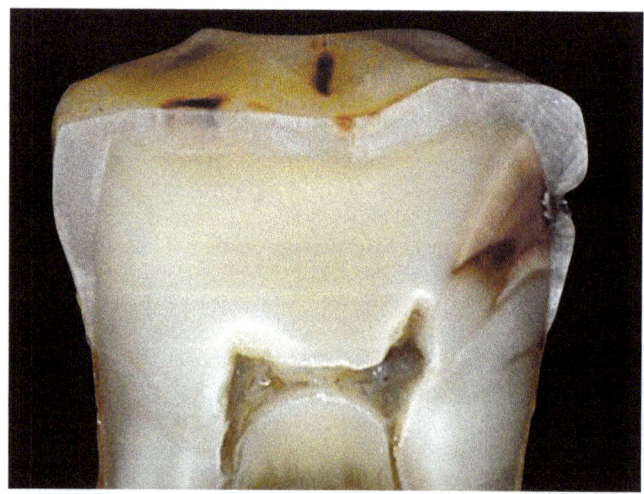

FIGURE 2.19: Photograph showing secondary and tertiary dentin.

TABLE 2.2: Difference between primary, secondary, and tertiary dentin.

	Primary	Secondary	Tertiary
Definition	Dentin formed before root completion	Formed after root completion	Formed as a response to any external stimuli such as dental caries, attrition, and trauma
Location	Found in all areas of dentin	It is not uniform, mainly present over roof and floor of pulp chamber	Localized to only area of external stimulus
Orientation of tubules	Regular	Irregular	Atubular

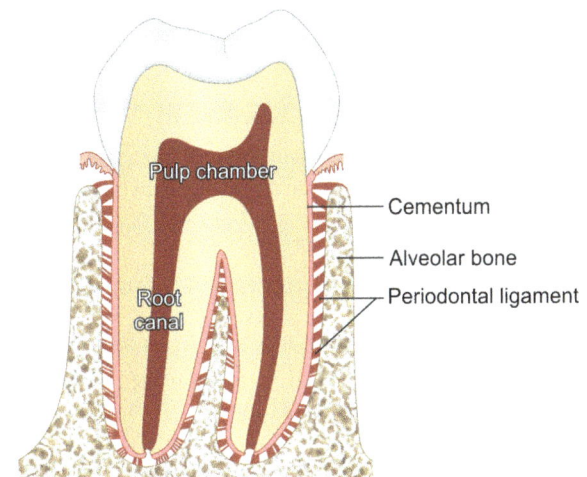

FIGURE 2.20: Schematic representation of dental pulp and periodontium.

Root Canal

It is the part of pulp cavity which extends from canal orifice to the apical foramen.

Functions

Formative
Formation of primary, secondary, and tertiary dentin.

Nutritive
It provides nutrition to dentin.

Innervative
Through the nervous system, pulp transmits pain, sensations of temperature and touch.

Defensive/Protective
Odontoblasts form reparative and sclerotic dentin in response to injury.

PERIRADICULAR TISSUE

Periradicular tissue consists of cementum, periodontal ligament and alveolar bone.

Cementum

Cementum can be defined as hard, avascular connective tissue that covers the roots of the teeth. It is light yellow in color and can be differentiated from enamel by its lack of luster and darker hue.

Composition
- Inorganic content—45 to 50% (by wt)
- Organic matter—50 to 55% (by wt)
- Water.

Acellular Cementum
- Covers the cervical third of the root
- Main function is anchorage.

Cellular Cementum
- Mainly found in apical third and interradicular
- Main function is adaptation.

Periodontal Ligament

Periodontal ligament is a unique structure as it forms a link between the alveolar bone and the cementum. Periodontal ligament houses the fibers, cells, and other structural elements such as blood vessels and nerves.

Alveolar Bone

Bone is specialized connective tissue which comprises inorganic phases that is very well-designed for its role as load-bearing structure of the body.

Significance of Periodontium

- Poor quality of restoration, for example, marginal discrepancy and roughness impairs the periodontal health
- Overhanging, over or under contoured restoration can result in food impaction, gingival inflammation, attachment loss, and bone loss.

FUNCTIONS OF TEETH (TABLE 2.3)

Mastication

Incisors—incisal edge of central and lateral incisors is used to punch and cut.

Canines—sharp cusp of canine helps in tearing and shearing of food.

Premolars and molars—two or three cusps of premolars and molars help in grinding of food.

TABLE 2.3: Types of teeth and their functions (**Fig. 2.21**).

Tooth	Name	Position	Function	Number
Incisors	Central and lateral incisors	Two teeth of each quadrant which are closest to midline	Biting, cutting, incision and shearing	08
Canine (Cuspid)	Canine	3rd tooth from midline in each quadrant	Cutting tearing, piercing and holding	04
Premolars (Bicuspid)	1st and 2nd premolars	4th and 5th teeth from midline	Tearing, holding and grinding	08
Molars	1st, 2nd and 3rd molars	6th, 7th, 8th teeth from midline	Grinding	12

Speech

Teeth are important in pronunciation of certain sounds and thus play vital role during speech.

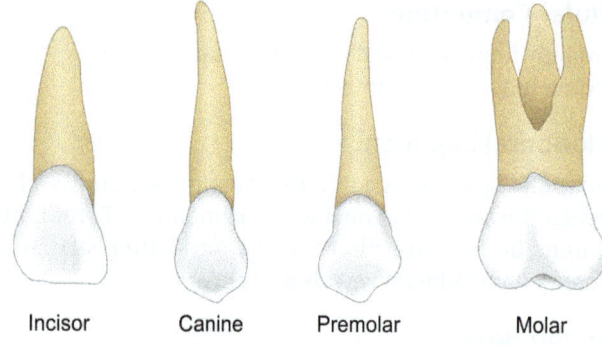

FIGURE 2.21: Image showing different types of teeth.

Esthetics

The form, alignment, and contour of anterior teeth play important role in maintaining esthetics of face.

Protection of Supporting Tissues

Teeth help in protection of supporting structures such as gingiva, periodontium, and alveolar bone.

PHYSIOLOGY FORM OF THE TEETH

Following are the protective functional forms of the teeth:
- Contour of teeth
- Marginal ridges
- Embrasures
- Interproximal area.

Contour of Teeth (Figs. 2.22A and B)

It is the convexity present on crown of a tooth. It is present on mesial, distal, buccal and lingual surfaces of the crowns of teeth.

Significance (Figs. 2.23A to C)

- Protects gingival tissue against bruising and trauma caused from food
- Prevents food being packed into gingival sulcus
- Normal deflection of food away from gingiva provides physiological stimulation of gingiva.

Problems with overcontouring or undercontouring of teeth
- **Overcontouring** Here restoration contains excessive restorative material which alters the normal contour of the tooth.

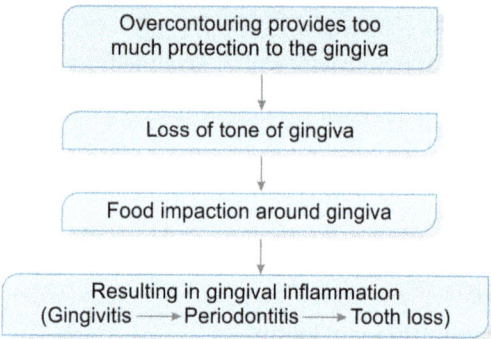

- **Undercontouring:** It means too little contouring, so that a space occurs between margins and the cavity walls. It leads to food impaction and trauma to the attachment apparatus.

Marginal Ridges (Fig. 2.24)

Marginal ridges are defined as rounded borders of enamel which form the mesial and distal margins of occlusal surfaces of premolars and molars and mesial and distal margins of lingual surfaces of the incisors and canines.

Importance

- Help in balancing of teeth in both the arches
- Improve the efficiency of mastication
- Prevent food impaction in interproximal areas.

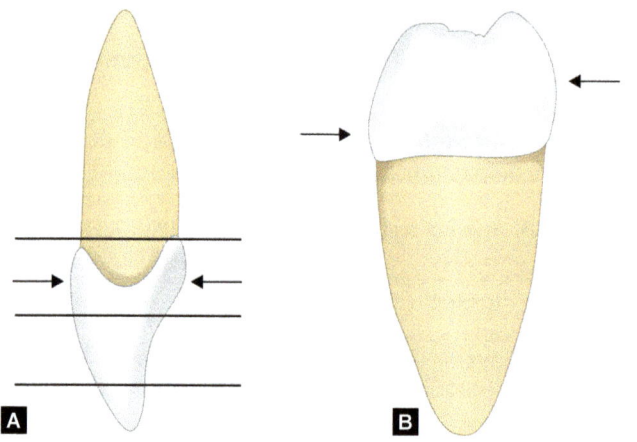

FIGURES 2.22A AND B: (A) Schematic representation of height of contour in anterior; (B) Posterior teeth.

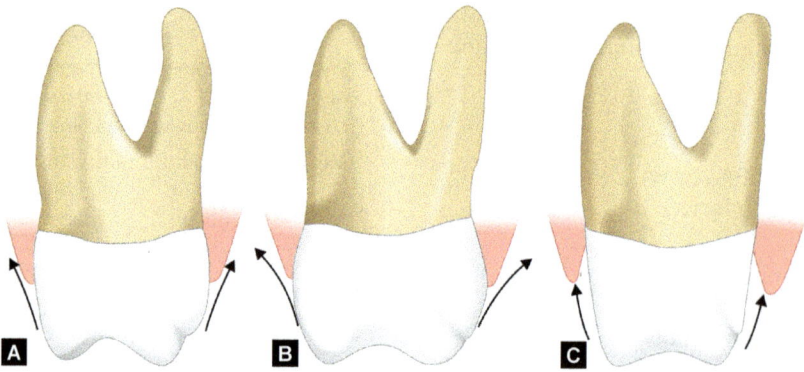

FIGURES 2.23A TO C: Schematic representation of normal, overcontour and undercontour. Arrows show the pathway of food during mastication: (A) Optimal contour allows adequate stimulation and protection of periodontium; (B) Overcontour causes deflection of food and thus under stimulation of gingiva; (C) Undercontour results in food impaction and trauma to periodontium.

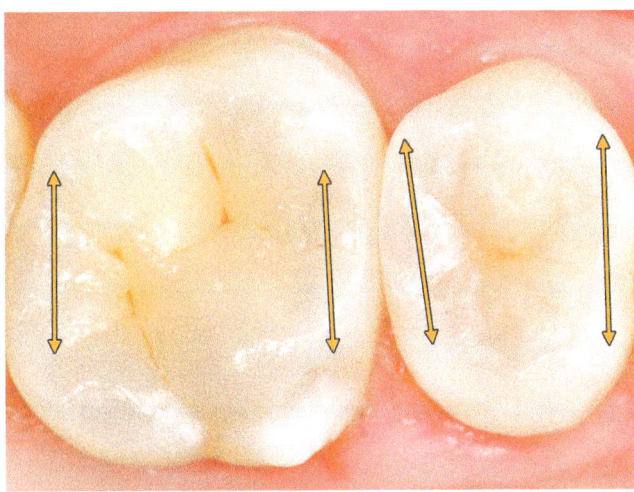

FIGURE 2.24: Marginal ridge (arrow) in molar and premolar.

Clinical Significance

- During restoration, marginal ridges should be restored in two planes, i.e., buccolingually and cervico-occlusally. Restoring marginal ridges in two planes prevent food lodgment which causes damage to the periodontium
- Restore adjacent marginal ridges at the same height.

Embrasures

Embrasures can be defined as V-shaped spaces that originate at proximal contact areas between adjacent teeth. These are named according to the direction in which they radiate. These are **(Figs. 2.25A and B)**:

- Labial/buccal and lingual embrasures: These are spaces that widen out from the area of contact labially or buccally and lingually
- Incisal/occlusal embrasures: These are spaces that widen out from area of contact incisally/occlusally
- Gingival embrasure: These are the spaces that widen out from the area of contact gingivally.

Functions

- Provides a spillway for food during mastication
- Prevents food from being forced through contact area.

Significance (Fig. 2.26)

- Correct size of embrasures provide escape of food from occlusal surfaces during mastication
- If embrasure size is decreased/absent, then additional forces are created in teeth and supporting structures a during mastication
- If embrasure size is enlarged, food impaction occurs in interproximal space by opposing cusp, resulting in damage to supporting tissues.

Interproximal Spaces (Figs. 2.27A and B)

Interproximal space is triangular-shaped area that is usually filled by gingival tissue. In this triangular area, the base is formed by alveolar process, sides by proximal surfaces of contacting teeth and apex is the contact area.

Proximal Contact Areas (Fig. 2.28)

- Each tooth in the arch has two contacting membranes adjoining it, one on mesial side and other on distal side.

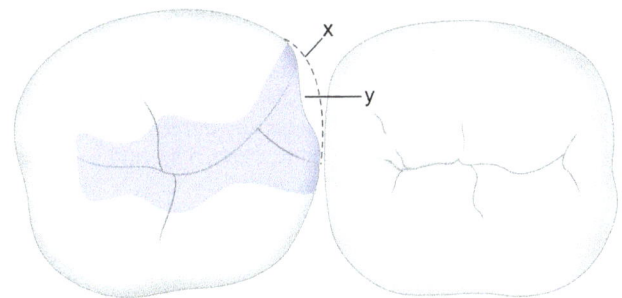

FIGURE 2.26: Embrasure. X–depicts a correct embrasure form; Y–depicts improper contour of restoration resulting in improper embrasure form.

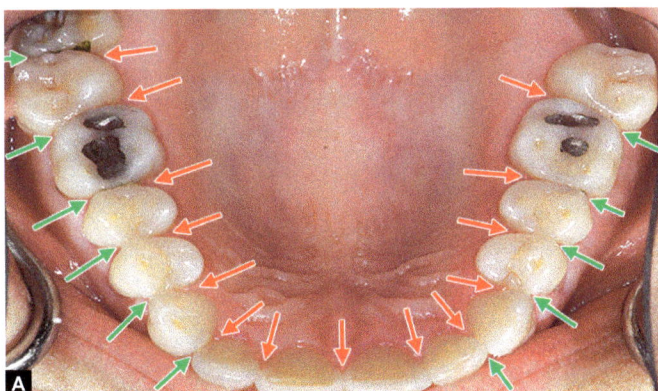

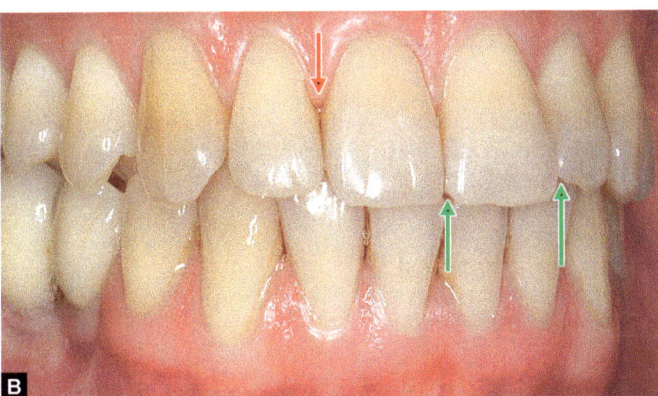

FIGURES 2.25A AND B: Photograph showing; (A) Palatal and lingual embrasures; (B) Buccal/lingual and incisal/gingiva embrasures.

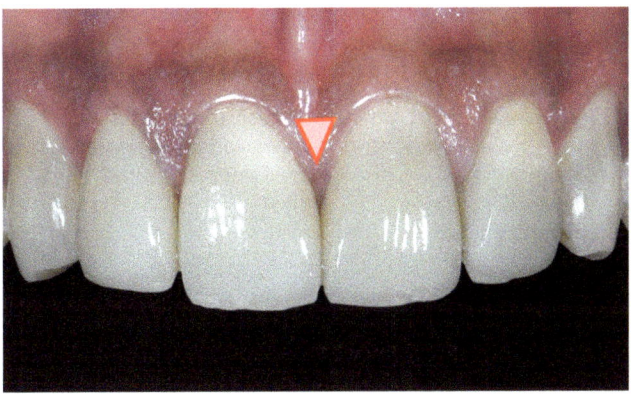

FIGURE 2.27A: Photograph showing interproximal space.

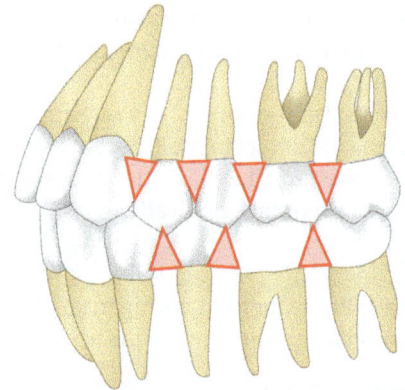

FIGURE 2.27B: Schematic representation of interproximal spaces.

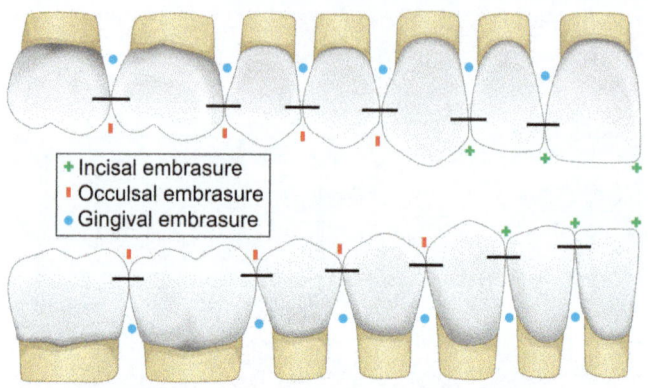

FIGURE 2.28: Schematic representation of proximal contact areas.

Proximal contact area denotes area of proximal height of contour of the mesial or distal surface of a tooth that contact sits adjacent tooth in the same arch

- **Importance of proper contact relation**
  - Stabilizes the dental arches by combined anchorage effect of all the teeth
  - Keeps food away from packing between the teeth
  - Protects interdental papillae.
- **Improper proximal contact area can result in:**
  - Food impaction
  - Periodontal disease
  - Carious lesions
  - Mobility of teeth.

CONCLUSION

The relationship between restoration and periodontal health of the teeth is inseparable; maintenance of gingival health constitutes one of the keys for tooth and dental restoration longevity. One should have thorough knowledge of relationship between periodontal tissues and restorative dentistry to ensure adequate form, function and esthetics.

MORPHOLOGY OF INDIVIDUAL TEETH

Maxillary Teeth			
Labial aspect	Lingual aspect	Proximal aspect	Incisal/Occlusal aspect
Central incisor			
■ Widest mesiodistally ■ Mesial outline is straight ■ Distal outline is convex ■ Mesioincisal angle is sharper than distoinicisal angle	■ Below cervical line, cingulum present ■ Palatal fossa present which is bordered by mesial and distal marginal ridge, incisal ridge and cingulum	■ Wedge triangular-shaped crown with base towards cervix and apex towards incisal ridge ■ Labial outline is convex, lingual outline is convex at cingulum, after this it becomes concave and then slightly convex again when it approaches linguoincisal ridge	■ Incisal edge is centered over the root, labial surface appears broad and flat, whereas lingual part shows cingulum
Lateral Incisor			
■ Rounded incisal edge and rounded incisal angles, mesially and distally ■ Mesioincisal angle can be as sharp as central incisor and distal outline is more rounded than central incisor	■ Palatal aspect cingulum and deep lingual fossa ■ Marginal ridges are more prominent than central incisor	■ Wedge triangular-shaped crown with base towards cervix and apex towards incisal ridge ■ Labial outline is convex, lingual outline is convex at cingulum. after this it becomes concave and then slightly convex again when it approaches linguoincisal ridge	May resemble central incisor or canine

Contd...

Contd...

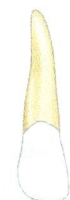 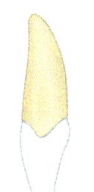 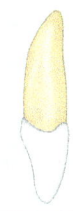 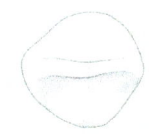

Canine

- Due to more development of middle lobe, labial ridge is seen
- Incisal edge ends to a point in form of cusp

- Cingulum is prominent or pointed and may appear as a cusp
- Marginal ridges are prominent and lingual ridge divides lingual fossa in mesial and distal lingual fossa

- Outline is wedge shape, labial surface appears convex, lingual outline shows convexity at cervical area, straight at middle third and again convex at incisal third

- Labial ridge present on labial surface, cingulum on lingual aspect
- Distal cusp ridge is longer than the mesial cusp ridge

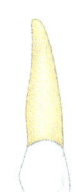 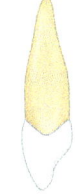 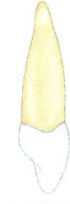 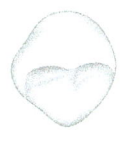

First Premolar

- Buccal ridge, buccal cusp is long and sharp, and thus resembles canine
- Mesial cusp slope is longer than distal cusp slope

- Palatal cusp is short and blunt as compared to buccal cusp

- Roughly trapezoidal in shape, mesial developmental depression and groove is present on mesial aspect
- Distal aspect is almost similar to mesial aspect except that there is no depression and deep developmental groove

- Resembles a six-sided hexagon, crown is wider on buccal aspect than on palatal aspect
- Central developmental groove divides the occlusal surface buccolingually

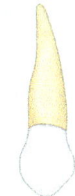 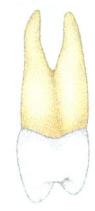 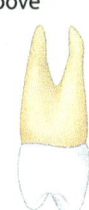 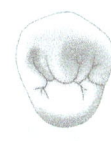

Second Premolar

- Crown is shorter, less pointed and more oblong in shape when compared to first premolar

- Both palatal and buccal cusps are of same dimensions and palatal surface is narrower than buccal surface

- Almost similar to 1st premolar except that no developmental groove or depression is found on mesial surface

- Outline is rounded or oval and central developmental groove is shorter and more irregular
- Multiple supplementary grooves radiate from central groove giving occlusal surface a wrinkled appearance

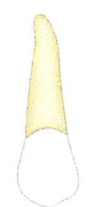 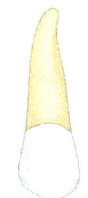 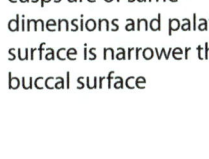 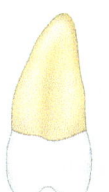 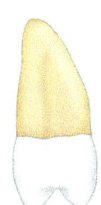 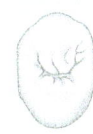

Contd...

Contd...

First Molar

■ Crown is trapezoidal in shape ■ Mesiobuccal cusp is broader than distobuccal cusp	■ Mesiopalatal cusp is the longest cusp ■ A fifth cusp, i.e., "Cusp of Carabelli" on the palatal surface of mesiopalatal cusp is seen	● On mesial aspect, outline is trapezoidal with small side occlusally	Rhomboidal or parallelogram ■ Mesiopalatal cusp is largest cusp, followed by mesiobuccal, distopalatal, distobuccal and fifth cusp in decreasing size ■ Triangular ridges of mesiopalatal and distobuccal cusp meet to form oblique ridge
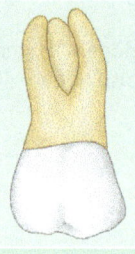	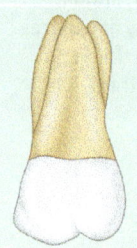	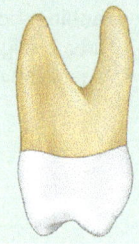 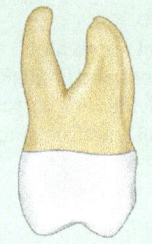	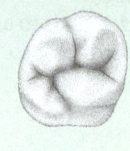

Second Molar

■ The crown is slightly shorter and narrower than first molar	■ It is mainly different from first molar due to shorter distopalatal cusp and absence of fifth cusp	● Crown length is less when compared to first molar	■ Heart shaped occlusal anatomy ■ More of supplementary grooves and pits are present than first molar
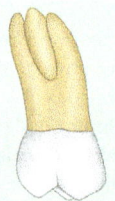	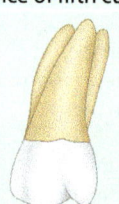	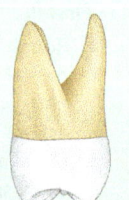 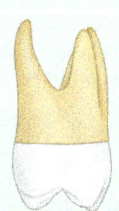	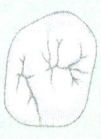

Mandibular Teeth

Central Incisor

■ Smallest tooth in arch ■ Bilaterally symmetrical	■ Cingulum present ■ Due to lingual convergence, crown is narrower on lingual side	■ Wedge shaped with incisal edge being lingual to long axis of the root	■ Bilaterally symmetrical and incisal edge is perpendicular to the line bisecting labiolingually
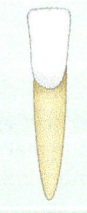	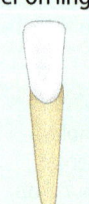	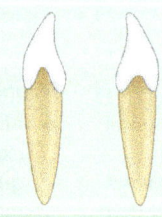	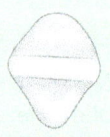

Lateral Incisor

■ Crown is tilted distally on the root, mesioincisal angle is sharp, whereas distoincisal angle is slightly rounded	■ Cingulum lies slightly distal to the long axis of the tooth	■ Incisal edge is twisted distolingually, i.e., distal portion is placed more lingually than mesial portion	■ Incisal edge is twisted distolingually. This twist corresponds to the curvature of mandibular arch
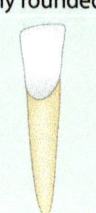	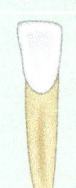	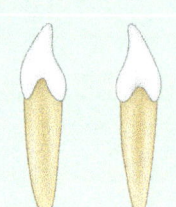	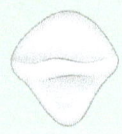

Contd...

Contd...

Canine

- Crown appears longer because of its narrowness than maxillary crown
- Mesial outline is almost straight and crown appears to be tilted distally because there is more of crown distal to long axis of root than mesial to it	- Lingual surface is flatter in comparison to maxillary canine, cingulum is not much prominent	- Due to less prominence of cingulum and less labiolingual thickness of crown, cusp appears more pointed with slender cusp ridge	- Cusp tip and mesial cusp ridge are lingually placed
- Tooth appears to have distolingual twist

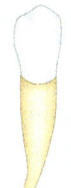 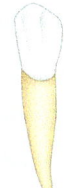  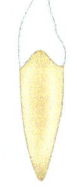 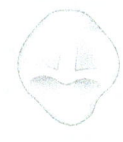

First Premolar

- Buccal cusp tip is pointed; mesial cusp slope is slightly shorter than distal cusp slope
- Buccal ridge is present from cervical margin to cusp tip	- Lingual cusp is small, with pointed tip
- Mesiolingual developmental groove is present which demarcates mesiobuccal and lingual lobe. It extends into the mesial fossa of occlusal surface	- Crown is tilted lingually
- Mesial marginal ridge merges with mesiolingual fossa
- Buccal triangular ridge slopes cervically at 45° from cusp tip towards center of occlusal surface. There is no developmental groove on distal marginal ridge	- Buccal ridge appears prominent
- Mesial fossa contains mesial developmental groove

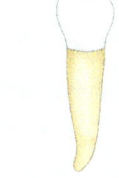 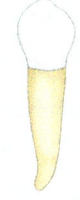 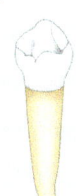 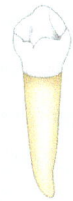 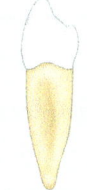 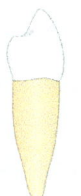 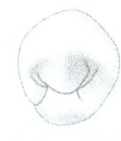

Second Premolar

- Crown appears as a square in shape and is smaller than 1st premolar	**Two forms are seen from this aspect:**
1. One buccal and one lingual cusp
2. One buccal cusp and two lingual cusps | **When compared with first premolar, in this:**
- Crown is wider buccolingually, buccal cusp is not so nearly centered over the root | **One buccal and one lingual cusp:**
- Rounded occlusal outline, buccal cusp is bigger than lingual cusp
- Central developmental groove extends mesiodistally and terminates in mesial and distal fossa

One buccal cusp and two lingual cusps:
- Square shape with buccal cusp being largest in size, followed by ML and DL
- Each cusp is separated by grooves which join to form a central pit and Y-shaped appearance
- Lingual development groove extends between two lingual cusps and ends on lingual surface of crown |

Contd...

Contd...

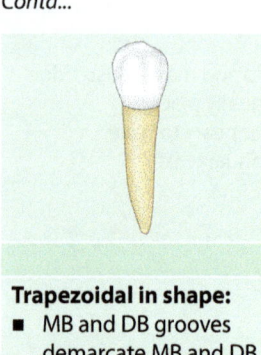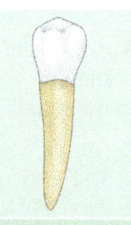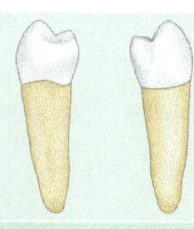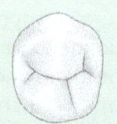

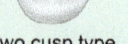 Two cusp type   Three cusp type

First Molar

Trapezoidal in shape:<ul><li>MB and DB grooves demarcate MB and DB cusp, DB and distal cusp</li><li>MB cusp is widest MD and distal cusp is smallest</li></ul>	<ul><li>ML cusp is widest mesiodistally</li><li>Lingual developmental groove demarcates ML and DL cusp</li></ul>	<ul><li>Mesial portion of tooth is broader than distal portion</li><li>Crown has lingual tilt with respect to long axis of root</li></ul>	**Hexagonal in outline:**<ul><li>MD> BL dimensions</li><li>Five cusps are seen, i.e., MB, DB, ML, DL and distal</li><li>Major fossa is central fossa which is present between buccal and lingual cusp ridges</li><li>Two minor fossae present are mesial and distal triangular fossa</li><li>Grooves present are central development groove, mesiobuccal distobuccal and lingual development groove</li></ul>

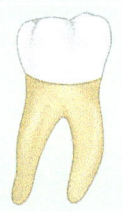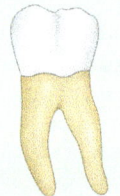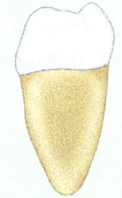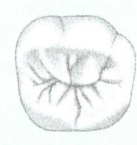

Second Molar

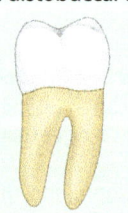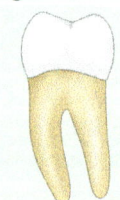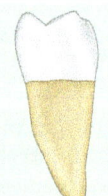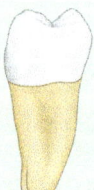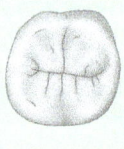

Crown is shorter when compared to first molar<ul><li>Buccal groove separates mesiobuccal and distobuccal cusp</li></ul>	<ul><li>Mesiolingual and distolingual cusps are seen, size of ML>DL cusp</li><li>Crown slightly converges on lingual side</li></ul>	<ul><li>Mesiolingual cusp is the largest cusp</li><li>Occlusal surface is constricted buccolingually</li></ul>	**Rectangular in shape:**<ul><li>MD>BL dimensions</li><li>Grooves mainly present are central groove, buccal groove and the lingual groove</li></ul>

■ VIVA QUESTIONS

Q.1 Which is the largest tooth?
Ans. Maxillary first molar.

Q.2 Which tooth has longest root?
Ans. Maxillary canine.

Q.3 Which tooth is widest mesiodistally?
Ans. Mandibular first molar.

Q.4 Which tooth is named as corner stone of mouth?
Ans. Canine.

Q.5 In which tooth cusp of Carabelli is present?
Ans. Maxillary first molar.

Q.6 In lower arch which tooth has five cusps?
Ans. Mandibular first molar.

Q.7 Which is the smallest cusp in mandibular first molar?
Ans. Distal.

Q.8 Which is the largest cusp of maxillary first molar?
Ans. Mesiopalatal.

Q.9 How can you differentiate maxillary right and left central incisor?
Ans.
- Mesial outline is straight
- Distal outline is rounded
- Mesioincisal angle is sharp and distoincisal angle is rounded

Tooth Nomenclature, Morphology, Anatomy and Physiology

- Curvature of cervical line towards incisal surface is more on mesial side than on distal side.

Q.10 Differentiate between right and left first maxillary premolar.
Ans.
- Mesial cusp ridge is longer than distal cusp ridge
- Mesial development groove is present in enamel of mesial marginal ridge
- Mesial development depression is present.

Q.11 How can you differentiate between right and left maxillary lateral incisor?
Ans.
- Distal outline is more rounded than mesial outline
- Distoincisal angle is more rounded than mesioincisal angle.

Q.12 What are differences between right and left maxillary canine?
Ans.
- Mesial cusp ridge is shorter than distal cusp ridge
- Curvature of cervical line is more on mesial side than on distal side.

Q.13 What are the differences between right and left maxillary first molar?
Ans.
- Cusp of Carabelli is present on palatal surface of mesiopalatal cusp
- Mesiopalatal cusp is the largest cusp
- Oblique ridge extends from mesiopalatal to distobuccal cusp.

Q.14 What are the differences between right and left maxillary second molar?
Ans.
- Mesiopalatal cusp is largest of all
- Occlusal surface shows tilt from mesial to distal.

Q.15 Differentiate right and left mandibular lateral incisor.
Ans.
- Mesial side longer than distal
- Incisal edge twisted distolingually
- Incisal edge slopes downwards in distal direction
- A deep concavity is present on distal side above the cervical line.

Q.16 What are the differences between right and left mandibular canine?
Ans.
- Mesial outline is almost straight and distal outline is convex
- Mesial cusp ridge is shorter than distal cusp ridge.

Q.17 What are the differences between right and left mandibular first premolar?
Ans.
- Occlusal surface slopes lingually
- Presence of mesiolingual groove which extends into mesial fossa of occlusal surface.

Q.18 Differentiate right and left second premolar.
Ans.
I. One buccal and one lingual cusp
- Curvature of cervical line is more on mesial side than on distal
- Distal marginal ridge is placed more cervically than mesial marginal ridge
- Mesial fossa is smaller than distal fossa.

II. One buccal and two lingual cusps
- Distolingual cusp is smaller than mesiolingual cusp
- Central fossa lies distal to the occlusal surface
- Distal groove is shorter then mesial groove.

Q.19 What are the differences between right and left mandibular first molar?
Ans.
- Mesiobuccal cusp is widest of all and distal cusp is smallest of all
- Occlusal surface shows distal tipping.

Q.20 Differentiate right and left mandibular second molar.
Ans.
- Crown shows distal tilt making occlusal surface to slope cervically from mesial to distal
- Crown shows distal and lingual taper.

Q.21 How can you differentiate maxillary first and second premolar?
Ans. Mesial cusp ridge is shorter than distal cusp ridge.

Q.22 Which tooth is bilaterally symmetrical?
Ans. Mandibular central incisor.

Q.23 What are important features of maxillary first molar?
Ans.
- First permanent tooth to erupt
- Most caries prone
- Location is at center of fully developed jaw anteroposteriorly
- Also called as 6 years molars because 1st molars erupt at the age of 6 years

Q.24 Name the protective functional form of the teeth.
Ans. The protective functional forms of the teeth are:
- Contour of teeth
- Marginal ridges
- Embrasures
- Interproximal area.

Q.25 What is the clinical significance of embrasure area?
Ans.
- Provides a spillway for food during mastication
- Prevents food from being forced through contact area.

Q.26 Define embrasures.
Ans. Embrasures can be defined as V-shaped spaces that originate at proximal contact areas between adjacent teeth. These are named according to the direction in which they radiate.

Q.27 Define marginal ridge.
Ans. Marginal ridges are defined as rounded borders of enamel which form the mesial and distal margins of occlusal surfaces of premolars and molars and mesial and distal margins of lingual surfaces of the incisors and canines.

Q.28 Discuss clinical significance of marginal ridge.
Ans.
- Help in balancing of teeth in both the arches
- Improve the efficiency of mastication
- Prevent food impaction in interproximal areas.

Q.29 What are problems with under contouring?
Ans. It means too little contouring, so that a space occurs between margins and the cavity walls. It leads to food impaction and trauma to the attachment apparatus.

Q.30 What are interproximal spaces?
Ans. Interproximal space is triangular-shaped area that is usually filled by gingival tissue. In this triangular area, the base is formed by alveolar process, sides by proximal surfaces of contacting teeth and apex is the contact area.

Q.31 What is significance of proper contact relation?
Ans.
- Stabilizes the dental arches by combined anchorage effect of all the teeth
- Keeps food away from packing between the teeth
- Protects interdental papillae.

Q.32 What is significance of marginal ridges
Ans.
- During restoration, marginal ridges should be restored in two planes, i.e., buccolingually and cervico-occlusally.
- Restoring marginal ridges in two planes prevent food lodgement which causes damage to the periodontium
- Restore adjacent marginal ridges at the same height.

Q.33 What are differences between maxillary first and second molar?
Ans.

Maxillary first molar	Maxillary second molar
Usually five cusps are present	Usually four cusps are present
Cusp of Carabelli is present	It is absent
Buccal cusps are equal in height	Distobuccal cusp is smaller in size
Oblique ridge is prominent	It is not prominent
Distopalatal cusp is large	It is smaller in size

Q.34 What are the differences between central and lateral incisor?
Ans.

Central incisor	Lateral incisor
Slightly more in dimensions (bigger size)	Smaller in dimensions (smaller size)
Mesiodistal dimensions more than labiolingual dimensions	Mesiodistal and labiolingual dimensions are almost same
Palatal fossa is large and shallow	Palatal fossa is small and deep
Palatal pit is not a common finding	Palatal pit is commonly seen
Mesioincisal angle is sharp	It is somewhat rounded
Distoincisal angle is slightly rounded	It is more rounded
Marginal ridges and cingulum are moderately prominent	Marginal ridge and cingulum are more prominent

Q.35 What are the differences between maxillary and mandibular canine?
Ans.

Maxillary canine	Mandibular canine
Buccolingual dimensions are more	Buccolingual dimensions are smaller than maxillary canine
Cingulum is more prominent	It is less prominent
Lingual fossa is quite deep	It is almost flat
In mesial and distal aspect cusp tip lies labial to long axis of root	Cusp tip lies lingual to line passing through cusp tip and long axis of root

Q.36 What are the differences between maxillary first and second premolar?
Ans.

First premolar	Second premolar
Buccal cusp is higher than palatal cusp	Both cusps are almost of similar height
Mesial and distal surfaces converge palatally	Mesial and distal sides are almost parallel
Mesial cusp slope is larger than distal cusp slope	Mesial cusp slope is shorter than distal cusp slope
Mesial marginal development groove is present	It is absent
Occlusal outline is almost hexagonal in shape	It is almost rounded or ovoid in shape

Q.37 Differentiate mandibular first and second premolar.
Ans.

First premolar	Second premolar
Buccal cusp is higher than palatal cusp	Both cusps are almost of similar height
Mesial and distal surfaces converge palatally	Mesial and distal sides are almost parallel
Mesial cusp slope is larger than distal cusp slope	Mesial cusp slope is shorter than distal cusp slope
Mesial marginal development groove is present	It is absent
Occlusal outline is almost hexagonal in shape	It is almost rounded or ovoid in shape

Q.38 What are the differences between mandibular central and lateral incisor?
Ans.

Central incisor	Lateral incisor
■ Bilaterally symmetrical	■ Asymmetrical
■ Mesioincisal and distoincisal angles are sharp	■ Distoincisal angle is more rounded than mesioincisal angle
■ Mesiodistal dimensions are less than lateral	■ Mesiodistal dimensions are more
■ Incisal edge is at right angle to labiolingual bisecting line	■ Incisal edge is twisted distolingually

Q.39 What are the differences between mandibular first and second molar?
Ans.

First molar	Second molar
■ Usually five cusps are present	■ Four cusps are present
■ Mesiodistal dimensions are more	■ Mesiodistal dimensions are less
■ Occlusal outline is almost hexagonal in shape	■ It is almost rectangular in shape
■ Main groove form Y-shaped pattern	■ Main groove forms + shaped pattern

Chapter 3: Carious and Non-carious Lesions of Teeth

Chapter Outline

- Etiology of dental caries
- Classification of dental caries
- Histopathology of dental caries
- Diagnosis of dental caries
- Recent methods of caries detection
- Caries risk assessment
- Prevention of dental caries
- Noncarious lesions of teeth
- Attrition
- Abrasion
- Erosion
- Abfraction
- Localized nonhereditary enamel hypoplasia
- Localized nonhereditary enamel hypocalcification
- Localized nonhereditary dentin hypoplasia
- Localized nonhereditary dentin hypocalcification

Loss of integrity of tooth surface may occur because of many reasons, carious and non-carious lesions being the most common.

Dental caries is one of the most prevalent chronic disease. It occurs as a result of an interaction between acid producing bacteria and fermentable carbohydrates. Acids present in the dental plaque may demineralize enamel and dentin.

Non-carious lesions like attrition, abrasion, abfraction, and other defects can affect the structural integrity of the tooth, contribute to dental sensitivity, influence pulp vitality and esthetics. Identifying the causative factors of tooth lesions is useful in establishing the diagnosis and patient treatment plan.

DEFINITIONS

- Microbial disease of the calcified tissues of the teeth, characterized by demineralization of calcified tissues and destruction of the organic substance of the teeth.
 —*Shafer*
- An infectious microbiological disease of teeth that results in localized dissolution and destruction of calcified tissues. —*Sturdevant*

ETIOLOGY OF DENTAL CARIES

Primary Factors

Tooth

- ***Susceptible areas on tooth***: Susceptible areas on tooth for caries are deep and narrow occlusal fissures, deep buccal or lingual pits, and exposed root. Also, enamel is quite thin at base of such deep pits and fissures
- ***Position of tooth***: If a tooth is out of position, rotated, or malaligned, it becomes difficult to clean, retains more food and debris, and thus becomes more prone to decay
- ***Biochemical structures of teeth:*** Surface enamel is more mineralized than subsurface enamel, and it also contains more fluoride than subsurface enamel. Therefore, in initial carious lesion, the subsurface enamel shows marked demineralization even though outer enamel is relatively intact. Lack of enamel maturation or presence of developmental defects, deficiency in minerals like calcium, phosphorus, fluorides, and hypoplasia make teeth more susceptible to tooth demineralization.

Substrate (Diet)

- ***Physical nature of diet***: More refined and less fibrous foods have low clearance from oral cavity and thus are more responsible for dental caries
- ***Chemical nature of diet***: Simple carbohydrates like glucose, fructose, and sucrose make the diet cariogenic. Complex carbohydrates are not easily fermentable and are thus less cariogenic
- ***Frequency of carbohydrate intake***: Greater the time lapse between acid attacks, better are the chances for the repair process (remineralization) to occur. This means lower the frequency of carbohydrate intake, lower is the risk of dental caries.

Bacteria

Streptococcus mutans is considered main causative factor for caries because of their ability to adhere to tooth surfaces, produce abundant amounts of acid, and survive and continue metabolism at low pH conditions.

Streptococcus mutans ferments the sucrose to produce the extracellular polysaccharide glucan, this glucan helps the ***S. mutans*** to adhere firmly to the tooth surface and inhibits diffusion of salivary buffers. By this, local environment becomes acidic which causes dissolution of tooth structure.

Time Period

Time period during which all above three principal factors, i.e., tooth, microorganisms, and substrate are acting jointly should be adequate to produce acidic pH which is critical for dissolution of enamel leading to carious lesion.

Modifying Factors

Saliva

- *Composition of saliva*: Under normal conditions, the tooth is continually in touch with saliva. Calcium and phosphate ions present in the saliva help in remineralization of the very early stages of carious lesion
- *pH of saliva*: The critical pH at which inorganic material of tooth begins to dissolve is 5.5; above this pH, saliva is saturated with Ca^{2+} and $PO4^{2-}$ ions
- *Viscosity of saliva:* Higher the viscosity of saliva, more is the incidence of dental caries
- *Antibacterial properties:* Lysozymes, lactoferrin, IgA, etc., present in saliva are responsible for antibacterial properties of saliva.

CLASSIFICATION OF DENTAL CARIES

Carious lesions can be classified in different ways:

Based on Anatomical Site

- *Pit and fissure caries* (**Fig. 3.1A**): Pit and fissure caries are seen in pit and fissures on occlusal surface of posterior teeth and buccal and lingual surfaces of molars and on lingual surface of maxillary anterior teeth
- *Smooth surface caries* (**Fig. 3.1B**): Smooth surface caries are seen on all smooth surfaces of teeth, viz. gingival third of buccal and lingual surfaces and proximal surfaces
- *Root caries* (**Fig. 3.1C**): Root caries occur on exposed root surface. These are most commonly seen in older patients.

Based on Whether Lesion is New One or Attacking

- *Primary caries* (**Fig. 3.2A**): It denotes lesions on unrestored surfaces
- *Recurrent/secondary caries* (**Fig. 3.2B**): Lesions developing adjacent to restorations are referred to as either recurrent or secondary caries.

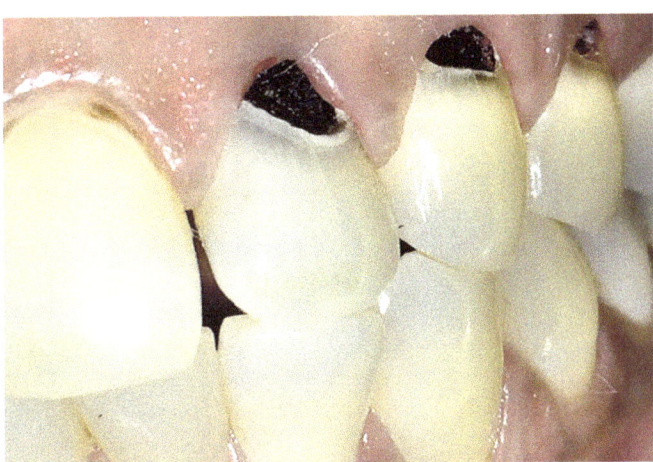

FIGURE 3.1C: Root caries.

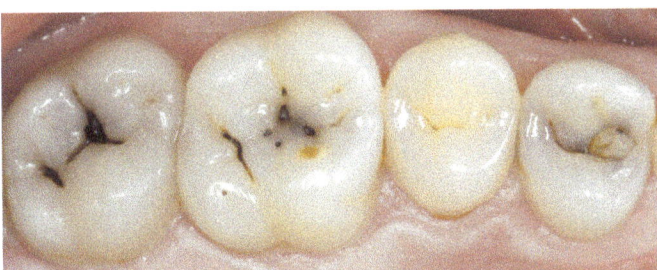

FIGURE 3.1A: Pit and fissure caries.

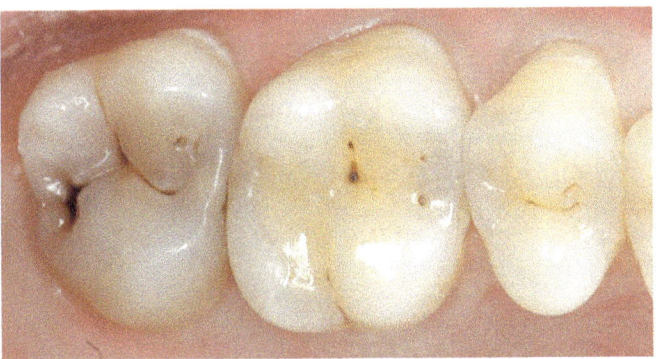

FIGURE 3.2A: Primary caries.

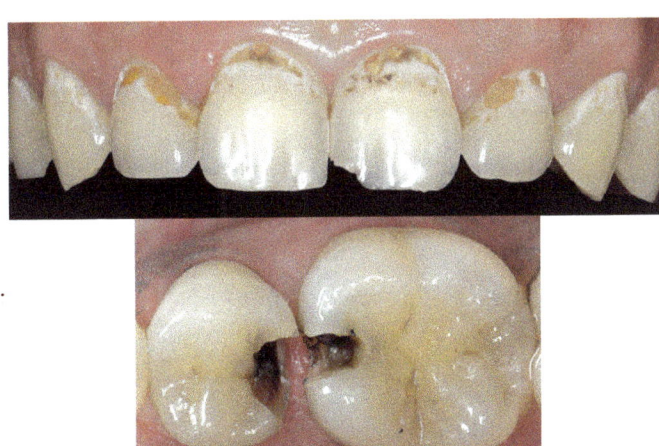

FIGURE 3.1B: Smooth surface caries.

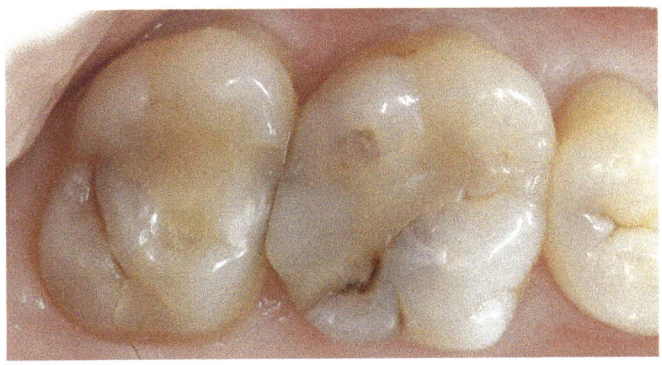

FIGURE 3.2B: Recurrent/secondary caries.

Based on Speed of Caries Progression

- *Acute caries:* Rapidly invading caries involving several teeth. If untreated, acute caries can result in pulp exposure. It is soft in consistency and light-colored
- *Chronic caries:* This is slowly progressing longstanding caries. It is hard in consistency and dark-colored
- *Rampant caries* (**Fig. 3.3**): Rampant caries is suddenly appearing, widespread, and rapidly burrowing type of caries resulting in early involvement of the pulp and affecting those teeth that are usually regarded as immune to caries
- *Arrested caries:* Arrested caries are caries which have become stationary or static and do not show tendency for further progression. These are seen in caries of occlusal surface with large open cavity which no longer retains food and becomes self-cleansing.

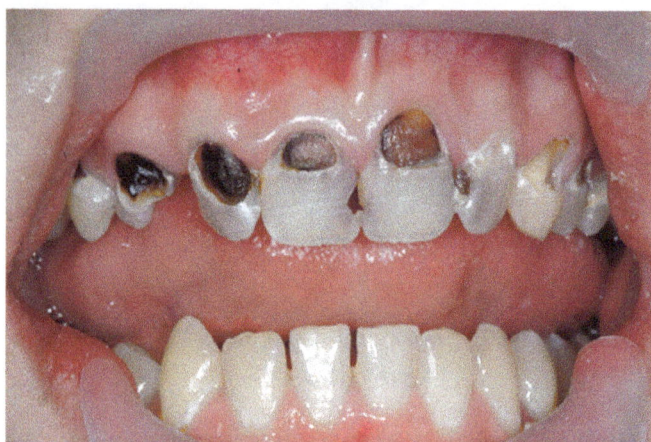

FIGURE 3.3: Rampant caries.

Based on Treatment and Restoration Design

- *Class I:* Pit and fissure caries occur in the occlusal surfaces of premolars and molars, the occlusal two-third of buccal and lingual surface of molars, and palatal surface of maxillary incisors (**Fig. 3.4A**)
- *Class II:* Caries on proximal surface of premolars and molars (**Fig. 3.4B**)
- *Class III:* Caries in the proximal surface of anterior teeth, not involving the incisal angles (**Fig. 3.4C**)
- *Class IV:* Caries in the proximal surface of anterior teeth involving the incisal angle (**Fig. 3.4D**)
- *Class V:* Caries on gingival third of facial and lingual or palatal surfaces of all teeth (**Fig. 3.4E**)
- *Class VI:* Caries on incisal edges of anterior and cusp tips of posterior teeth without involving any other surface (**Fig. 3.4F**).

Based on Number of Tooth Surfaces Involved

- *Simple caries:* Caries involving only one tooth surface is termed as simple caries
- *Compound caries:* If two surfaces are involved, it is termed as compound caries
- *Complex caries:* If more than two surfaces are involved, it is called as complex caries.

Based on Tooth Surface to be Restored

This classification uses initials of the involved tooth surfaces to be restored.

- O: Occlusal surface
- M: Mesial surface
- D: Distal surface
- F: Facial surface
- B: Buccal surface
- L: Lingual surface

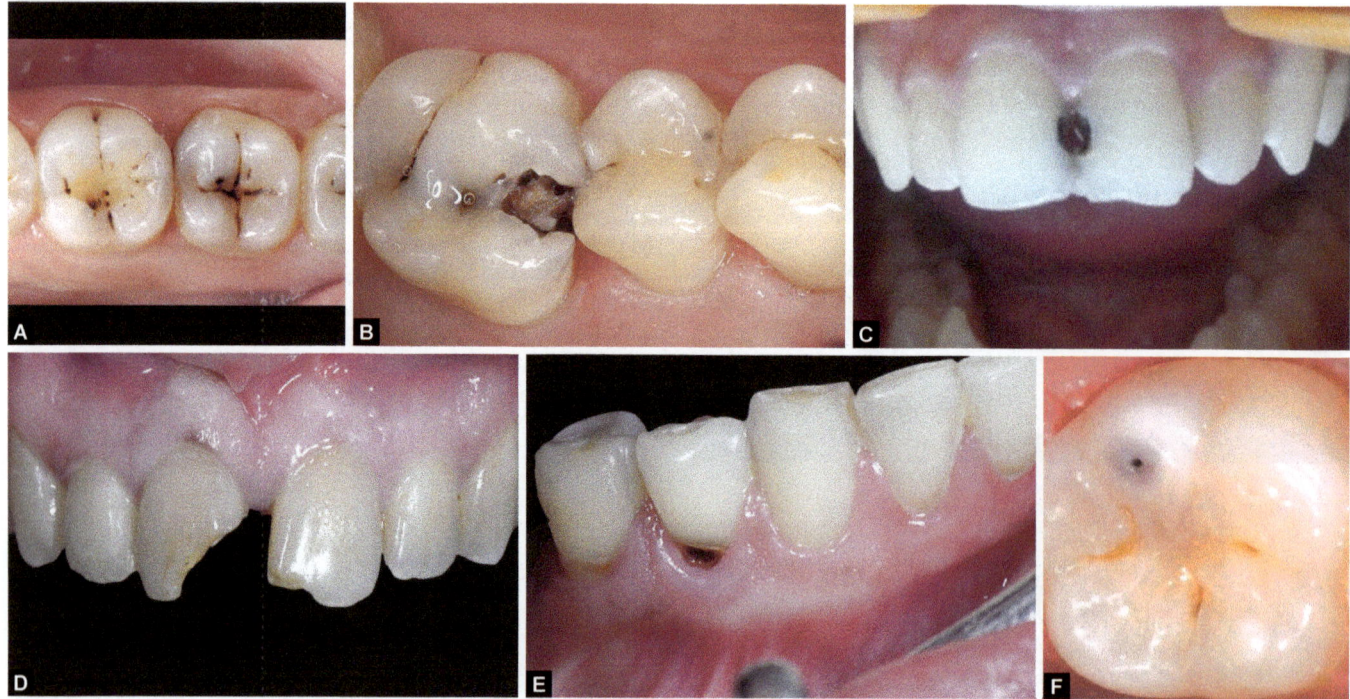

FIGURES 3.4A TO F: (A) Class I dental caries; (B) Class II dental caries; (C) Class III dental caries; (D) Class IV dental caries; (E) Class V dental caries; (F) Class VI dental caries.

HISTOPATHOLOGY OF DENTAL CARIES

Enamel Caries

Caries begin once bacterial plaque gets deposited in pits and fissures. Caries start on lateral walls of tissues which eventually fuse at base of fissure. Later, these pits and fissures become storehouse of bacteria causing dissolution of remaining enamel and later spread of caries in dentin.

Incipient Enamel Caries

These are covered with dental plaque. When plaque is removed and tooth is dried, incipient caries appears opaque and turn translucent on wetting.

Cavitation

If enamel lesion advances further, demineralization progresses resulting in cavitation, i.e., break in enamel. By this, bacteria gain entry into deeper tooth structure.

Zones of Enamel Caries (Fig. 3.5)

Different zones are seen before complete disintegration of enamel. Early enamel lesion seen under polarized light reveals four distinct zones of mineralization. Starting from surface, proceeding toward DEJ, the zones of enamel caries are as following:

- *Surface zone:*
  - This zone is least affected by caries
  - Greater resistance probably due to greater degree of mineralization and greater fluoride concentration
  - It is less than 5% porous
  - Its radiopacity is comparable to adjacent enamel.
- *Body of the lesion:*
  - Largest portion of the incipient caries
  - Found between the surface and the dark zone
  - It is the area of greatest demineralization making it more porous.
- *Dark zone*:
  - It lies adjacent and superficial to the translucent zone
  - Usually present and thus referred as positive zone
  - Called dark zone because it does not transmit polarized light
  - Formed due to demineralization.
- *Translucent zone:*
  - Represents the advancing front of the lesion
  - Ten times more porous than sound enamel
  - Not always present.

Dentinal Caries

When enamel caries reaches the dentino-enamel junction, it spreads rapidly laterally because it is least resistant to caries. Spread of caries is more in dentin as compared to enamel because of:
- Decreased calcification
- Dentinal tubules act as a tract along which microorganisms travel to pulp.

Zones of Dentinal Caries (Fig. 3.6)

Caries in dentin form a triangular shape with base toward DEJ and apex toward pulp with five distinct zones.

Beginning from the pulpal side, zones of dentinal caries are as following:

Zone 1: Normal Dentin

It is deepest layer with normal collagen, odontoblastic processes, and intertubular dentin.

Zone 2: Subtransparent Dentin

- Intertubular dentin is demineralized
- There are no bacteria in this zone. Hence, this zone is capable of remineralization.

Zone 3: Transparent Dentin

No bacteria are seen and collagen crosslinking is intact. Therefore, this zone is capable of remineralization.

Zone 4: Turbid Dentin

- Dentinal tubules contain bacteria
- Dentin is not self-repairable because of less mineral content.

Zone 5: Infected Dentin

- Outermost zone
- Consists of decomposed dentin filled with bacteria

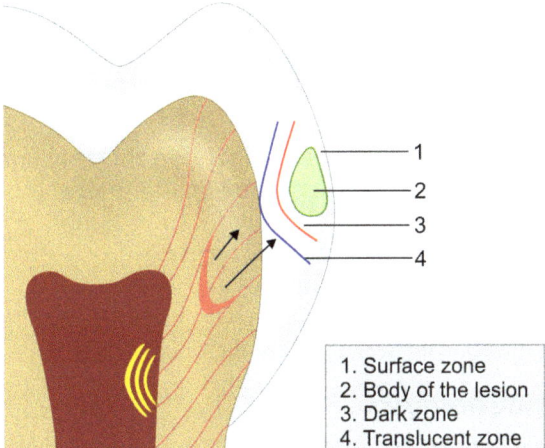

FIGURE 3.5: Schematic representation of zones of enamel caries.

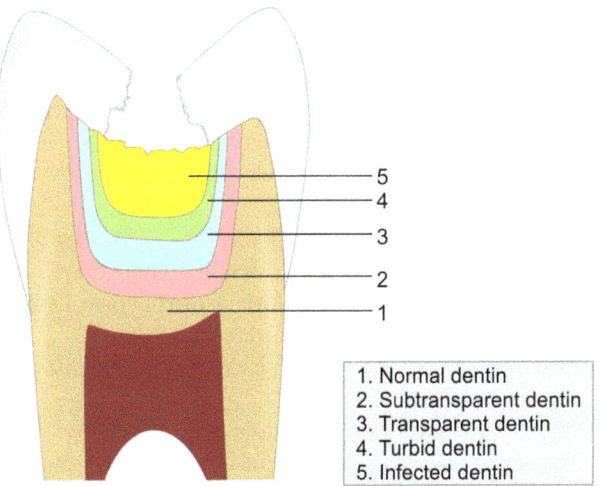

FIGURE 3.6: Zones of dentinal caries.

- It must be removed during tooth preparation
- Clinically, zones 2 and 3 constitute the affected dentin and zones 4 and 5 form infected dentin.

DIAGNOSIS OF DENTAL CARIES

Visual Examination

Visual examination is based on the criteria like cavitation, surface roughness, opacification and discoloration of clean and dried teeth under adequate light source.

Tactile Examination

Here explorer is used to detect softened tooth structure. Explorer is used with gentle pressure just to blanch a fingernail without causing any pain.

Radiographic Examination

For detecting caries radiographically, conventional, intraoral, periapical and bitewing radiographs are used. Radiographic diagnosis of pits and fissures decay is difficult in earlier stages because decalcified, radiolucent tooth structure is less as compared to the healthy surrounding tooth structure. Bitewing radiographs are preferably used to detect interproximal caries. Root caries appear as diffuse radiolucent areas with ill-defined borders on proximal aspects of teeth in the cervical areas.

Ultraviolet Illumination

Natural fluorescence of enamel is decreased in carious areas because of less mineral content. Carious lesion appears dark spot against a fluorescent background.

RECENT METHODS OF CARIES DETECTION

- *Digital dental radiography:* It results in low radiation dose, better contrast and resolution of the images
- *Digital imaging fiberoptic transillumination (DIFOTI).* Light from DIFOTI probe is positioned on the tooth, tooth is illuminated, and resultant images are captured by a digital electronic charge-coupled device (CCD) camera and displayed on computer.

CARIES RISK ASSESSMENT

Assessment of a caries risk at screening or initiation of therapy allows better appraisal of caries activity and refinement of the treatment planning. For example, children at high-risk of caries require intense prevention to primarily prevent caries initiation and secondarily to arrest caries progression.

High Caries Risk

A patient is said to be at high caries risk, if there is:
- One new lesion on smooth surface during past 1 year
- New carious lesion on root surface
- Patient on medication which causes hyposalivation
- Systemic disorder
- Past dental history with multiple restorations
- Exposure to sugary snacks for more than three times a day
- Senility.

Factors commonly seen in patients with high caries risk:
- *Status of oral hygiene:*
  - Poor oral hygiene
  - Nonfluoridated toothpaste
  - Low frequency of tooth cleaning
  - Orthodontic treatment
  - Partial dentures.
- *Dental history:*
  - History of multiple restorations
  - Frequent replacement of restorations.
- *Medical factors*:
  - Medications causing xerostomia
  - Gastric reflux
  - Sugar-containing medications
  - Sjögren's syndrome.
- *Behavioral factors:*
  - Bottle feeding at night
  - Eating disorders
  - Frequent intake of snacks
  - More sugary foods
  - Nonfluoridated toothpaste.
- *Socioeconomic factors:*
  - Low education status
  - Poverty
  - No fluoride supplement.

PREVENTION OF DENTAL CARIES

Dietary Measures

- **Avoid excessive intake of sugary and sticky foods**, such as cakes, biscuits, jams, and sweets
- **Intake of raw fruits and vegetables** helps in increasing the salivary flow, thereby removal of food debris from the oral cavity
- **Fats** form a protective barrier on enamel or carbohydrate surface, so that it becomes less available for bacteria. They also speed up the clearance of carbohydrate from oral cavity, thus decreasing cariogenic potential.

Oral Hygiene

Oral hygiene can be maintained by toothbrushing, interdental cleaning by dental floss, tape, and interdental brushes.

Chemical Measures

- *Chlorhexidine gluconate:* Chlorhexidine binds to the bacterial cell wall and interferes with membrane transport systems
- *Fluorides:* Fluoride ions increase the resistance of hydroxyapatite in enamel and dentin to dissolution by plaque acids
- *Effects of fluorides:* Fluorides cause:
  - Formation of fluorapatite
  - Induces remineralization
  - Inhibits bacterial metabolism.

Fluoride Products

- *Professional topical fluorides:* Commonly used products under professional applications are:

- **2.72% acidulated phosphate fluoride (APF) gel** contains 12,300 ppm fluoride. It is made from sodium fluoride and 0.1 M phosphoric acid
- **2% sodium fluoride gel:** It contains 9,200 ppm fluoride.

Methods of Use
- Administer 0, 1, 2, 3, and 4 times a year as indicated by caries risk level
- Isolate the teeth and apply gel for 4 minutes
- Advise patient to avoid rinsing, drinking, or eating for 30 minutes after application
- Apply at age of 3, 7, 11 and 13 years of age and 4 applications each year at one-week interval
- *Fluoride varnish:* Duraflor is commonly used fluoride varnish which contains 5% NaF
- *Mouthrinses:* Daily rinsing with 0.05% NaF (226 ppm F), and use of 0.2% NaF (900 ppm F) once every 2 weeks has shown to be effective
- *Dentifrices:* Dentifrices are considered as principal means of delivering topical fluoride.

Application of Remineralizing Agents
Commonly used agents are dicalcium phosphate dihydrate (DCPD), calcium carbonate, casein phosphopeptide (CPP), and amorphous calcium phosphate (ACP) complexes.

Mechanism of Action of CPP-ACP
CPP stabilizes calcium phosphate in solution and increases the level of calcium phosphate. Thus, CPP-ACP nanocomplexes act as a reservoir of calcium and phosphate ions so as to have supersaturation state with respect to tooth enamel and buffer plaque pH.

NONCARIOUS LESIONS OF TEETH
Several categories of tooth surface loss exist including erosion, attrition, abrasion, and abfraction, etc. There can be many causes of these conditions including bruxism, clenching, dietary factors, habits, lifestyle, incorrect tooth brushing, abrasive dentifrices, and aging.

ATTRITION (FIG. 3.7)

Definition
Attrition may be defined as the physiologic wearing away of a tooth as a result of tooth-to-tooth contact during mastication, and parafunctional movements. It is most often seen on the occlusal, incisal, and proximal surfaces of teeth.

Etiology of Attrition
Attrition of teeth is a normal physiological process.
However, several factors can cause excessive or pathological occlusal wear.
- *Parafunctional habits:* Bruxism is a parafunctional, habit of grinding or clenching the upper and lower teeth against each other
- *Developmental anomalies:* Amelogenesis imperfecta and dentinogenesis imperfecta predispose teeth to rapid wear

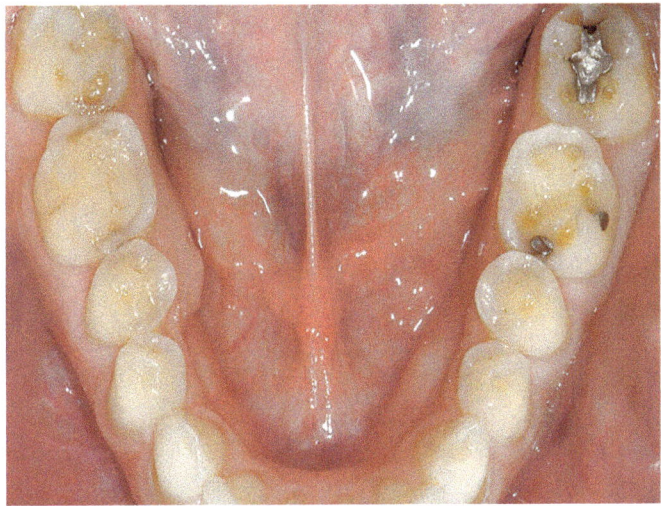

FIGURE 3.7: Attrition of occlusal aspect of posterior teeth.

- *Iatrogenic:* Occlusal prematurities due to faulty restorations can be uncomfortable for the patient which can make him grind his teeth against each other
- *Occupation:* Attrition can occur when a person is exposed to an atmosphere of abrasive dust and cannot avoid getting the material into his/her mouth.

Features
- There is appearance of a small polished facet on a cusp tips or ridges or a slight flattening of incisal edges
- Attrition may be entirely asymptomatic, or there may be dentin hypersensitivity secondary to loss of the enamel layer
- Loss in posterior and occlusal stability, so mechanical failure of restoration occurs.

ABRASION (FIG. 3.8)
Abrasion is a pathologic wearing away of tooth surface through some abnormal mechanical process, habits, and abrasive substance. Abrasion usually occurs on exposed root surfaces of teeth, but under certain circumstances it may be seen on other surfaces, such as on incisal or proximal surfaces.

Etiology of Abrasion
Various etiological factors are:
- *Faulty oral hygiene practice:* The common cause of abrasion is the faulty use of toothbrush carrying dental abrasive. Toothbrush can cause wear particularly if used in horizontal direction
- *Abnormal oral habits:* Abrasion can be caused due to certain habits like:
  - Habitual holding of pins in teeth may result in notching of incisal edges of maxillary incisors
  - Chewing tobacco can cause generalized occluding surface abrasion
  - Forcing toothpicks, interproximal brushing can cause proximal surface abrasion.

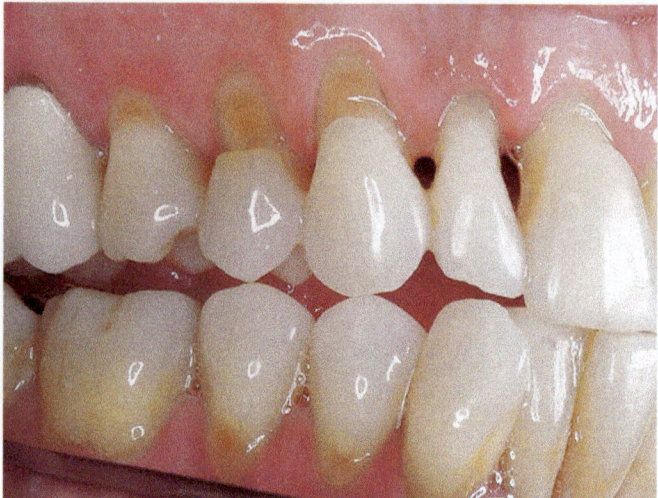

FIGURE 3.8: Abrasion cavities present on maxillary canine, 1st and 2nd premolars showing wedge shaped defects.

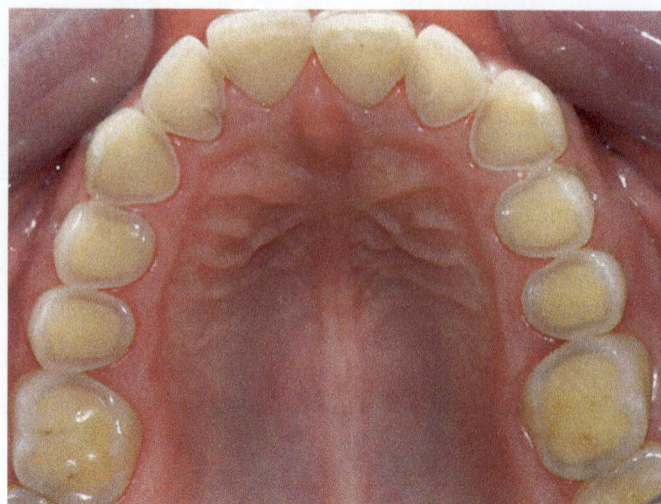

FIGURE 3.9: Clinical picture of erosion.

Clinical Features
- It is V-shaped or wedge-shaped defect on the CEJ in teeth with some gingival recession with angle of the V being sharp one
- Exposed dentin is smooth and polished
- Lesion may be extremely sensitive to cold, touch or air.

EROSION (FIG. 3.9)

Definition
Erosion can be defined as the loss of tooth structure resulting from chemical process in the absence of specific microorganisms.

Etiology of Erosion
- *Intrinsic erosion:* It occurs due to involvement of endogenous acids, mainly due to regurgitation of gastric acid into the oral cavity. This may occur in following conditions:
  - Eating disorders like anorexia nervosa and bulimia nervosa
  - Vomiting
  - Recurrent vomiting
  - Psychogenic vomiting syndrome
  - Gastrointestinal disorder
  - Peptic ulcer.
- *Extrinsic erosion:* Occurs due to acids from:
  - Environmental origin like professional wine tasters, battery, electroplating chemical manufacturer, and swimmers
  - Dietary origin: It is by high intake of citrus fruit and juices, carbonated beverages, and pickled foods
  - Medicinal origin: Aspirin, vitamin C, iron tonics, and acidic mouthwashes can cause extrinsic erosion.

Clinical Features
- Erosion affects upper teeth more than lower teeth, especially attacking the facial surface of cuspids and premolars
- These are rounded lesions with no demarcation so explorer can easily pass without interruption between lesions and surrounding teeth
- Surface of lesion is glazed
- Loss of surface characteristics of enamel in young children
- Dentin sensitivity to physical, chemical, and mechanical stimuli may be present
- Teeth with erosion do not tend to retain plaque.

ABFRACTION (FIG. 3.10)

Abreak means "to break away" and the term is derived from the Latin words "ab", or "away" and "fractio", or "breaking". Here, tooth substance loss occurs due to biomechanical loading forces that result in flexure and ultimate fatigue of enamel and dentin at a location away from loading.

Etiology of Abfraction
- When a tooth is hyperoccluded, the masticatory forces are transmitted to this tooth, which transfers this energy to the cervical region
- Lateral force produces compressive stress on the side toward which the tooth bends and the tensile stress is on the other side. These stresses create microfractures in the enamel or dentin at the cervical region. These fractures are perpendicular to the long axis of the tooth leading to a localized defect around the CEJ. The lesion is formed by combined bending and deformations. This leads to alternating tensile and compressive stresses, resulting in weakening of the enamel and dentin. If the forces reach up to a fatigue limit, the tooth cracks or breaks **(Flowchart 3.1)**.

Clinical Features
- Abfraction is very common on the anterior and premolar teeth, because of their smaller size on buccal or lingual surfaces due to the direction of the occlusal or incisal loads

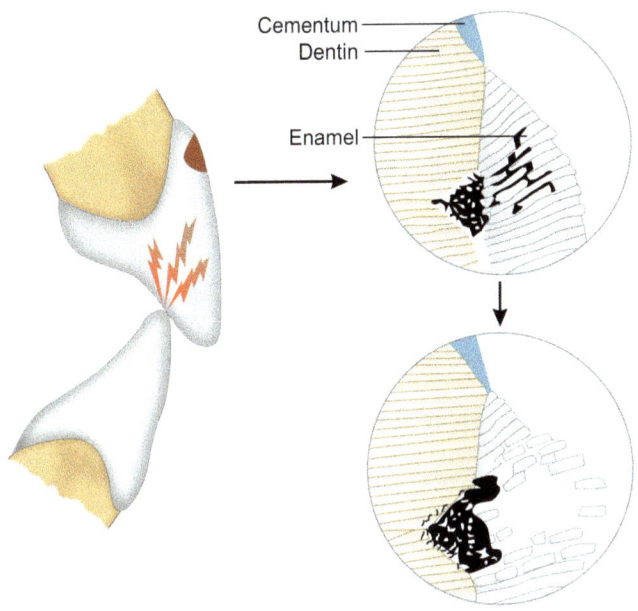

FIGURE 3.10: Abfraction. Fracture of tooth due to lateral forces.

FLOWCHART 3.1: Loss of tooth structure in abfraction.

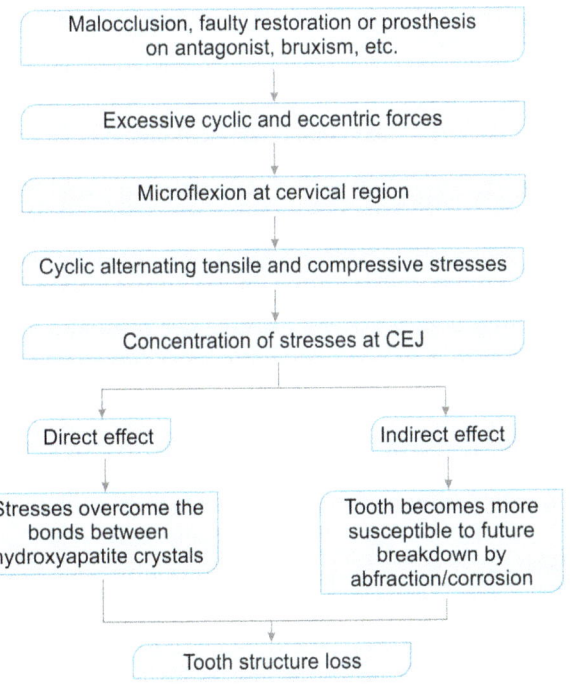

- Abfraction lesion appears as a wedge-shaped defect with sharp line angles. In the early stages, it may appear as minor irregular crack or fracture line in cervical region of the tooth. But in later stages, it appears as groove extending into the dentin.

LOCALIZED NONHEREDITARY ENAMEL HYPOPLASIA

During amelogenesis, ameloblasts that are responsible for formation of enamel, if they are injured, it will result in defective formation of enamel matrix. This will ultimately result in defective enamel formation. When the teeth erupt, these defects will be evident in the crown portion of the tooth

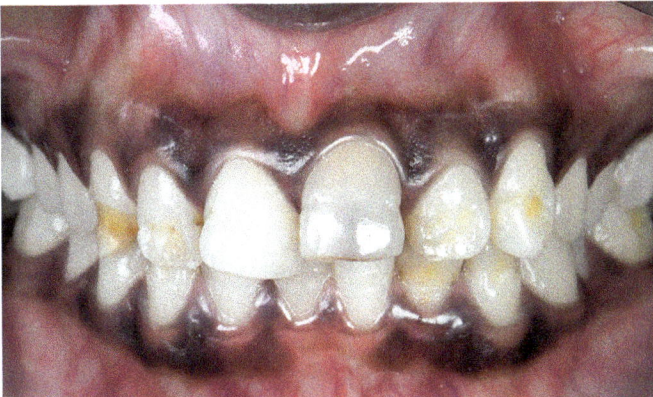

FIGURE 3.11: Amelogenesis imperfecta.

and this is called localized nonhereditary enamel hypoplasia (**Fig. 3.11**).

Etiology
- ***Systemic disorders:*** Nutritional deficiency such as deficiencies of vitamin A, C, and D and hypocalcemia
- ***Birth injuries:*** If birth is traumatic, then there may be alteration of formation of enamel which leads to enamel hypoplasia
- ***Localized infection:*** These include periapical infections of the preceding deciduous tooth (Turner's hypoplasia), etc.
  - Fluorides: Ingestion of fluoride containing drinking water during the time of tooth formation may cause mottled enamel. Enamel hypoplasia may range from white flecks to pitting and brownish staining of enamel.

LOCALIZED NONHEREDITARY ENAMEL HYPOCALCIFICATION (FIG. 3.12)

These are the defects of the enamel which are ectodermal in origin. These usually occur when ameloblasts are injured during mineralization of enamel. If mineralization of enamel matrix is affected in the calcification stage, it leads to nonhereditary enamel hypocalcification. The highest incidence of hypocalcification is on the anterior teeth of the upper and lower jaws.

Clinical Features
- These areas are chalky and can be easily stained
- The shades of teeth may range from chalky to yellow or brown, dark brown, and/or grayish.

LOCALIZED NONHEREDITARY DENTIN HYPOPLASIA

Their function and products (dentin) can be disturbed by environmental irritation, leading to deficient or complete absence of dentin matrix deposition. If ameloblasts are damaged, it means no enamel in that area but in odontoblasts, there will be no dentin temporarily but dentin deposition will be resumed as soon as other cells of pulp start depositing it. In these cases, defect will be isolated within the dentin substance and this situation does not require any treatment.

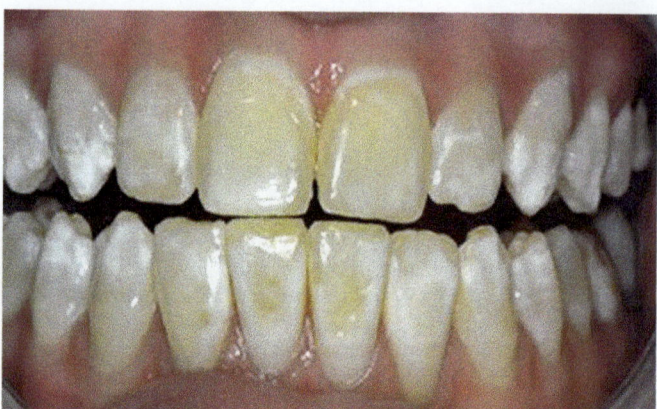

FIGURE 3.12: Hypocalcification.

LOCALIZED NONHEREDITARY DENTIN HYPOCALCIFICATION

In some cases, during the formative stage, if odontoblasts are disturbed, it may result in total absence or faulty deposition of dentin. If dentin matrix is deposited and fails to calcify, it will results in localized dentin hypocalcification. Dentin in such cases is soft, easily penetrable, and less resilient.

VIVA QUESTIONS

Q.1 Define dental caries.
Ans. It is defined as multifactorial, transmissible, infectious oral disease caused primarily by complex interaction of cariogenic oral flora with fermentable dietary carbohydrates on the tooth surface over time.

Q.2 Which bacteria cause dental caries?
Ans. Dental caries is a multibacterial diseases in which single bacteria cannot be said as the causative factor, though the most commonly associated bacterias with dental caries are **S. mutans** and **L. acidophilus**.

Q.3 What are characteristic features of cariogenic bacterias?
Ans. Cariogenic microorganisms are aciduric (capable of living in acid environment) and acidogenic (capable of producing acid).

Q.4 What is role of plaque in developing dental caries?
Ans. Plaque is a tenacious membrane formed around the teeth, mainly consisting of microorganisms. These microorganisms produce acids which reduce pH of plaque, and dissolve mineral content of enamel and thus, initiate caries.

Q.5 If bacteria are present in mouth, will they initiate caries?
Ans. For caries to occur, fermentable carbohydrates need to be present around the teeth so that bacteria can utilize food particles for energy by breakdown of carbohydrate molecules. This produces acid byproducts which initiate the dental caries.

Q.6 What are most commonly affected parts of teeth?
Ans.
- Deep pits and fissures
- Gingival recession cases
- Below contact area.

Q.7 Classify dental caries.
Ans. **According to their anatomical site**
- Pit and fissure caries
- Smooth surface caries
- Root caries.

According to whether it is a new lesion or recurrent carious lesion
- Primary caries
- Recurrent caries
- Residual caries.

According to speed of caries progression
- Acute dental caries
- Rampant caries
- Chronic dental caries.

Based on treatment and restoration design
- Class I
- Class II
- Class III
- Class IV
- Class V
- Class VI.

Q.8 What are pit and fissure caries?
Ans. These occur on occlusal surface of posterior teeth and buccal and lingual surfaces of molars and on lingual surface of maxillary incisors.

Q.9 What are acute and chronic caries?
Ans. Acute caries travel towards the pulp at a very fast speed. Chronic caries travel very slowly towards the pulp.

Q.10 What are rampant caries?
Ans. It is the name given to multiple active carious lesions occurring in the same patient, frequently involving surfaces of teeth that are usually caries free.

Q.11 What are smooth surface caries?
Ans. These occurs on gingival third of buccal and lingual surfaces and on proximal surfaces.

Q.12 What are primary caries?
Ans. Primary caries denotes lesions on unrestored surfaces.

Q.13 What are recurrent caries?
Ans. Lesions developing adjacent to restorations are referred to as either recurrent or secondary caries.

Q.14 What are residual caries?
Ans. Residual caries are those which remains in the prepared tooth surface even after placing the restoration.

Q.15 What is Graham Mount's classification of caries?
Ans. This classification system is based on two simple parameters:
1. Location of carious lesion
2. Size of carious lesion

Cavity site	Size 1 (Minimal)	Size 2 (Moderate)	Size 3 (Enlarged)	Size 4 (Extensive)
Site 1 Pit and fissure	1.1	1.2	1.3	1.4
Site 2 Contact area	2.1	2.2	2.3	2.4
Site 3 Cervical region	3.1	3.2	3.3	3.4

Q.16 What are different reasons of non-carious loss of tooth surface?
Ans. Erosion, attrition, abrasion, and abfraction, etc.

Q.17 Define attrition
Ans. Attrition may be defined as the physiologic wearing away of a tooth as a result of tooth-to-tooth contact during mastication, and parafunctional movements. It is most often seen on the occlusal, incisal, and proximal surfaces of teeth.

Q.18 What is etiology of attrition?
Ans. Though it is a physiological process, but parafunctional activity like bruxism can cause excessive occlusal wear. Occlusal prematurities due to faulty restorations can be uncomfortable for the patient which can make him grind his teeth against each other.

Q.19 Define abrasion.
Ans. Abrasion is a pathologic wearing away of tooth surface through some abnormal mechanical process, habits, and abrasive substance.

Q.20 What is etiology of abrasion?
Ans. Faulty oral hygiene practice, toothbrush can cause wear particularly if used in horizontal direction. Abnormal oral habits like habitual holding of pins in teeth may result in notching of incisal edges, chewing tobacco and forcing toothpicks can cause proximal surface abrasion.

Q.21 Define erosion.
Ans. Erosion can be defined as the loss of tooth structure resulting from chemical process in the absence of specific microorganisms.

Q.22 What is etiology of erosion?
Ans.
- Intrinsic erosion due to involvement of endogenous acids, eating disorders like anorexia nervosa, bulimia nervosa, vomiting, gastrointestinal disorder and peptic ulcer.
- Extrinsic erosion occurs due to acids from, environmental origin like professional wine tasters, battery, electroplating chemical manufacturer, and swimmers. Dietary origin by high intake of citrus fruit and juices, carbonated beverages, and pickled foods.

Q.23 What are clinical features of erosion?
Ans. Erosion affects facial surface of teeth. Lesions have rounded appearance with no demarcation, surface of lesion is glazed and sensitive.

Chapter 4: Dental Materials

Chapter Outline

- Classification of dental materials
- Properties of dental materials to be considered
- Dental cements
- Zinc oxide-eugenol cement
- Ethoxybenzoic acid reinforced cement
- Polymer reinforced zinc oxide-eugenol cement
- Zinc phosphate cement
- Zinc silicophosphate cements
- Calcium hydroxide
- Zinc polycarboxylate cement/zinc polyacrylate cement
- Glass ionomer cements
- Composition
- Setting reaction of glass ionomer cement
- Dental amalgam
- Clinical considerations
- Steps to reduce mercury exposure in the dental clinic
- Adhesive dentistry
- Definitions
- Enamel bonding
- Dentin bonding
- Evolution of dentin-bonding agents
- Composites
- Classification of composites
- Cast metal alloys
- Components of cast gold alloys
- Classification of cast gold alloys
- Waxes

Dental materials are especially fabricated materials which are designed to be used in dentistry. Many metals, nonmetals, resins, ceramics, organic and inorganic materials are used to replace or alter the tooth structure in form of dental materials.

CLASSIFICATION OF DENTAL MATERIALS

Classification According to Use

- Preventive (materials which primarily prevent or inhibit tooth decay)
  - Pit and fissure sealants
- Restorative (materials used to repair or replace the tooth structure)
  - Cements
  - Composites
  - Amalgam
  - Ceramics
  - Cast metals.
- Auxiliary (used for fabrication of prosthesis or appliances but don't become part of these devices)
  - Etchants
  - Waxes
  - Impression materials
  - Bleaching trays
  - Gypsum products.

PROPERTIES OF DENTAL MATERIALS TO BE CONSIDERED

- Physical properties
  - Coefficient of thermal expansion
  - Opacity
  - Translucency
  - Thermal and electrical conductivity
  - Hue, value and chroma.
- Mechanical properties
  - Compressive strength
  - Tensile strength
  - Shear strength
  - Malleability and ductility
  - Hardness.
- Biological properties
  - Allergy
  - Toxicity
  - Biocompatibility.
- Chemical properties
  - Setting reaction
  - Tarnish and corrosion
  - Chemical solubility and disintegration
  - Galvanic reaction.

DENTAL CEMENTS

Dental cement is the dental material which forms a hardened mass by mixing two components and are used as restorative materials, pulp protective materials underneath restorations and as luting cements for restorations. These components are available as powder and liquid or as two paste system.

Uses of Dental Cements

- As temporary restorations
- As permanent restorations
- For temporary luting

Dental Materials

- For permanent luting
- As root canal sealers
- For pulp protection as liners and bases.

Classification of Dental Cements based on Composition

- Conventional cement
  - Zinc oxide eugenol (ZOE) cement
  - Zinc phosphate cement
  - Glass ionomer cement
  - Polycarboxylate cement.
- Resin–base cement
  - Resin cement
  - Resin-modified glass ionomer cement.

ZINC OXIDE-EUGENOL CEMENT (FIG. 4.1)

Zinc oxide-eugenol cement is one of the oldest used cements. It has soothing action on pulpal tissues and eugenol has topical anesthetic properties therefore, it is also termed as an obtundent material. Though other cements are also used for temporization, but zinc oxide- eugenol cement is used most commonly because it is much less irritating to the pulp and produces better marginal seal than zinc phosphate.

Composition of Zinc Oxide-eugenol Powder

Sl. No.	Component	Percentage (%)	Purpose
1.	Zinc oxide (ZnO)	69.0%	Reactive ingredient
2.	White rosin	29.3%	Reduces brittleness
3.	Zinc stearate	1.0%	Catalyst
4.	Zinc acetate (acts as accelerator)	0.7%	Accelerator

Composition of Liquid

Sl. No.	Component	Percentage (%)	Purpose
1.	Eugenol	85.0%	Reactor
2.	Olive oil	15.0%	Plasticizer

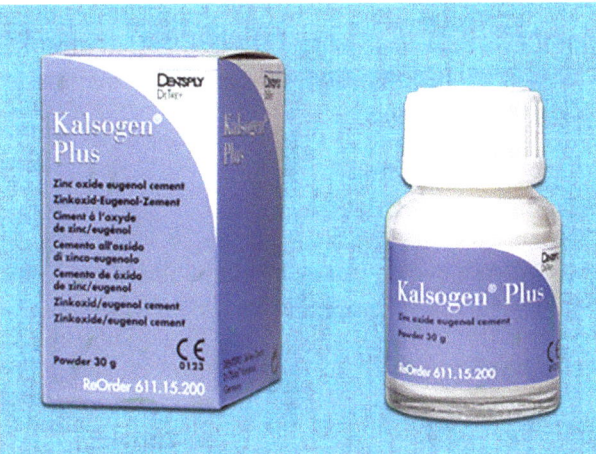

FIGURE 4.1: Zinc oxide-eugenol.
(*Courtesy:* Dentsply India)

Setting Reaction of Zinc Oxide-eugenol Cement

- On mixing powder and liquid, the zinc oxide hydrolysis occurs and subsequent reaction take place between zinc hydroxide and eugenol to form a chelate, zinc eugenolate
- *First reaction:*
$$ZnO + H_2O \rightarrow Zn(OH)_2$$
- *Second reaction:*
$$Zn(OH)_2 + 2HE \rightarrow ZnE_2 + 2H_2O$$
- Water is needed for the reaction and it is also a byproduct of the reaction. So, reaction progresses more rapidly in humid conditions
- Because zinc eugenolate rapidly hydrolyzes to form free eugenol and zinc hydroxide, it is one of the most soluble cements. To increase the strength of the set material, changes in composition can be made to the powder and liquid.

ETHOXYBENZOIC ACID REINFORCED CEMENT

- In this cement, ethoxybenzoic acid (EBA) chelates with zinc forming zinc benzoate
- Addition of fused quartz, alumina, and dicalcium phosphate improves mechanical properties of cement.

Composition of Ethoxybenzoic Acid Reinforced Cement

Sl. No.	Component	Percentage (%)	Purpose
1.	Zinc oxide (ZnO)	70%	Reactive ingredient
2.	Alumina	30%	Increases strength
3.	Fused quartz and calcium	30%	Improve mechanical properties

Composition of Liquid

1.	Eugenol	37.5%
2.	Ortho- ethoxybenzoic acid	62.5%

Effects of EBA on Eugenol Cement

- Increase in compressive and tensile strength
- More powder can be incorporated to achieve standard consistency
- Decrease in setting time (if concentration is <70%).

POLYMER REINFORCED ZINC OXIDE-EUGENOL CEMENT

In this mixture, resin helps in improving strength, smoothness of the mixture, and decreases flow, solubility, and brittleness of the cement.

Composition of Polymer Reinforced Zinc Oxide-eugenol Cement

Sl. No.	Component	Percentage (%)	Purpose
1.	Zinc oxide	80%	Reactive ingredient
2.	Polymethyl–methacrylate	20%	Increases strength
3.	Traces of zinc stearate, zinc acetate		

Composition of Liquid

| 1. | Eugenol | 85% | Reactor |
| 2. | Acetic acid | 15% | Accelerator |

Manipulation of zinc oxide-eugenol (ZOE) cement: ZOE cement is available as:
- Powder and liquid system
- Paste-paste system.

Manipulation of Powder and Liquid System (Fig. 4.2)

- Powder is measured and dispensed with a scoop whereas liquid is dispensed as drops on glass slab
- Powder is divided in main bulk increment, followed by smaller increments
- Start the mixing by incorporating half of the powder into the liquid with a heavy folding motion and pressure
- When powder particles are wet with liquid, add the remaining powder to the mixture and continue to use a heavy folding motion to attain a putty consistency
- For base, when mixing is done, bring the mixture together and roll it. One should be able to pick up the mixture without deformation.

Paste-paste system: In this, two pastes are dispensed in equal lengths on paper pad. Two pastes have different colors, and mixing is done till a homogeneous color is obtained.

Factors Affecting Working and Setting Time

- Higher the powder: Liquid ratio, faster the material sets
- Cooling of glass slab slows down the setting reaction
- Setting time of this cement is long but since water accelerates the setting reaction, it sets faster in mouth than outside.

Advantages	Disadvantages
▪ Least irritating cement	▪ Highly soluble
▪ Good short-term sealing	▪ Low strength
	▪ Low compressive strength

ZINC PHOSPHATE CEMENT

Zinc phosphate cement is one of the oldest and most widely used cements. It was first introduced in 1878 and still used today because of excellent clinical track record. Its ADA specification number is 8.

The Types of Zinc Phosphate Cement

- **Type I**: Used for cementation. It forms the film thickness of less than 25 μm.
- **Type II**: Used as base. It results in film thickness between 25 μm and 40 μm.

Composition of Zinc Phosphate Cement

Sl. No.	Component	Percentage (%)	Purpose
1.	ZnO	90.2%	Main ingredient
2.	MgO	8.2%	Increases compressive strength
3.	SiO_2	1.4%	Aids in calcination process
4.	Bi_2O_3	0.1%	Imparts smoothness to the mixed cement
5.	Miscellaneous (BaO, Ba_2SO_4, and CaO)	0.1%	

All the ingredients are sintered at temperatures between 1000°C and 1400°C into a cake that is subsequently ground into fine powder

Composition of Liquid

1.	Phosphoric acid	38.2%	Main reactive ingredient
2.	Water	36.0%	
3.	Aluminum or zinc phosphate	16.2%	
4.	Zinc	7.1%	Buffer
5.	Aluminum	2.5%	Buffer

Setting Reaction (Fig. 4.3)

Setting reaction is a two-stage process. In first part, zinc oxide powder reacts with phosphoric acid to form zinc phosphate and water. This zinc phosphate reacts with more zinc oxide forming hopeite (hydrated zinc phosphate). Aluminum prevents crystallization and permits the formation of an amorphous cement.

Manipulation of Cement

- Working time ~ 5 minutes
- Setting time ~ 2.5–8 minutes.
  Mixing on a cooled glass slab allows the heat produced in the reaction to dissipate more easily and slow the chemical reaction, thus increasing the working time. Care must be taken not to cool the slab below the dew point or water condensation will form and affect the properties of the cement.

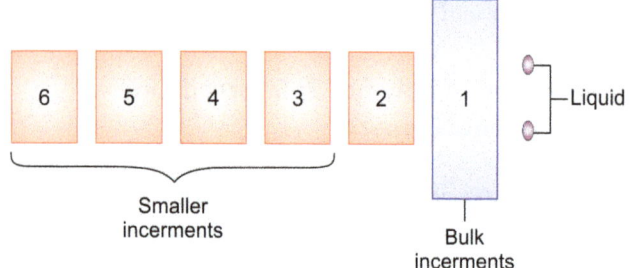

FIGURE 4.2: Distribution of powder and liquid for manipulation of ZOE cement.

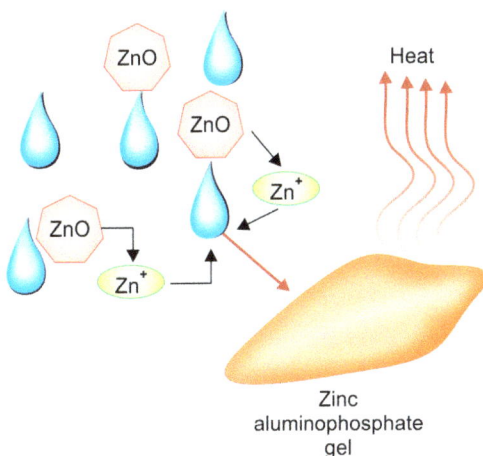

FIGURE 4.3: Setting reaction of ZOE cement.

Since setting reaction is an exothermic type, the heat liberated while setting further accelerates the setting rate. So, it is very important to dissipate the heat using chilled glass slab, mixing smaller increment for initial mixing of cement on large area of glass slab
- Powder is divided into 5–8 increments of different sizes **(Fig. 4.4)**
- *First two increments are smaller in size so as to:*
  - Achieve the slow neutralization of the liquid
  - Control the reaction by decreasing exothermic heat of reaction
- *Middle increments are larger in size:*
  - To saturate the liquid to form zinc phosphate
  - Because of presence of less amount of unreacted acid, this step is not affected by heat released from the reaction.
- *In the end, the smaller increments* of powder are added so as to:

Achieve Optimum Consistency

- While dispensing, the liquid bottle should be held vertical and close to the powder. Repeated opening of the liquid bottle or early dispensing of the liquid prior to mixing should be avoided because evaporation of liquid can result in changes in water/acid ratio which can further result in decrease in pH and an increase in viscosity of the mixed cement. If the liquid is cloudy or crystals are present in the bottle, it should be discarded as the concentration of the acid has been changed and it is no longer optimal
- For base or temporary restoration, consistency should be such that it can be rolled into a ball without sticking.

Mechanical Properties

- Strength depends on its powder to liquid ratio; zinc phosphate cement achieves 75% of its ultimate strength within 1 hour
- Good compressive strength of cement is 104 MPa
- Low tensile strength—5.5 MPa
- Modulus of elasticity is 13.7 gigapascals. This high MOE makes the cement quite stiff and resistant to elastic deformation
- Retention of cement by mechanical interlocking and not by chemical interaction.

Biocompatibility

Because of presence of phosphoric acid, acidity of cement is quite high (pH is 2.0) making it irritable to pulp

Advantages	Disadvantages
Long record of clinical acceptability	Low initial pH, irritant to pulp
High compressive strength	Lack of an adhesion to tooth structure
Thin film thickness	Lack of anticariogenic effect
	Soluble in water

ZINC SILICOPHOSPHATE CEMENTS

It is hybrid cement which is combination of zinc phosphate cement with silicate cement and is also known as silicophosphate cement. Most commonly used cement is silicophosphate cement that consists of 90% silicate cement powder and 10% zinc phosphate cement powder.

Composition

- Powder contains an acid soluble silicate, zinc, and magnesium oxides
- Liquid consists of phosphoric acid.

Properties of Zinc Silicophosphate Cements

- Translucent and more esthetic than zinc phosphate cement
- Anticariogenic because of fluoride release from this cement
- Has sufficient strength and low solubility.

CALCIUM HYDROXIDE

Calcium hydroxide has high alkaline pH (12.5). Its alkaline pH helps in neutralization of acids produced by the microorganisms and irritating acidic component of restorative base and materials. Calcium hydroxide also provides antibacterial properties.

Calcium hydroxide is available in:
- Powder form **(Fig. 4.5A)**
- Quick-setting paste form (Dycal) **(Fig. 4.5B)**.

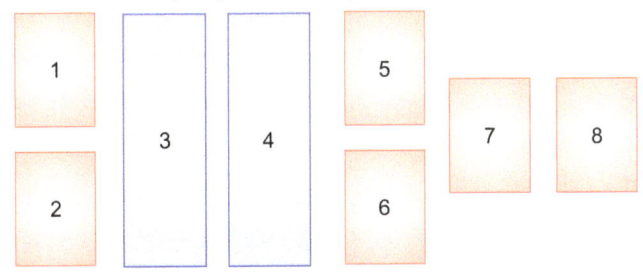

FIGURE 4.4: Division of powder into 5–8 small increments. First two increments are smaller in size so as to have slow neutralization of liquid and control the reaction. Middle increments are larger in size to saturate the liquid and form bulk and finally smaller increments of powder are added so as to achieve optimum consistency.

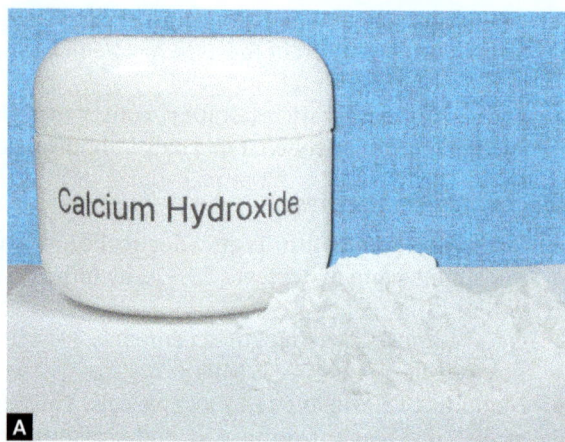
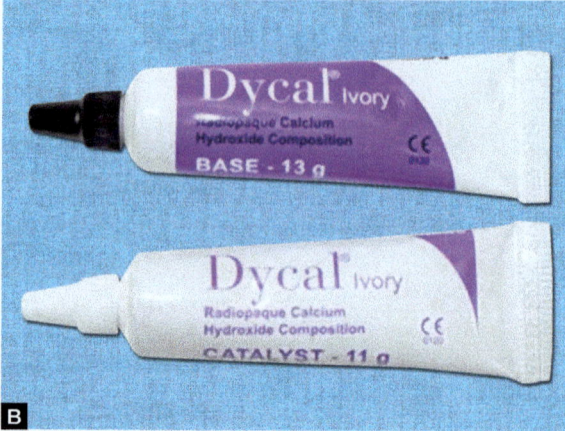

FIGURES 4.5A AND B: Calcium hydroxide.

Mixing Calcium Hydroxide Cement

- Dispense equal amount of base and catalyst onto the mixing pad
- Using calcium hydroxide applicator or spoon excavator, mix the cement for 10–15 seconds until a uniform color is achieved. Place the cement in the deepest portion of cavity.

Uses of Calcium Hydroxide

- As liner and sub-base
- For direct and indirect pulp capping
- In pulpotomy
- For apexification
- As root canal sealer.

ZINC POLYCARBOXYLATE CEMENT/ZINC POLYACRYLATE CEMENT (FIG. 4.6)

It was one of the first chemically adhesive dental materials introduced in the 1960s. It bonds to tooth structure because of chelation reaction between carboxyl groups of cement and calcium present in tooth structure.

Its ADA specification number is 96.

Composition of Zinc Polycarboxylate Cement/Zinc Polyacrylate Cement

Sl. No.	Component	Percentage (%)	Purpose
1.	Zinc oxide	85–96%	Main reactive ingredient
2.	Stannous fluoride	4%	Improves the set, leaches fluoride— anticariogenic
3.	Magnesium oxide	4–10%	Preserves white color
4.	Silica	0–2%	Improves sintering process
5.	Alumina	<5%	Forms complexes with acid

Composition of Liquid

Sl. No.	Component	Percentage (%)	Purpose
1.	Polyacrylic acid	32–43%	Main ingredient
2.	Itaconic acid/maleic acid	32–43%	

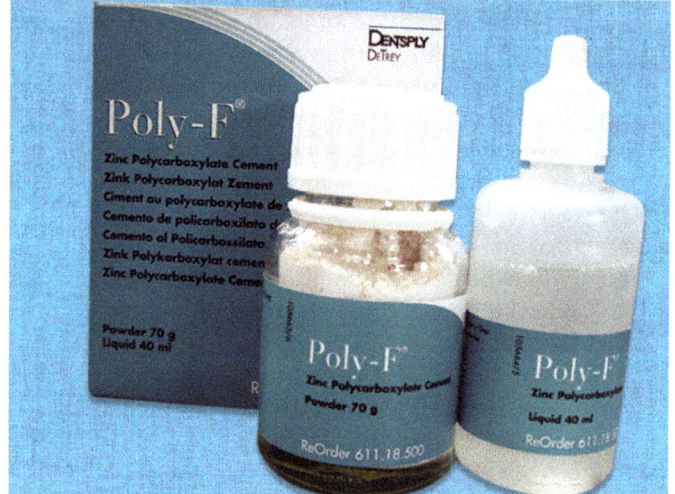

FIGURE 4.6: Zinc polycarboxylate cement.
(*Courtesy:* Dentsply)

Manipulation of Zinc Polycarboxylate Cement

- Liquid is dispensed just before mixing of the cement as the loss of water from liquid can result in increase in its viscosity. While dispensing the liquid bottle should be held vertical, so that liquid comes out under its own weight
- Mix first-half of powder to liquid to obtain the maximum length of working time. Mixed cement should be adapted to tooth till it is glossy in appearance. It shows presence of unreacted acid groups which are available for bonding.

Setting Reaction

When the zinc oxide and polyacrylic acid come into contact, a salt (zinc polyacrylate) matrix is formed only on the surface of the zinc oxide particles. Polyacrylic acid chains cross-link through the zinc ions of the zinc oxide. The set material has cores of zinc oxide within the zinc polyacrylate matrix binding the unreacted zinc oxide cores together.

The mixed cement goes through a rubbery phase as it is setting and it should not be disturbed during this phase because otherwise adhesive bond of the cement will be ruptured. This can cause microleakage if cement is pulled away from the tooth surface. The cement should not be disturbed until it can be removed cleanly from the margin of a cemented restoration.

Properties

- *Working time and setting time*:
  - Working time ~ 2.5 minutes
  - Setting time ~ 6-9 minutes.
- *Adhesive to tooth structure*:
  - Polyacrylic acid bonds with calcium ion via the carboxyl group. Adhesion depends on the unreacted carboxyl group.
- *Mechanical properties*:
  - Compressive strength is less than zinc phosphate cement ~ 55-67 MPa
  - Tensile strength ~ 2.4-4.4 MPa
  - Low modulus and is, therefore, slightly more elastic and less likely to fracture under heavy load.
- *Solubility*: It is low in water. But in acidic environment with pH of less than 4.5, solubility increases. Reduction in P:L ratio also increases solubility
- *Biological considerations*: pH of the liquid is 1.7 but increases rapidly after mixing. Zinc polycarboxylate is biocompatible because of the following reasons:
  - Size of polyacrylic acid molecule is bigger, this makes it difficult to enter into dentinal tubules.
- pH of the cement rises more rapidly when compared to that of zinc phosphate.

Advantages	Disadvantages
■ Adhesion to tooth structure	■ Short working time (2-3 minutes)
■ Rapid rise in pH upon cementation	■ Does not resist plastic deformation under high masticatory stresses
■ Biocompatible	

GLASS IONOMER CEMENTS

Glass ionomer cement (GIC) was introduced to dentistry in 1972 by Wilson and Kent. It is described as hybrid of dental silicate cements and zinc polycarboxylates where phosphoric acid of silicate cements is replaced by polyacrylic acid of zinc polycarboxylates.

Classification According to Skinners

- *Type I:* Luting cements
- *Type II:* Restorative cements
- *Type III:* Liner or base.

COMPOSITION

Conventional GIC

Glass ionomer is an acid-soluble calcium fluoroaluminosilicate glass, i.e., an ion leachable glass.

Composition of Glass Ionomer Powder

Sl. No.	Component	Percentage (%)	Purpose
1.	Silica	29	Forms mass of the cement
2.	Alumina	16	
3.	Aluminum fluoride	5	i. Acts as flux and decreases fusion temperature
4.	Calcium fluoride	34	ii. Improves translucency
5.	Sodium aluminum fluoride	5	iii. Improves strength and wearing characteristics
6.	Aluminum phosphate	9.9	i. Improves translucency
			ii. Adds body to mix cement
7.	Lanthanum, barium, and strontium	Traces	Radiopacifiers

Composition of Liquid

1.	Polyacrylic acid	45	Main component—contributing for formation of cement matrix
2.	Water	50	Reaction medium—essential part of cement structure helps in ionic exchange reaction
3.	Modifiers like: Itaconic acid, maleic acid	5	Prevents gelation of liquid which is formed due to hydrogen bond of two polyacrylic chains

These raw materials are fused at a temperature of 1,100-1,500°C to form uniform glass. This glass is then ground to powder having particle size of 15-50 μm.

Metal Reinforced Glass Ionomer Cements (Fig. 4.7)

Silver Alloy Admix Glass Ionomer Cement

In this, silver amalgam alloy is mixed with glass powder in ratio of 1:7. This cement has improved strength but poor resistance to abrasion and poor esthetics.

Cermet Cement

Cermet is manufactured by sintering and grinding of silver powder and glass ionomer powder at temperature of 800°C. It has improved compressive and tensile strength, greater abrasion resistance, and radiopacity when compared to conventional GICs, e.g., ketac silver.

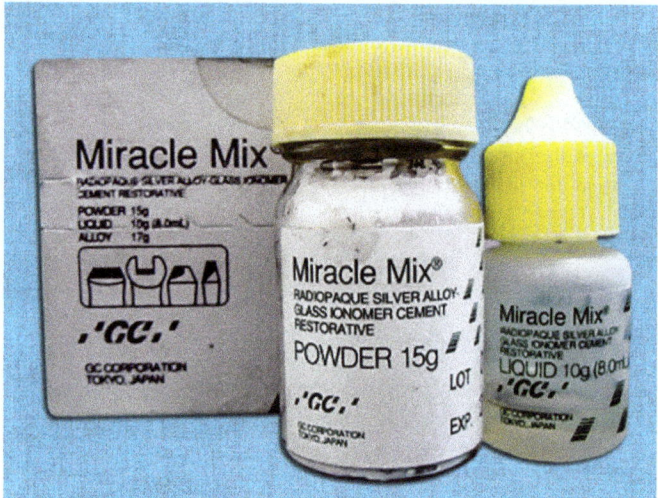

FIGURE 4.7: Miracle mix.

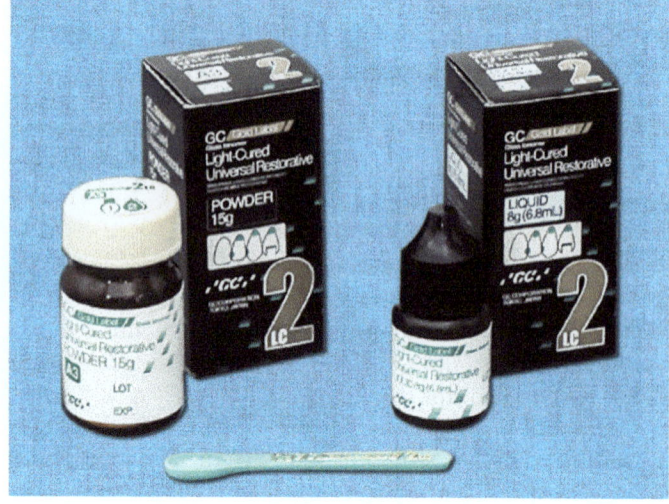

FIGURE 4.8: Resin-modified glass ionomer cement.

Resin-modified Glass Ionomer Cement (Fig. 4.8)

Powder
Fluoroaluminosilicate glass particles along with photoinitiator or chemical initiator.

Liquid
- Polyacrylic acid modified with methacrylate groups and HEMA monomers (15-25%)
- Water.

Advantages
- Improved physical properties
- Less technique sensitive
- Improved handling.

Manipulation of the Cement
- For mixing, dispense powder and liquid on mixing paper pad **(Fig. 4.9A)**. Always dispense powder before liquid to minimize loss of water due to evaporation
- Hold the bottle upright to ensure consistent sized drops while dispensing the liquid **(Fig. 4.9B)**
- Divide the powder into two equal portions **(Fig. 4.9C)**
- Mix first portion of powder with liquid for 10-15 seconds, then add 2nd half of powder and mix for another 15-20 seconds in folding motion by gently but rapidly folding powder into the liquid **(Fig. 4.9D)**
- The objective is to wet the particles, and not dissolving them. Mixing should be completed within 40-60 seconds
- Working time for glass ionomer cement is 60-90 seconds
- For restoration, bring the mix together. One should be able to pick up the mix without sticking to the instrument **(Fig. 4.9E)**
- For luting consistency, "1 inch" string should be formed when flat surface of spatula is pulled from the mixed cement **(Fig. 4.9F)**.

Loss of gloss/slump test: Final mixed cement should have glossy appearance. Loss of gloss shows end of working time. It is 60-90 seconds for conventional cement.

SETTING REACTION OF GLASS IONOMER CEMENT

Setting Reaction of Autocure Glass Ionomer Cement
It is an acid–base reaction between powder and liquid **(Fig. 4.10)**.
- Powder and liquid are mixed
- Surface of glass ionomers is attacked by H^+ ions
- Polyacid attacks the glass particles to release Ca^{2+} and Al^{3+}, F^- and Na^+
- Initially, calcium ions and later aluminum ions cross-link with polyacrylic acid to form calcium and aluminum polysalts
- Acid attacks Ca^- rich sites and metal ions migrate into aqueous phase of cement towards polyacrylic acid chains
- Cross linking of chains occur resulting in gelation and formation of calcium polyacrylate
- The salts hydrate to form gel matrix and surround the unreacted part of glass particles
- Final set cement consists of unreacted glass surrounded by silica gel bound together by matrix of hydrated calcium and aluminum polysalts.

Advantages	Disadvantages
■ Adhesion to tooth structure because of chemical bonding to enamel and dentin through ion exchange	■ Brittle and have low fracture resistance when compared to composite restorations
■ Biocompatible because large-sized polyacrylic acid molecules prevent the acid from producing pulpal response	■ Low wear resistance when compared to composite restorations
■ Anticariogenic because of fluoride release	■ Sensitive to moisture contamination and desiccation soon after placement, which can affect physical properties and esthetics
■ Good color matching and translucency makes it esthetic	
■ Glass ionomers show less solubility than other cements	

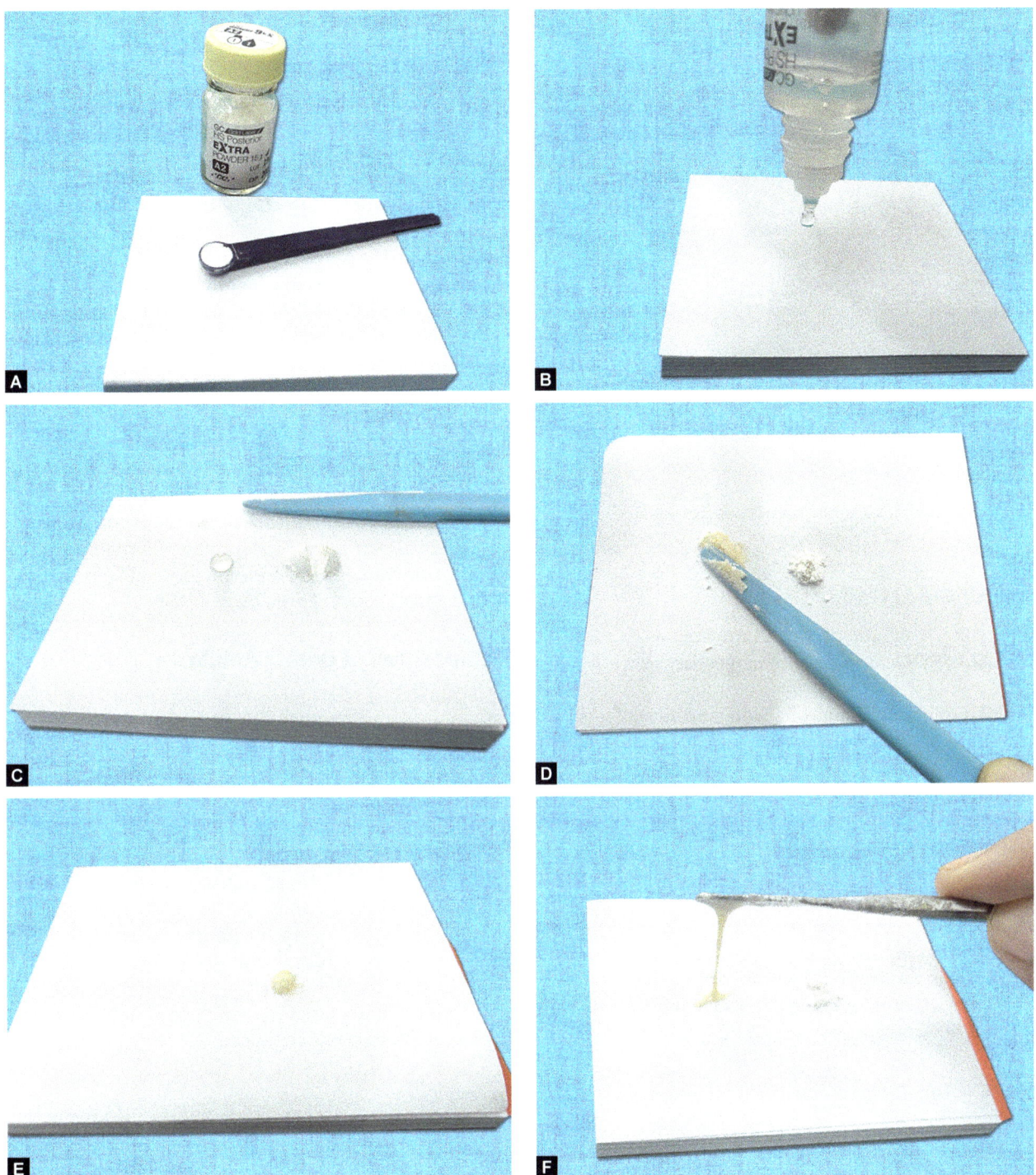

FIGURES 4.9A TO F: (A) For mixing, dispense powder and liquid on mixing paper pad; (B) Hold the bottle upright to ensure consistent sized drops while dispensing the liquid; (C) Divide the powder into two equal portions; (D) Mix first portion of powder with liquid for 10–15 seconds, then add 2nd half of powder and mix for another 15–20 seconds in folding motion; (E) For restoration, one should be able to pick up the mix without sticking to the instrument; (F) For luting consistency, "1 inch" string should be formed when flat surface of spatula is pulled from the mixed cement.

Indications	*Contraindications*
■ As pit and fissure sealants ■ As liners and bases ■ As luting agents ■ For restorations of small class I (buccal and palatal pits), III and V Lesions ■ In high caries risk patients	■ In stress-bearing areas like class I, class II, and class IV preparations because glass ionomers lack fracture toughness ■ In patients with xerostomia because restorations can become opaque, brittle, and disintegrate over a short period of time ■ In mouth breathers because restoration may become opaque, brittle, and may fracture over time ■ In areas requiring esthetics like veneering of anterior teeth

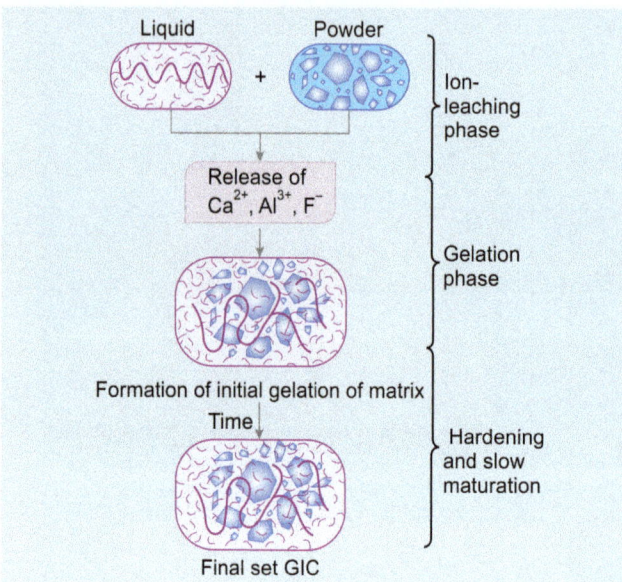

FIGURE 4.10: Setting reaction of glass ionomer cement.

DENTAL AMALGAM

- **Alloy:** Alloy is a union of two or more metals
- **Amalgam:** Amalgam is an alloy of mercury with any other metal
- **Dental amalgam:** Dental amalgam is an alloy of mercury with silver, tin, and varying amounts of copper, zinc, and other minor constituents
- **Dental amalgam alloys:** Dental amalgam alloys are silver-tin alloys with varying amounts of copper, zinc, and other metals.

Classification of Dental Amalgam

- **Based on shape of particles**
  - *Irregular:* In this, shape of particles is irregular, and may be in the shape of spindles or shavings
  - *Spherical:* In this, shape of particle is spherical with smooth surface
  - *Spheroidal:* In this, shape of particle is spheroidal with irregular surface
- **Based on copper content**
  - *Low copper alloy:* Contains copper in range of 2 to 6%
  - *High copper alloy:* Contains copper in the range of 12 to 30%.
- **Based on zinc content**
  - *Zinc-containing alloys:* In these, zinc is in range of 0.01–1%
  - *Zinc-free alloys:* Contain less than 0.01% of zinc.
- **Based on the presence of alloyed metals**
  - *Binary alloys:* Contain two metals, i.e., silver and tin
  - *Ternary alloys:* Contain three metals, i.e., silver, tin, and copper
  - *Quaternary alloys:* Contain four metals, i.e. silver, tin, copper, and zinc
  Out of these, quaternary alloys are most acceptable.
- **Based on whether alloy is unicompositional or admixed**
  - *Single composition or unicompositional:* Each particle of alloy has same chemical composition
  - *Admixed alloys:* These are physical blend of lathe-cut and spherical particles.

Composition of Dental Amalgam

Amalgam consists of amalgam alloy and mercury. Amalgam alloy is composed of silver-tin alloy with varying amounts of copper, zinc, indium, and palladium.

Table 4.1 shows the Composition of amalgam alloys. **Table 4.2** summarizes the differences between high and low copper amalgam alloys.

In general, amalgam alloy consists of silver 40% (minimum), tin 32% (maximum), copper 30% (maximum), zinc 2% (maximum), and traces of indium or palladium. In *preamalgamated alloys,* 3% mercury is used, which reacts more rapidly when mixed with silver-tin alloy.

Mercury used for dental amalgam is purified by distillation. **Table 4.3** is showing the effects of constituent metals on properties of amalgam.

TABLE 4.1: Composition of amalgam alloys (percentage of elements by weight).

Alloy	Silver %	Tin %	Copper %	Zinc %	Indium %	Palladium %
Low copper	65–70	26–28	2–5	0–2	0	0
High copper						
i. Admixed	40–70	26–30	13–30	0–1	0	0
ii. Unicompositional	40–60	0–30	13–30	0	0–1	0–1

TABLE 4.2: Difference between high copper and low copper alloys.

	High copper alloys	Low copper alloys
Copper content	12–30%	<6%
Mercury required for amalgamation	Less	More
Dormant phase	It is Cu_6Sn_5, i.e., η phase	It is Ag_2Hg_3, i.e., γ1 phase
Tarnish and corrosion	It is due to copper-rich phase, i.e., Cu_6Sn_5(η)	It is due to gamma-2 phase, i.e., Sn_8Hg(γ2)

TABLE 4.3: Effects of constituent metals on properties of amalgam.

Silver	Tin	Copper	Zinc	Palladium	Indium
▪ Increases strength and setting expansion ▪ Reduces setting time ▪ Decreases flow	▪ Increases setting time ▪ Reduces strength, hardness, and setting expansion	▪ Reduces tarnish and corrosion ▪ Strengthening effect on the set amalgam	▪ Scavenges the available oxygen to prevent oxidization of alloy during manufacturing ▪ On contamination with moisture, delayed or secondary expansion occurs	Improves the corrosion resistance and mechanical properties	Decreases amount of mercury required to wet alloy particles

Types of Amalgam Alloy Powder

Lathe-cut is made by cutting of alloy from a pre- homogenized ingot, which was heat treated at 420°C for many hours. Fillings are then reheated at 100°C for 1 hour for aging of the alloy.

Spherical (spheroidal) alloy is formed when molten alloy is sprayed into a column filled with inert gas; this molten metal solidifies as fine droplets of alloy.

Admixed alloy is when different size or shape of amalgam powder particles are mixed together to increase filling efficiency.

Single composition is that alloy in which every particle of alloy is having same shape, size, and composition.

Dispersion modified, high copper alloys are that, in which high copper alloy is mixed with conventional alloy.

Setting Reaction/Amalgamation Reaction

Lathe-cut Low Copper Alloys

On mixing amalgam alloy with mercury, the alloy particles get dissolved in the mercury. Mercury reacts with alloy particles to form two products, i.e., the silver-mercury phase and tin-mercury phase. After this reaction, the unreacted particles are embedded in the matrix of reaction products with mercury. The reaction is as follows:

$$Ag_3Sn + Hg \longrightarrow Ag_2Hg_3 + Sn_8Hg + \text{unreacted } Ag_3Sn$$
$$(\gamma) \qquad\qquad (\gamma_1) \qquad (\gamma_2) \qquad\qquad (\gamma)$$

In lathe-cut low copper amalgams both γ_1 and γ_2 form a continuous network. Since γ_2 phase is least corrosion-resistant phase, its distribution in reaction product is important.

Admixed High Copper Alloys

For high copper alloys, the reaction is different. It occurs in two phases. The initial reaction is similar to that of low copper alloys, i.e.,

$$(\gamma)\, Ag_3Sn + Ag\text{-}Cu + Hg \longrightarrow (\gamma_1)\, Ag_2Hg_3 + (\gamma)\, Sn_8Hg$$
$$+ \text{unreacted } Ag_3Sn + Ag\text{-}Cu$$

Second phase of reaction involves the silver–copper phase (Ag-Cu).

It reacts with g (Ag_3Sn) and mercury to form Ag_2Hg_3, Sn_8Hg and Cu_6Sn_5 phase. The mercury released from Sn_8Hg (g_2 phase) reacts with silver to form Ag_2Hg_3 (g1) phase.

$$Sn_8Hg + Ag\text{-}Cu \longrightarrow Cu_6Sn_5 + Ag_2Hg_3 + Ag_3Sn$$
$$(\gamma) \qquad (\eta_1) \qquad\qquad (\gamma_1) \qquad\qquad (\gamma)$$

This reaction goes on. After one week, the g_2 phase reacts completely with eutectic and replaces all the g_2 phase by g and g_1 phase.

Unicompositional High Copper Alloy

Difference in admix type and the unicompositional alloys is that, in latter, the eutectic phase, i.e., Ag-Cu phase is absent and the reaction is directly with silver, copper and tin phases. In these, only silver reacts with mercury and the tin remains bound to copper.

$$Ag_3Sn + Cu_3Sn + Hg \longrightarrow Cu_6Sn_5 + Ag_2Hg_3$$
$$(\gamma) \qquad (\epsilon) \qquad\qquad (\eta) \qquad (\gamma_1)$$

Final phase formed is Cu_6Sn_5 (γ). There is no Sn_8Hg (γ_2) phase.

Table 4.4 shows different phases of silver amalgam setting reaction.

TABLE 4.4: Phases of silver amalgam.

Code	Component
(γ) gamma	Ag_3Sn (Silver–tin phase) strongest phase
(γ1) gamma 1	Ag_2Hg_3 (Silver–mercury phase) noblest phase
(γ2) gamma 2	Sn_8Hg (Tin–mercury phase): Least resistant to tarnish and corrosion and weakest phase
(ϵ) epsilon	Cu_3Sn (Copper–tin phase)
(η) eta	Cu_6Sn_5 (Copper–tin phase) More corrosion resistant and stronger than gamma-2 phase

Indications	Contraindications
▪ In moderate to large class I and II preparations ▪ For restoration of class V lesions where esthetic is not required ▪ As a postendodontic restoration to restore the access cavity ▪ To restore fractured cusp using pin and slot	▪ When esthetics is main concern ▪ Small class I and class II preparations ▪ Grossly decayed teeth

Advantages	Disadvantages
■ Easy to manipulate and less technique sensitive ■ Self sealing of interface of amalgam and tooth due to formation of corrosion products ■ High compressive strength ■ Biocompatible ■ Good wear resistance ■ Economical	■ Unesthetic ■ Requires extensive tooth preparation ■ Corrosion and tarnish causing discoloration of tooth ■ Being metallic restoration, it transmits thermal sensation to the pulp ■ Marginal degradation is seen in low copper alloys ■ Amalgam has poor tensile strength thus making it a brittle material ■ Results in galvanic current in association with gold restoration or even in same restoration with non-uniform condensation

Manipulation of Amalgam Restoration

Mercury-alloy Ratio

Mercury-alloy ratio should be according to type of alloy used. Eames preferred 1:1 ratio of alloy/mercury for best results. Lathe-cut amalgam alloys require more (45%) of mercury to wet than the spherical alloys (40%).

Trituration

Purpose of trituration is to remove oxide layers from alloy particles so as to coat each alloy particle with mercury, resulting in a homogeneous mass for condensation. Trituration can be done by hand or mechanical means. Mechanical method is done with the help of automatic amalgamator **(Fig. 4.11A)** and hand method of trituration is done with the mortar and pestle **(Fig. 4.11B)**.

Time for which the trituration is done, speed, and force applied for trituration, affect the quality of trituration. Trituration can produce following three types of mixes **(Figs. 4.12A to C)**:
1. ***Normal triturated mix:*** This is a shiny mix which is plastic in consistency, appears as homogeneous mass and convenient to handle.
2. ***Over-triturated mix:*** This mix is "warm", shiny, and hard due to premature setting of amalgam. This mix is difficult to condense in prepared cavity.
3. ***Under-triturated mix:*** This mix is dry and crumbly which is very weak and dull in appearance and difficult to manipulate.

Mulling

Mulling of the amalgam can be done manually or mechanically. By hand, it can be done by squeezing the freshly mixed amalgam collected in the chamois skin. Mechanical mulling is done in the amalgamator by triturating it for 2–3 seconds.

Insertion of Amalgam

Use amalgam carrier to carry amalgam alloy into the preparation and condense it with flat surface of condenser

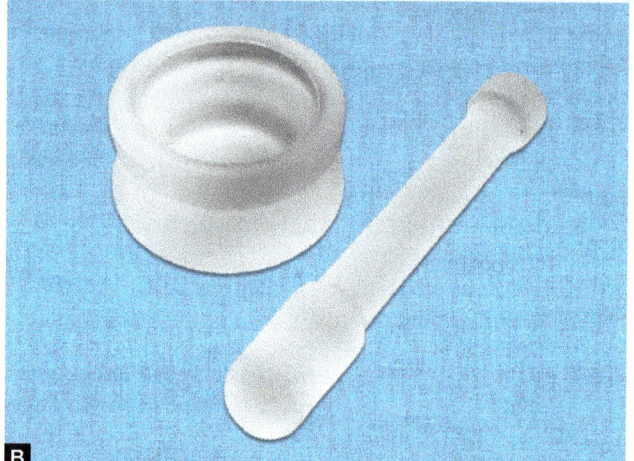

FIGURES 4.11A AND B: (A) Amalgamator; (B) Mortar and pestle.

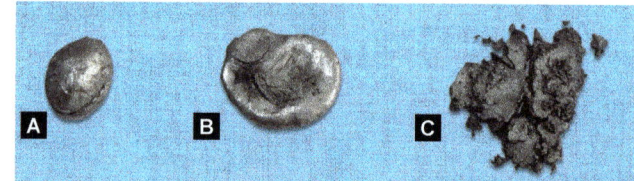

FIGURES 4.12A TO C: (A) Normal triturated is shiny homogenous mass with plastic consistency; (B) Overtriturated mix is shiny and hard due to premature setting of amalgam; (C) Undertriturated mix is dry, crumbly and dull in appearance.

After it, add next increment and again condense it till level of amalgam reaches preparation margins **(Figs. 4.13A to E)**

Condensation

Condensation is done by using different shapes of condensers like round, elliptical, trapezoid, and parallelogram. Working end of condenser should be serrated so as to avoid slipping away of amalgam while manipulation.

Precarve Burnishing (Fig. 4.13F)

Precarve burnishing is done soon after condensation to improve the marginal integrity of restoration and reduce the mercuric content of amalgam.

Carving (Fig. 4.13G)

Carving is done to produce anatomical contours and functional occlusion for the restoration. Commonly used

Dental Materials

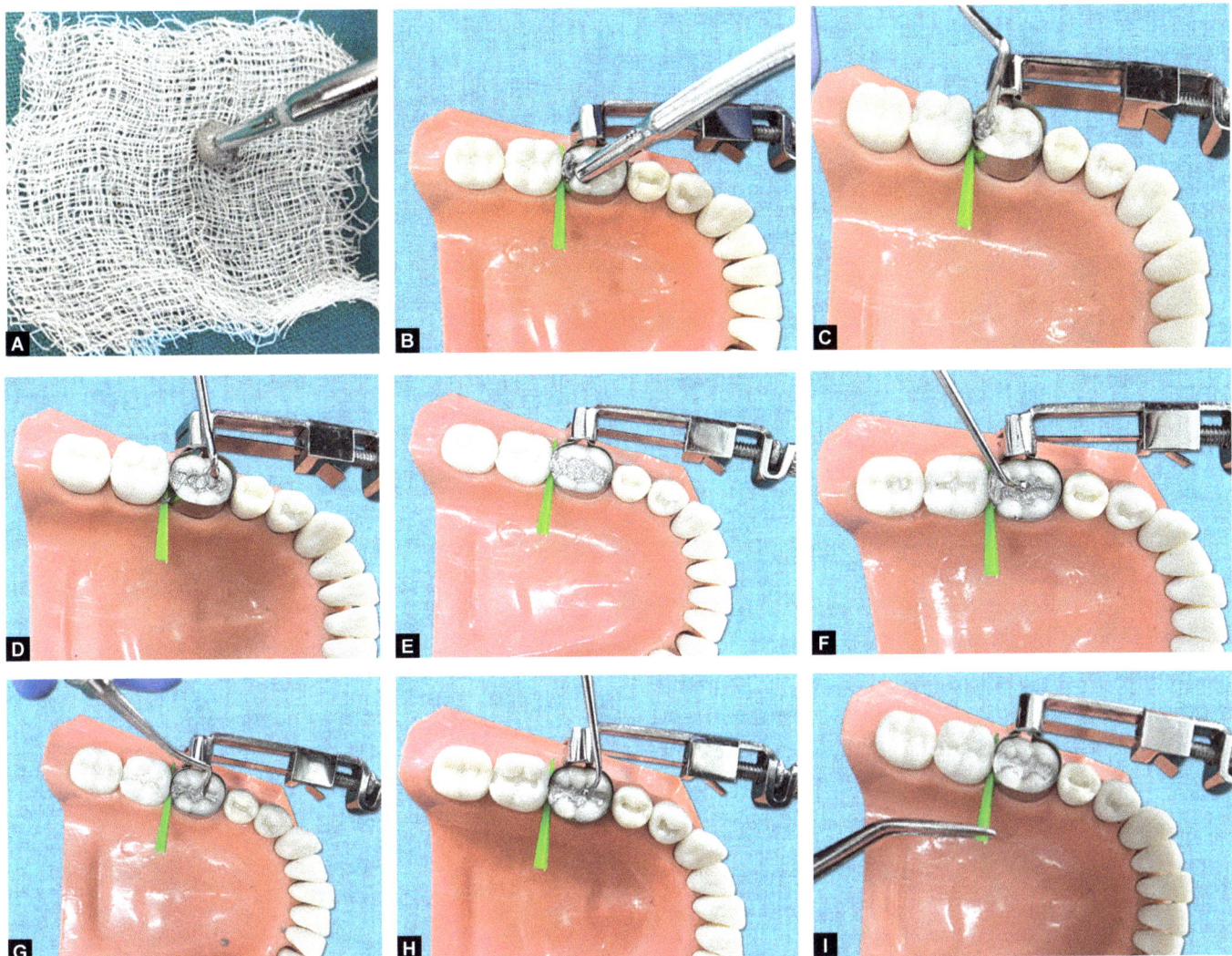

FIGURES 4.13A TO I: (A and B) Use amalgam carrier to carry amalgam alloy into the preparation; (C) Condense it with flat surface of condenser; (D and E) After it, add next increment and again condense it till level of amalgam reaches preparation margins; (F) Precarve burnishing; (G) Carving; (H) Postcarve burnishing; (I) Finished amalgam restoration.

carvers are Hollenback carver, Frahm's carver (diamond-shaped) and cleoid-discoid carver.

Postcarve Burnishing (Fig. 4.13H)

It is done after completion of carving to reduce surface roughness and improve marginal seal.

Finishing and Polishing (Fig. 4.13I)

Finishing and polishing should be done after 24 hours of placement of amalgam restoration. Premature finishing and polishing will interfere with crystalline structure of hardening amalgam, resulting in weakening of the restoration.

CLINICAL CONSIDERATIONS

Plastic Deformation (Creep)

- Creep is time-dependent response of an already set material to stress in form of plastic deformation
- Creep is undesirable because it causes amalgam to flow out over the margins resulting in marginal deterioration and fracture
- Increased condensation pressure reduces creep because it reduces residual mercury level.

Tarnish and Corrosion

Tarnish is the surface discoloration of metal or alteration of surface finish or luster. Corrosion is actual deterioration of a metal by reaction with its environment.

When amalgam comes in contact with dissimilar metal (gold restoration), amalgam undergoes ***galvanic corrosion*** due to large difference in electromotive force of two materials.

Thermal Conductivity

Because of good thermal conductivity, amalgam can transmit temperature changes readily to the pulp. Therefore, it should be placed in tooth after adequate pulp protection like sealing dentinal tubules by applying varnish to walls or placing base on pulpal floor.

Marginal Ditching (Fig. 4.14)

Marginal ditching is breakdown of amalgam at the margins due to fracture or poor seal because of improper cavity margins.

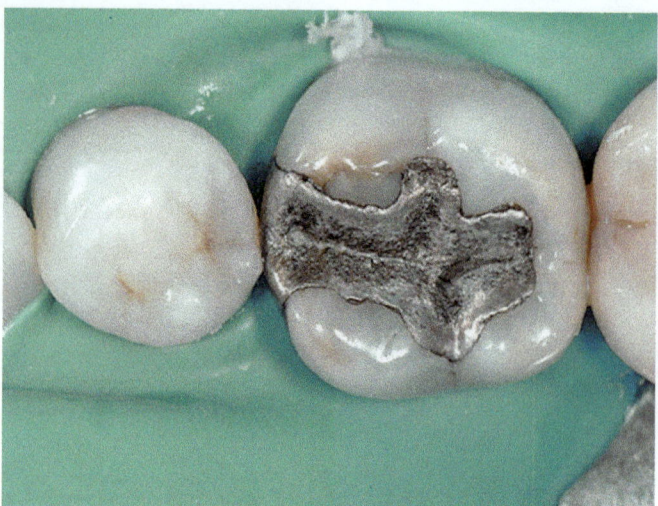

FIGURE 4.14: Marginal ditching.

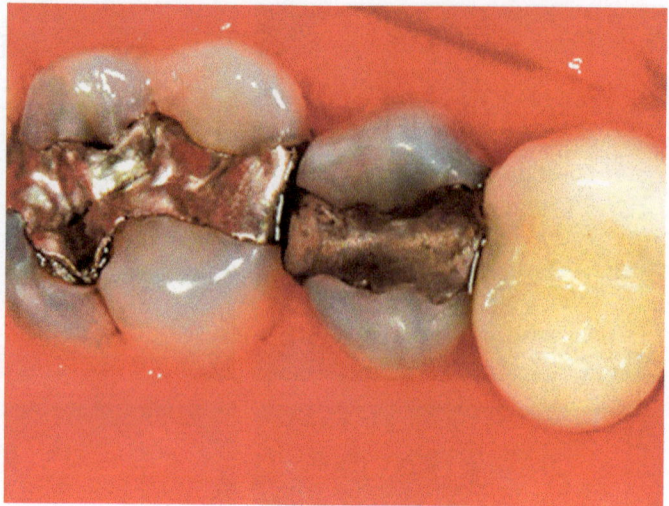

FIGURE 4.15: Fracture of restoration.

Fracture or Tooth or Restoration

Fracture of tooth or restoration can occur because of lack of resistance and retention form. Such restorations need to be replaced **(Fig. 4.15)**.

Improper Proximal Contacts

Improper contact in form of open contact leads to food impaction and further periodontal problem. Such restorations need to be replaced.

STEPS TO REDUCE MERCURY EXPOSURE IN THE DENTAL CLINIC

- Mercury should be stored in tight container
- Avoid spilling of mercury while trituration
- Ventilation should be good to minimize air contamination.
- Avoid direct exposure of the mercury with skin as it may cause hypersensitivity reactions
- Scrap amalgam during insertion and condensation should be carefully collected and stored under water, glycerin or spent X-ray fixer solution in tightly capped jar
- Mercury- contaminated cotton rolls should be stored in a tightly capped plastic container for separate disposal
- Clean the mercury-contaminated instruments.

ADHESIVE DENTISTRY

Dentistry has seen enormous advancements in field of adhesive dentistry for past two decades. The availability of adhesive materials permits the placement of esthetic restorations like composite resins, aesthetic inlays and veneers, etc.

DEFINITIONS (FIG. 4.16)

Adhesion or Bonding

Adhesion is defined as the forces or energies between atoms or molecules at an interface that hold two phases together.

Adhesive

A material that can join substances together, resist separation and transmit loads across the bond is an adhesive. The material to which it is applied is adherend.

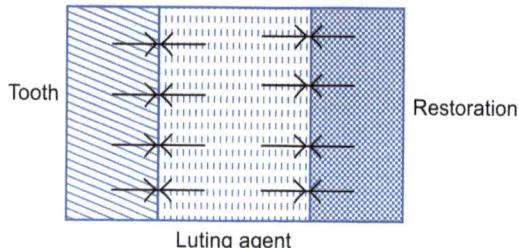

FIGURE 4.16: Schematic representation showing the role of adhesive cement for tooth and restoration.

Factors Affecting Adhesion

- Cleaner the surface, greater is the adhesion. Presence of saliva, blood, moisture, oil, etc., reduces adhesion
- More surface energy of adherend results in better adhesion
- Smaller the contact angle is, better is the adhesion **(Fig. 4.17)**
- Lesser the water content, better is the adhesion.

ENAMEL BONDING

Buonocore, in 1955, was the first to reveal the adhesion of acrylic resin to acid etched enamel. Etching is the process of increasing the surface reactivity by demineralizing the superficial calcium layer and thus creating the enamel tags. These tags are responsible for micromechanical bonding between tooth and restorative resin.

Steps for Enamel Bonding

Step 1: Perform oral prophylaxis procedure using nonfluoridated and oil less prophylaxis pastes.

Step 2: Clean and wash the teeth. Isolate to prevent any contamination from saliva or gingival crevicular fluid.

Step 3: Apply acid etchant in the form of liquid or gel for 10–15 seconds.

Step 4: Wash the etchant continuously for 10–15 seconds.

Step 5: Note the appearance of a properly etched surface. It should give a frosty white appearance on drying.

Dental Materials

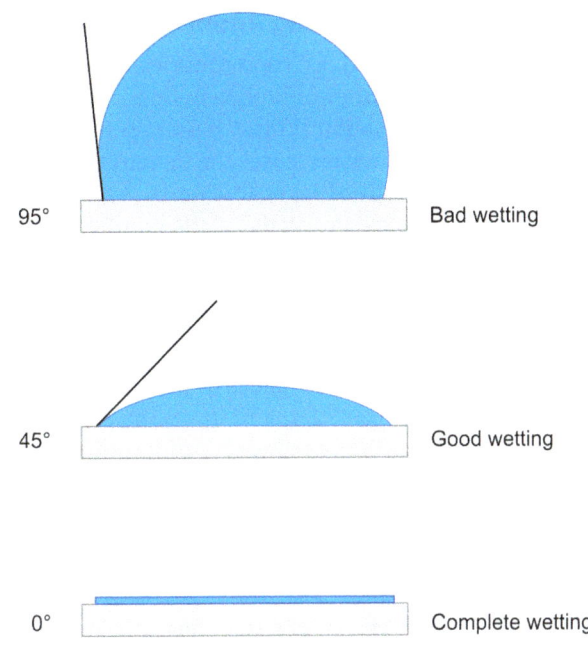

FIGURE 4.17: In this figure we can see that smaller the contact angle, better is the adhesion, resulting in complete wetting.

Step 6: If any sort of contamination occurs, repeat the procedure.

Step 7: Now apply bonding agent and low viscosity monomers over the etched enamel surface.

Step 8: Finer network of numerous resin micro- and macrotags is formed within the enamel surface which constitutes the fundamental mechanism of enamel-resin adhesion **(Fig. 4.18)**.

DENTIN BONDING

Bonding to dentin is difficult because of difference in morphologic, histologic and compositional differences from enamel.

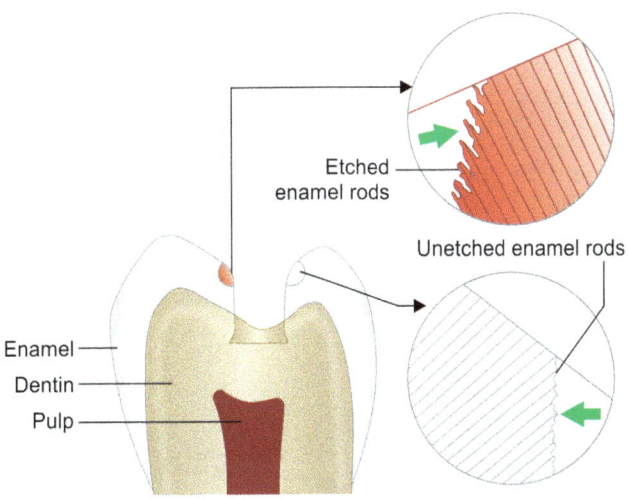

FIGURE 4.18: Schematic representation of the etched and unetched enamel rods.

Dentin Adhesive Systems Consist
- Primer
- Bonding agent.

Primer
Primer is a hydrophilic, low viscosity resin which is usually bifunctional monomer in a volatile solvent like acetone or alcohol. Monomers commonly used in primers are HEMA, NPG-GMA, PMDM, BPDM, etc.

Dentin-bonding Agent
It forms chemical bond to inorganic and organic or both the components. It is bifunctional structure, i.e., it has both hydrophilic and hydrophobic ends. Hydrophobic end is methacrylate which copolymerizes with composite resin, hydrophilic end has monomer like HEMA.

EVOLUTION OF DENTIN-BONDING AGENTS

First Generation Dentin-bonding Systems
In this, NPG-GMA was supposed to chelate with calcium of dentin to form water resistant chemical bond to dentin. These products ignored the smear layer.

Second Generation Dentin-bonding Systems
Here, phosphate groups, or carboxylic acid groups present in bonding agents bond to calcium of dentin but not much success was achieved.

Third Generation Dentin-bonding Systems
These were designed not to remove the entire smear layer but to modify it by applying mild acids to allow penetration of acidic monomer. These resulted in better bond strength as compared to 1st and 2nd generation.

Fourth Generation Dentin-bonding Agents
These bonding agents applied concept of total etching of enamel and dentin simultaneously using 37% phosphoric acid to remove the smear layer. In this resin of dentin-bonding agent micromechanically interlocks with intertubular dentin and surrounding collagen fibers. These involve etching, priming and adhesive agent application.

Fifth Generation Dentin-bonding Agents
In these agents, the primer and adhesive resin are combined in one bottle. In fourth generation bonding system is available in two bottles, one primer and other adhesive, fifth generation dentin-bonding agents are available in one bottle only **(Fig. 4.19)**. These involve two steps, application of etchant and combined primer + bonding agent.

Mechanism of Bonding in Total Etch Technique
It involves complete removal of smear layer by total etching of enamel and dentin. Thus, resin of dentin-bonding agent micromechanically interlocks with intertubular dentin and surrounding collagen fibers forming a hybrid layer.

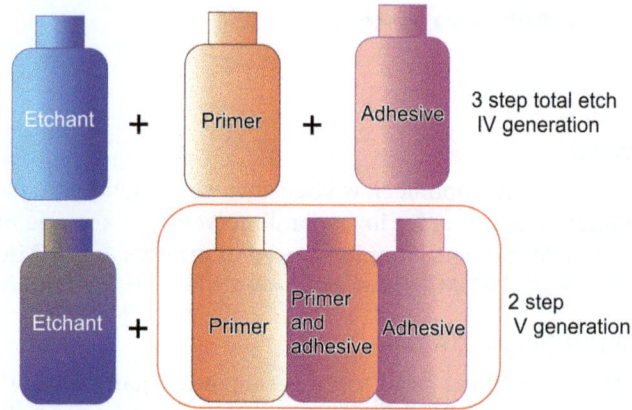

FIGURE 4.19: Schematic representation showing the difference in 4th and 5th generation bonding agents. Note that in the 4th generation primer and adhesive are present in separate bottles, whereas in the 5th generation, primer and adhesive are combined in single bottle.

Sixth Generation Dentin-bonding Agents/Self-etch Primers (Fig. 4.20)

In sixth generation etching step is eliminated, here, self-etch primers and bonding are used. Sixth generation bonding agents are of two types:

Self-etching Primer and Adhesive/Two Step/Non-rinsing Conditioner

It is available in two bottles; primer and adhesive and primer is applied prior to the adhesive.

Self-etching Adhesive/All-in-One System

It is available in two bottles; primer and adhesive. A drop from each bottle is taken, mixed and applied to the tooth surface.

Seventh Generation Dentin-bonding Agents All-in-One System (Fig. 4.21)

These bonding agents require no mixing, thus avoiding any mistakes in mixing. These are less technique sensitive and easy to use.

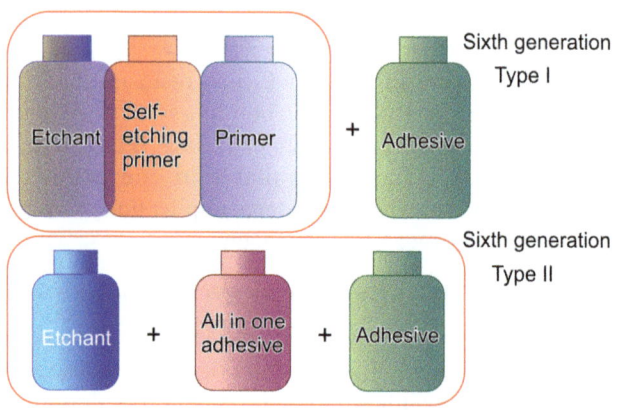

FIGURE 4.20: Sixth generation dentin-bonding agent.

Eighth Generation Bonding Agent (Fig. 4.22)

It was introduced in 2010, by voco America. It's all in one step: they limit the number of bottles to one like the seven generation so reducing clinical time. It uses nanosize fillers. The use of nanosize fillers increases the penetration of resin monomers and the hybrid layer thickness, which in turn improves the mechanical properties of the bonding systems. It has longer shelf life.

Mechanism of Bonding in Self-etch Primers

In self etch primers, as soon as the decalcification process starts, infiltration of the empty spaces by the dentin-bonding agent is initiated.

Figure 4.23 shows the mechanism of bonding in total etch and self-etch primers.

Generations of dentin bonding agents							
Properties	1st	2nd	3rd	4th	5th	6th	7th	8th
Etching	?	Yes	Yes	Yes	Yes	No	No	No
Conditioning	No	No	Yes	Yes	Yes	Yes	No	No
Removal of smear layer	?	No	Yes	Yes	Yes	No	No	No
Hybrid layer	No	No	No	Yes	Yes	Yes	Yes	Yes
No. of steps	2/3	3	3	3–4	2	2	1	1

COMPOSITES

Composite refers to a solid formed from two or more distinct phases that have been combined to produce properties superior to or intermediate to those of individual components.

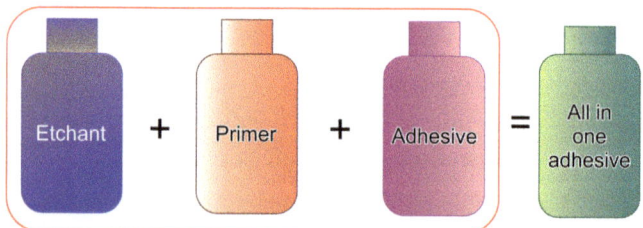

FIGURE 4.21: Schematic representation showing 7th generation bonding agent.

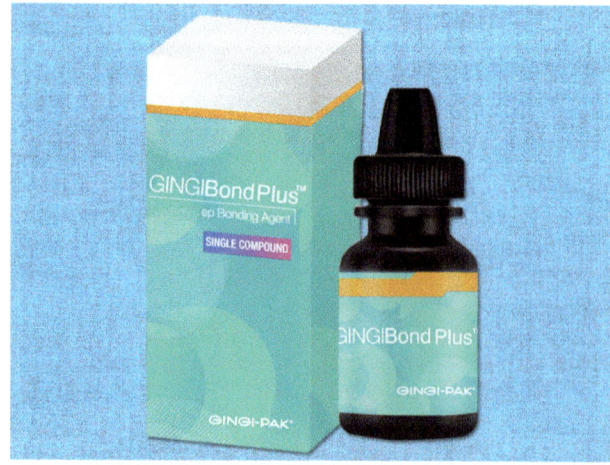

FIGURE 4.22: Eight generation bonding agent.

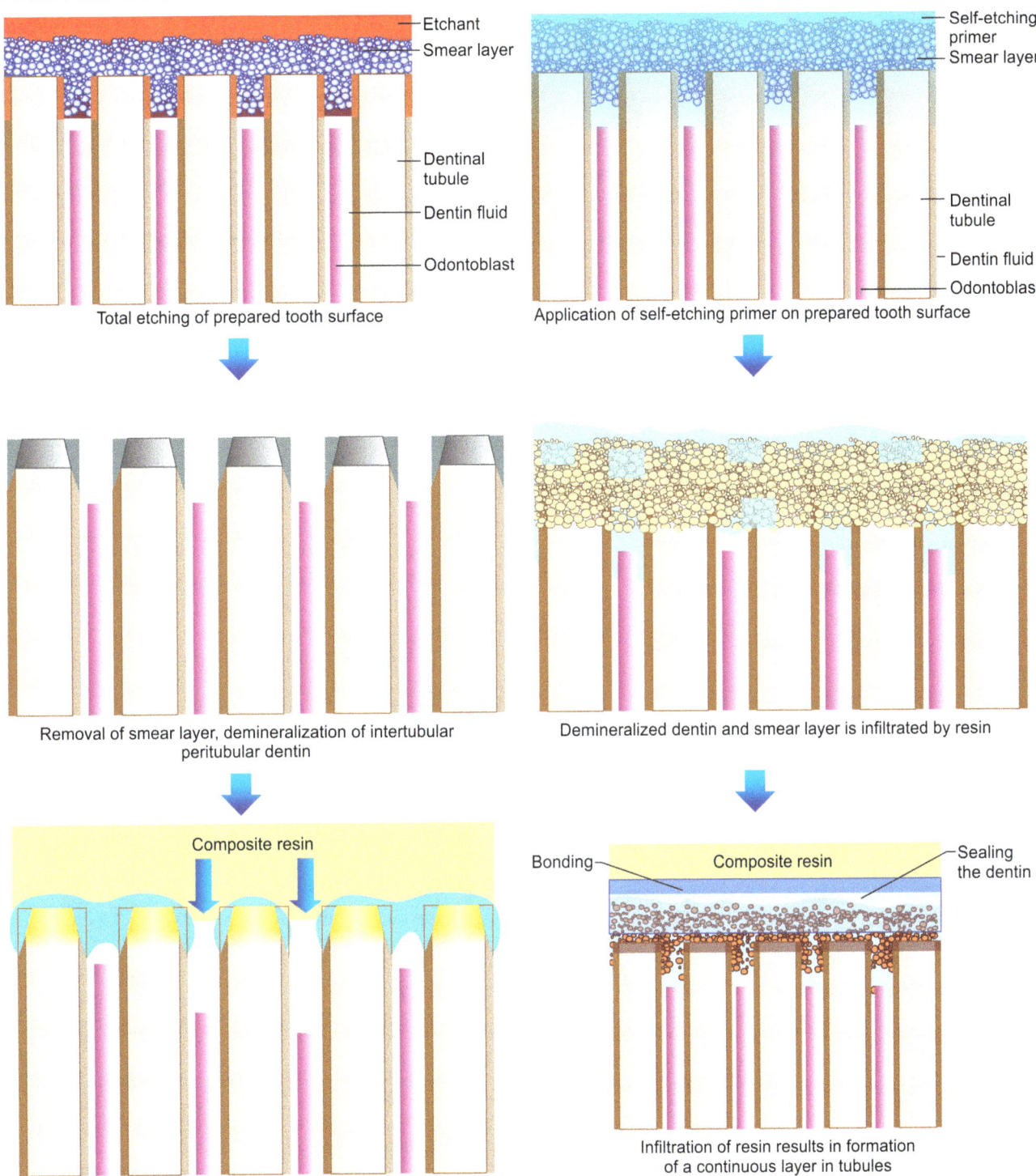

FIGURE 4.23: Schematic representation showing mechanism of bonding of total etch and self etch primers.

Composition of Dental Composites

Resin Matrix (Fig. 4.24)

Resin matrix consists of polymeric mono-, di-, or trifunctional monomers like Bis-GMA or UDMA. It represents the backbone of composite resin system.

Fillers

Dispersed phase of composite resins is made up of an inorganic filler material. Commonly used fillers are silica, quartz, barium glass, etc. Within the limits, greater is the percentage of filler particles, better are the physical properties of composites. Composites with large filler particle size show rough surface texture, decreased curing depth, and scattering of light, so appear opaque and tend to stain. Composites with small filler particle size show smooth surface texture, increased curing depth, and less scattering of light, so appear less opaque and show high esthetics.

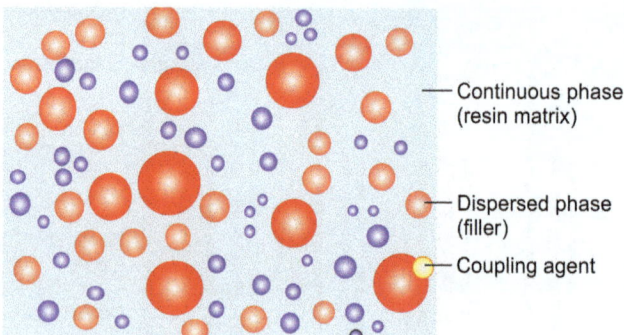

FIGURE 4.24: Schematic representation showing the arrangement of resin matrix, fillers and coupling agents in dental composites.

Silane Coupling Agents

Coupling agents bind filler particles to the organic resin. These are composed of bifunctional molecules. The silane group chemically bonds to the inorganic materials and ethoxy and methoxy group of coupling agents bind to the resin molecules of matrix.

Activator-initiator Agents

Polymerization of composite resin takes place by release of free radicals which can be done either by chemical reaction or light activation.

Initiator-activator system used in various types of composites.

Sl. No.	Types of composite	Initiator	Activator
1.	Chemically-cured composite	Benzoyl peroxide	N, N-dimethyl-p-toluidine
2.	Light-cured composite		
	▪ Ultraviolet light-activated composite	0.1% Benzoin methyl ether	Tertiary amine
	▪ Visible light-cured composite	0.06% camphorquinone	Dimethylaminoethyl methacrylate

Inhibitors

These agents inhibit the free radical generation by spontaneous polymerization of the monomers.

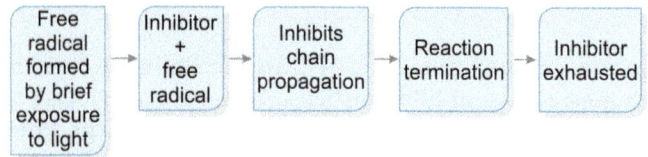

Coloring Agents

Coloring agents like titanium oxides and aluminum oxides are used to give shades.

CLASSIFICATION OF COMPOSITES

According to Skinner

- Macrofilled/traditional or conventional composites—8-12 μm
- Small particle-filled composites—1-5 μm
- Microfilled composites—0.04-0.4 μm
- Hybrid composites—0.6-1 μm

Classification according to polymerization shrinkage

- Self-curing
- Light curing:
  - Ultraviolet light curing
  - Visible light curing
- Dual curing.

Macrofilled/Traditional or Conventional Composites

- Average particle size of macrofilled composite resin ranges from 8 to 12 μm
- Filler content is 75% by weight
- Exhibits a rough surface texture because of the relatively large size and extreme hardness of the filler particles
- Physical and mechanical performance is better than unfilled acrylic resins
- Poor polishability and more prone to staining.

Small Particle-filled Composites

- Average particle size ranges from 1 to 5 μm
- Filler content is 65%
- Superior polishing and texturing properties
- Good abrasion and wear resistance
- Decreased polymerization shrinkage.

Microfilled Composites

- Average particle size ranges from 0.04 to 0.4 μm
- Filler content is 30-40% by weight
- Small particle size results in smooth polished surface which is resistant to plaque, debris, and stains
- Because of less filler content, physical properties are inferior
- Highly polishable and esthetic
- Low wear resistance.

Hybrid Composites

- Hybrid composites are named so because they are made up of glasses of sizes
- Filler content in these composites is 75-80% by weight
- Mixture of fillers is responsible for their physical properties similar to those of conventional composites with the advantage of smooth surface texture
- Excellent polishing and texturing properties
- Good abrasion and wear resistance
- Nanofill and nanohybrid composites have average particle size smaller than that of microfilled composites. These are highly polishable and have high wear resistance.
- Microhybrid composites have filler content of 56-66% by volume with average particle size of 0.4-0.8 μm. They have

better polishability and surface finishing and because of presence of large filler content, microhybrid composites have improved physical properties and wear resistance than microfilled composites.

Newer Composite Resins

Flowable Composite Resin

- Here filler content is 60% by weight with particle size ranging from 0.02 to 0.05 µm
- Low filler loading is responsible for decreased viscosity of composites
- Penetration into every irregularity of preparation due to low viscosity
- High flexibility, so less likely to be displaced in stress concentration areas
- More susceptible to wear in stress-bearing areas
- Weaker mechanical properties.

Condensable (Packable) Composites

- Condensable/packable composites have improved mechanical properties and handling characteristics similar to amalgam so it can be packed into posterior tooth preparation
- In this, ceramic inorganic fillers are present in silanated network of ceramic fibers
- Filler content in packable composites ranges from 48 to 65% by volume with average particle size ranging from 0.7 to 20 µm
- Deeper depth of cure is due to light conducting properties of ceramic fibers. Each increment of composite can be condensed like amalgam and cured to a depth of over 4 mm
- Increased wear resistance because of presence of ceramic fibers.

Expanding Matrix Resins Composites

- Composites show polymerization shrinkage on curing which can result in marginal leakage, postoperative sensitivity, and secondary caries
- To reduce these effects, Spiro orthocarbonates (SOCs) are added in composites because they expand on polymerization
- Epoxy resins contract 3.4% and SOCs expand 3.6%. Both are mixed to achieve desired expansion.

Compomers (Polyacid Modified + Composite Resins)

- Compomers provide combined advantages of composites (term "Comp" in their name) and glass ionomer ("Omers" in their name)
- Composition includes dimethacrylate monomer, silicate glass containing filler and photo-initiator
- They are available in single paste, light enable material in syringe or compules
- They offer optimal esthetics, polishing and are easy to use
- However they are technique sensitive with limited fluoride release.

Advantages	Disadvantages
■ Conservation of tooth structure	■ Polymerization shrinkage
■ Good esthetics	■ More expensive than amalgam
■ Low thermal conductivity	■ Technique sensitive
■ Mechanical bonding to tooth structure	■ Low wear resistance
■ Controlled working time	■ High linear coefficient of thermal expansion
■ Restoration can be completed in one dental visit	
■ No galvanism	

CAST METAL ALLOYS

Cast metal restorations were introduced in dentistry about 100 years ago. Most of the cast metal restorations are made from alloys formed by combination of gold with other metals such as silver, copper, zinc, platinum, and palladium. Cast metal alloys are used to make inlays, onlays, crowns, bridges, removable cast partial dentures and dentures.

COMPONENTS OF CAST GOLD ALLOYS

Element	Function
Gold	■ Primary constituent ■ Provides yellow color, density, nobility and castability
Copper	■ Second most important constituent ■ Increases hardness and strength ■ Imparts reddish color
Silver	■ Lightens the color ■ Decreases nobility
Platinum and palladium	■ Increases hardness and strength ■ Whitens the alloy
Zinc	■ Scavenger for oxygen, i.e., deoxidizer

CLASSIFICATION OF CAST GOLD ALLOYS

In 1927, the Bureau of Standard divided gold casting alloys into type I to IV, according to their use.

Type I (Soft)

- Soft, weak, ductile and easily burnishable
- Gold content ranges between 75% and 83%
- Simple inlays in class I, III or V cavities.

Type II (Medium)

- Harder and stronger than type I
- Gold content ranges from 70 to 75%
- Used for three quarter crowns, pontics and full crowns.

Type III (Hard)

- Used in high stress areas
- Gold content ranges from 65 to 70%

- High stress inlays, full crowns, pontics, and short span FPDs.

Type IV (Extra Hard)
- Used in very high stress areas
- Gold content is 60%
- High stress inlays, bars and clasps and long span FPDs.

WAXES
- Waxes are thermoplastic materials which are normally solids at room temp but melt, without decomposition to form mobile liquids.
- They are primarily used to form patterns prior to casting, impression making, bite registration, etc.

Properties of Waxes
- Waxes have a melting range rather than melting point, for example paraffin wax melts between 500°C-700°C of temperature
- Waxes have very high coefficient of thermal expansion. Thus, a small changes in temperature can cause a sufficient change in dimensions
- Waxes have low thermal conductivity, thus sufficient time must be allowed both to heat them uniformly throughout and to cool them to room temperature
- Waxes are usually brittle, wide melting ranges cause greater ductility.

Inlay Casting Wax (Fig. 4.25)
- It is a specialized dental wax that can be applied to dies to form direct or indirect patterns
- ADA specification number is 4
- It is available in blue, green, ivory, or deep purple colors. Dark color provides contrast with die material and thus helps in better identification and finishing of the margins
- It is of two types:
  1. *Type I:* Medium wax—used for direct pattern
  2. *Type II*: Soft wax—used for indirect technique.

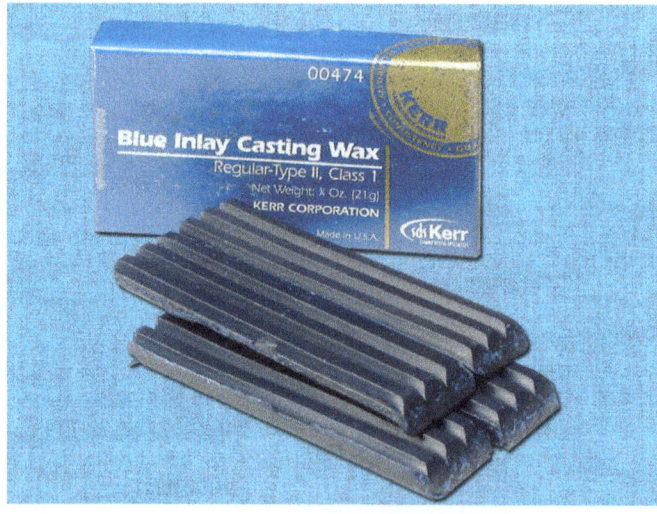

FIGURE 4.25: Photograph showing blue inlay wax.

Composition
- Paraffin wax: 40-60%
- Carnuba wax: 25%
- Ceresin: 10%
- Gum Dammer : 1%
- Candelilla wax and synthetic waxes.

VIVA QUESTIONS

Q.1 **Define dental cements.**
Ans. These are the materials made from two components, powder and liquid, mixed together.

Q.2 **What are uses of dental cements?**
Ans.
- As temporary restoration
- For luting
- As root canal sealer
- For pulp protection
  - Bases
  - Liners.

Q.3 **What is composition of ZOE cements?**
Ans.
- Powder
  - Zinc oxide (ZnO)—69.0%
  - White rosin—29.3%
  - Zinc stearate—1.0%
  - Zinc acetate (acts as accelerator)—0.7%
- Liquid
  - Eugenol—85.0%
  - Olive oil—15.0%

Q.4 **Why is ZOE not used with resins?**
Ans. Zinc oxide eugenol is not used with resins because eugenol interferes with polymerization process of resins.

Q.5 **How does setting of ZOE cement take place?**
Ans. On mixing powder and liquid, the zinc oxide hydrolysis and subsequent reaction take place between zinc hydroxide and eugenol to form a chelate, zinc eugenolate.

Q.6 **Why should the liquid bottle be kept perpendicular to glass slab/paper pad while dispensing?**
Ans. It lets the liquid fall under its own weight.

Q.7 **What are types of zinc phosphate cement?**
Ans.
- *Type I:* Used for cementation. It forms the film thickness of less than 25 μ
- *Type II:* Used as base. It results in film thickness between 25 and 40 μ.

Q.8 **What is composition of zinc phosphate cement?**
Ans.
- Powder
  - ZnO—90.2%.
  - MgO—8.2%
  - SiO_2—1.4%
  - Bi_2O_3—0.1%
  - Miscellaneous—BaO, Ba_2SO_4, CaO
- Liquid
  - Phosphoric acid – 38.2%
  - Water – 36.0%

Dental Materials

- Aluminum or zinc phosphate — 6.2%
- Zinc — 7.1%
- Aluminum — 2.5%

Q.9 Why zinc phosphate powder is mixed in increments?
Ans. Powder is divided into 5–8 increments.
- Initial increments are smaller in size so as to:
  - Achieve the slow neutralization of the liquid
  - Control the reaction
- Middle increments are larger in size:
  - To saturate the liquid to form zinc phosphate
  - Because of presence of less amount of unreacted acid, this step is not affected by heat released from the reaction
- In the end, the smaller increments of powder are added so as to: Achieve optimum consistency.

Q.10 What is composition of zinc polycarboxylate cement?
Ans. Powder is similar to that of zinc phosphate cement powder.
Liquid is an aqueous solution of 32–43% polyacrylic acid.

Q.11 Why is zinc polycarboxylate cement biocompatible?
Ans.
- Size of polyacrylic acid molecule is bigger, this makes it less favorable to disperse into the dentinal tubules
- pH of the cement rises more rapidly when compared to that of zinc phosphate.

Q.12 Why GIC is called hybrid cement?
Ans. Glass ionomer cement is also described as hybrid of dental silicate cements and zinc polycarboxylates where phosphoric acid of silicate cements is replaced by polyacrylic acid of zinc polycarboxylates.

Q.13 What is composition of glass ionomer cement?
Ans.
- Silica — 41.9%
- Alumina — 28.6%
- Aluminum fluoride — 1.6%
- Calcium fluoride — 15.7%
- Sodium fluoride — 9.3%
- Aluminum phosphate — 3.8%
- Polyacrylic acid (itaconic acid, maleic acid) — 40–55%
- Tartaric acid — 6–15%
- Water — 30%

Q.14 What is composition of miracle mix?
Ans. *Powder:* Physical blend of silver alloy and glass powder in 1:7 ratio.
Liquid: Glass ionomer cement liquid.

Q.15 What is composition of cermet cement?
Ans. *Powder:* Sintering of silver powder and glass powder, 5% titanium oxide.
Liquid: Glass ionomer cement liquid.

Q.16 What is composition of resin-modified GIC?
Ans. *Powder:* Fluoroaluminosilicate glass particles along with photoinitiator or chemical initiator.
Liquid: 15-25% resin component in the form of HEMA
Polyacrylic acid copolymer along with photoinitiator and water.

Q.17 How does setting of glass ionomer take place?
Ans. It occurs in three different but overlapping stages:
1. Ion-leaching phase
2. Hydrogel phase
3. Polysalt gel phase.

Q.18 What are mechanical properties of GIC?
Ans. Glass ionomer cements have high compressive strength, high modulus of elasticity but low fracture toughness, flexure strength and wear resistance. All these make GICs hard but brittle material.

Q.19 What makes the GIC biocompatible?
Ans.
- Polyacrylic acid present in the liquid is a weak acid
- Dissociated hydrogen ions present in GIC are further bound to the polymer chains electrostatically
- Long polymer chains tangle in one another. This prevents their penetration into dentin tubules.

Q.20 What will happen if GIC is exposed to air/desiccation after mixing?
Ans.
- If desiccation occurs during initial setting of cement, it retards the setting reaction since water plays an important role in setting reaction
- If desiccation occurs in later stages, it prevents increase in strength of cement because hydration of silica-based hydrogel and polycarboxylates cannot occur. It can also result in crazing, decreased esthetics and early deterioration of the cement.

Q.21 How does GIC adheres to tooth structure?
Ans. GIC bonds to tooth structure by chelation of carboxyl groups of the cement and calcium of the tooth structure.

Q.22 Why GIC bonds better to enamel than dentin?
Ans. Since enamel has higher percentage of inorganic content, bonding of GIC to enamel is stronger than to dentin.

Q.23 What are advantages of GIC?
Ans.
- Adhesion
- Biocompatible
- Anticariogenic
- Conservative tooth preparation
- Esthetic
- Low solubility.

Q.24 What are different pulpal irritants?
Ans.
- Bacterial
- Traumatic

- Iatrogenic
- Idiopathic.

Q.25 What are factors affecting pulp while tooth preparation?
Ans.
- Pressure
- Heat
- Vibration
- Remaining dentin thickness
- Speed
- Nature of cutting instruments.

Q.26 What are uses of varnish?
Ans.
- Reduces microleakage
- In case of amalgam restoration, varnish improves the sealing ability of the amalgam
- Reduces postoperative sensitivity
- Prevents discoloration of tooth.

Q.27 Why do we use varnish?
Ans.
- To seal the dentinal tubules
- To act as barrier to protect the tooth from chemical irritants from cements
- To reduce microleakage around restorations.

Q.28 Which materials are used for varnish?
Ans. Varnish is an organic copal or resin gum suspended in solutions of ether or chloroform.

Q.29 How is varnish applied?
Ans. Varnish is applied on cavity walls using a small cotton pellet.

Q.30 Where is use of varnish contraindicated?
Ans.
- Beneath GIC as varnish interferes the bonding
- With restorative resins because varnish dissolves in monomer and also interfere with the polymerization of resins.

Q.31 What are functions of cavity liners?
Ans.
- Protect pulp from chemical irritants by sealing ability
- Stimulate formation of reparative dentin.

Q.32 Which materials are used as cavity liners?
Ans.
- Zinc oxide eugenol liners
- Calcium hydroxide
- Flowable composites
- Glass ionomers.

Q.33 What are bases?
Ans. Bases are used as pulp protective materials and they provide thermal insulation, encourage recovery of injured pulp from thermal, mechanical or chemical trauma, galvanic shock and microleakage.

Q.34 What is pH of calcium hydroxide?
Ans. 12.5.

Q.35 What should be the thickness of base?
Ans. 0.5–2.0 mm.

Q.36 Which materials are used as bases?
Ans. Zinc oxide eugenol, zinc phosphate cement, GIC and calcium hydroxide.

Q.37 Should base be applied to gingival seat?
Ans. No. Since it will be open to external margin, the base might get dissolved/disintegrated because of action of saliva resulting in microleakage and thus, secondary caries.

Q.38 Where should be the varnish applied?
Ans. 2–3 coats of varnish should be applied on all the prepared surfaces, viz; walls and floors including margins of preparation.

Q.39 What is the film thickness of varnish?
Ans. 5–10 micrometers.

Q.40 What is a sub-base?
Ans. It is given at the deepest portion of the tooth preparation for reparative dentin formation. Commonly used material as sub-base is calcium hydroxide.

Q.41 Name tooth colored restorations.
Ans. GIC, Composites and ceramic restorations.

Q.42 Where is calcium hydroxide used?
Ans.
- Direct pulp capping
- Indirect pulp capping
- Pulpotomy
- Apexogenesis
- Apexification
- As root canal sealer
- Intracanal medicament.

Q.43 Where should be base applied?
Ans. On pulpal floor and axial wall.

Q.44 What are adhesive cements?
Ans. Cements which form chemical bonding to tooth structure are called adhesive cements. For example, GIC and zinc polycarboxylate cement.

Q.45 Define composite resin restoration?
Ans. Composite refers to a solid formed from two or more distinct phases that have been combined to produce properties superior to or intermediate to those of individual components.

Q.46 What is components of dental composite?
Ans. Resin matrix, fillers, coupling agent, activator-initiator agents, inhibitors, coloring agents.

Q.47 What are the types of composite according to curing mechanism?
Ans. Chemically cured and light cured. Under light cured, there are ultraviolet light activated composite and visible light-cured composite.

Q.48 What is the main advantage of composite over unfilled direct filling resins?
Ans. Lower co-efficient of thermal expansion.

Dental Materials

Q.49 What are different types of composite according to fillers particle size?

Ans.
- Macrofilled/traditional or conventional composites— 8–12 µm
- Small particle-filled composites—1–5 µm
- Microfilled composites—0.04–0.4 µm
- Hybrid composites—0.6–1 µm.

Q.50 What are the recent advancements in composite resin?

Ans. Flowable composite, condensable (Packable) composites, expanding matrix resins composites, compomers, etc.

Q.51 What is the advantage of using visible light for light cure resin?

Ans.
- It can cure resins through enamel.
- It can cure greater depth of resin as compared to UV light.

Chapter 5: Instruments Used in Operative Dentistry

Chapter Outline

- Materials used for manufacturing cutting instruments
- Classification
- Nomenclature by GV black
- Parts of hand cutting instruments
- Instrument formula
- Different instrument designs
- Description of various instruments
- Hand cutting instruments
- Restorative instruments
- Instrument grasps
- Finger rests
- Methods of use of instruments
- Rotary cutting instruments
- Handpieces
- Dental burs
- Diamond abrasive instruments
- Matricing
- Matrix
- Classification
- Tofflemire universal matrix band retainer (designed by Dr BR Tofflemire)
- Separation of teeth

INTRODUCTION

Various hand and rotary instruments are used for diagnosis, tooth preparation and for insertion, compaction, and finishing of the restoration. Commonly used instruments are mouth mirrors, probe, tweezer, carvers, plastic carrier, condensers, etc.

MATERIALS USED FOR MANUFACTURING CUTTING INSTRUMENTS

Material	Stainless steel	Caron steel	Stellite
Composition	Chromium—18% Carbon—1% Iron—81.4%	Carbon—1% Manganese—0.2% Silicon—0.2% Iron—98.4–98.6%	Cobalt—65–90% Chromium—35% Trace amounts-Tungsten, Molybdenum, Iron
Advantages	Chromium present in alloy reduces corrosion by depositing an oxide layer on surface of metal. Remains lustrous under most conditions	Harder than stainless steel	High resistance to acid hardness
Disadvantages	Tendency to dull with time	Prone to corrosion	
Uses	Mainly used for working points and cement instruments		Manufacture of mixing and restorative instruments

CLASSIFICATION

Sturdevant's Classification

- Cutting
  - Excavators
    - Ordinary hatchet
    - Hoe excavator
    - Angle former
    - Spoon excavator.
  - Chisels
    - Straight
    - Curved/Wedelstaedt
    - Binangle
    - Enamel hatchet
    - Gingival marginal trimmer.
  - Others
    - Knives
    - Files
    - Carvers; Discoid-Cleoid.
- Noncutting
  - Amalgam condenser
  - Mirrors
  - Explorer
  - Probes.

NOMENCLATURE BY GV BLACK

- **Order:** Function or purpose of the instrument, e.g., excavator, condenser
- **Suborder:** Position, mode or manner of use, e.g., push, pull
- **Class:** Design or form of the working end, e.g., hatchet, spoon excavator
- **Subclass:** Shape of the shank, e.g., binangle, contra angle.

These names are combined to give a complete description of the instrument. Naming of an instrument generally moves from 4 to 1, for example, binangle hatchet excavator.

■ PARTS OF HAND CUTTING INSTRUMENTS

Each hand instrument is composed of three parts (Fig. 5.1):
1. Handle or shaft
2. Shank
3. Blade or nib.

Handle or Shaft
- Handle is used to hold the instrument
- It can be small, medium or large, smooth or serrated for better grasping and developing pressure (Fig. 5.2).

Shank
- Shank connects the handle to the blade
- It tapers from the handle down to the blade and is normally smooth, round or tapered
- The shank may be straight or angled. Angulation of instrument is provided for access and stability. Depending on number of angles, shank can be classified as *straight* (no angle), *monoangle* (one angle), *biangle* (two angles), *triple-angle* (three angles), and *quadrangle* (four angles) (Fig. 5.3).

Balancing
Balancing of an instrument is achieved by designing the angles of shank so that cutting edge of blade lies within 2–3 mm of long axis of the handle. This principle of instrument design is also called as *contra-angling* (Figs. 5.4A and B).

Advantages of Balancing of Instruments
- Prevents rotation of instruments when in use
- Generates maximum force at tip of the instrument
- Improves accessibility and visibility of operating site.

Blade or Nib
- Blade is working part of the instrument which is connected to the handle by shank. **For cutting instruments**, blade is beveled to create the cutting edge. Depending on bevels, instruments can be single beveled, bibeveled, triple beveled or circumferential beveled
- **For noncutting instruments,** working part is termed as nib which is used to place, condense, and burnish the material in the tooth.

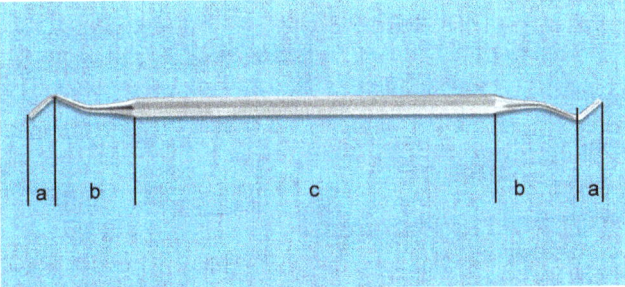

FIGURE 5.1: Parts of hand cutting instrument, a. cutting edge/blade, b. shank, c. shaft/handle.

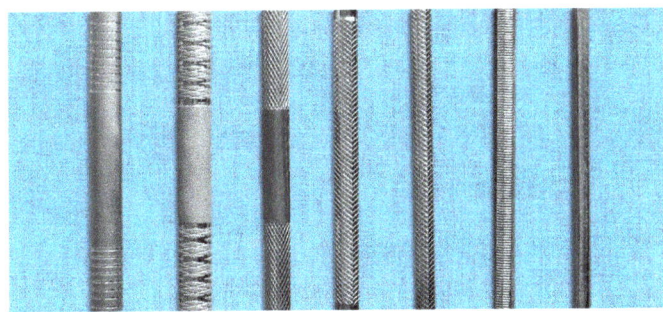

FIGURE 5.2: Different designs of handle of instrument.

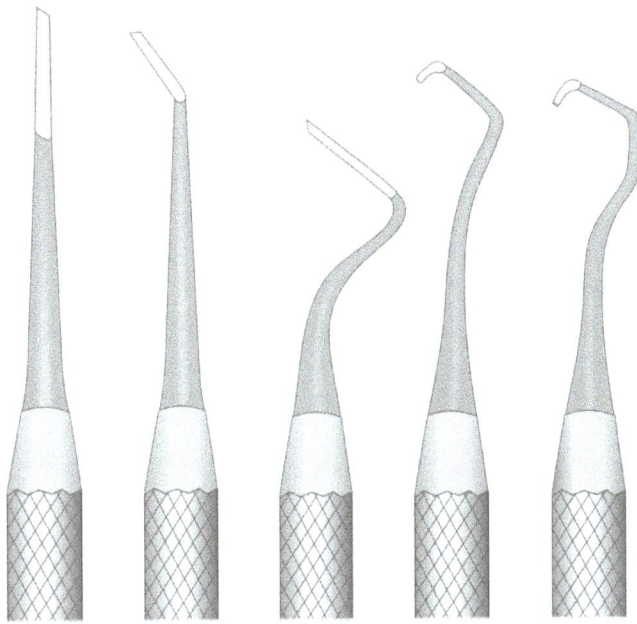

FIGURE 5.3: Instruments with different shank designs.

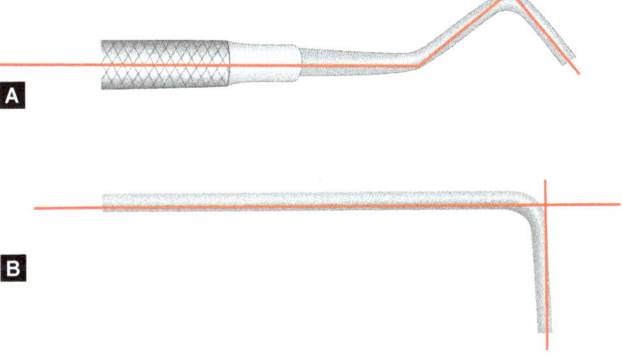

FIGURES 5.4A AND B: (A) Balancing of instrument means cutting edge of blade lies within 2–3 mm of long axis of the handle; (B) Lack of balancing of instrument.

■ INSTRUMENT FORMULA

Greene Vardiman Black established an instrument formula for describing dimensions of blade, nib or head of instrument, and angles present in shank of the instrument. Formula is usually printed on the handle consisting of a code of three or four numbers separated by spaces.

1 centigrade is equal to 1/100th of a circle, i.e., 1/100 × 360 = 3.6°.

Four-number Formula (Fig. 5.5)

It is used for the instruments in which primary cutting edge is not at right angle to long axis of the blade, e.g., *gingival margin trimmer* and *angle former*.

- **1st number:** Blade width—expressed in 1/10th of mm
- **2nd number:** Primary cutting-edge angle, i.e., angle between the primary cutting edge and handle of the instrument and is expressed in centigrade **(Fig. 5.6)**
- **3rd number:** Blade length—expressed in mm
- **4th number:** Blade angle—it is the angle between long axis of the blade and the long axis of the handle, it is expressed in centigrades.

Example of a Four-number Formula

Instrument with formula 15-95-8-12 **(Fig. 5.7)** represents the following:

- **1st number**—blade width—15 × 1/10 = 1.5 mm
- **2nd number**—primary cutting edge angle—95°
- **3rd number**—blade length, i.e., 8 mm
- **4th number**—blade angle—12°.

Three-number Formula (Fig. 5.8)

It is used for the instruments in which cutting edge is at right angle to the long axis of the blade, e.g., enamel hatchet.

- **1st number**—blade width—expressed in 1/10th of mm

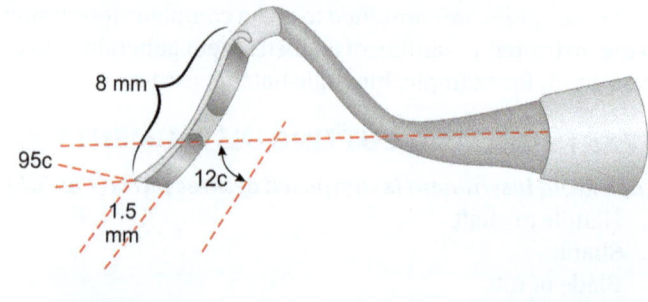

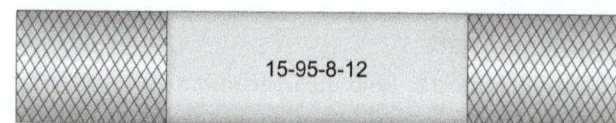

FIGURE 5.7: Schematic representation of an instrument with four-number formula (15-95-8-12).

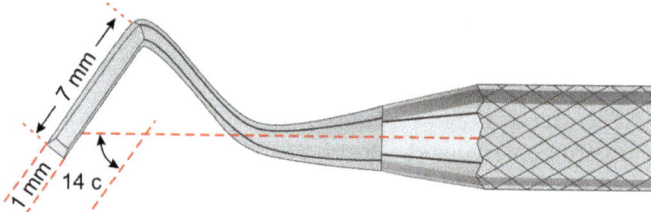

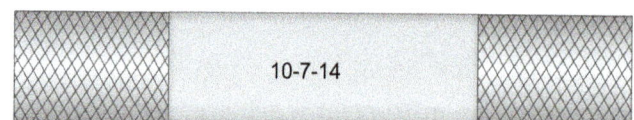

FIGURE 5.8: Schematic representation of three-number formula.

- **2nd number**—blade length—expressed in mm
- **3rd number**—blade angle—it is the angle between long axis of the blade and the long axis of the handle, it is expressed in centigrades.

Most instruments have 3 number formula. An instrument having instrument formula of 15-8-14 indicates following:

- **1st number** is blade width, i.e., 15 × 1/10 = 1.5 mm
- **2nd number** is blade length, i.e., 8 mm
- **3rd number** is blade angle, i.e., 14 degree centigrade.

DIFFERENT INSTRUMENT DESIGNS

Bevels in Cutting Instruments

Single-beveled Instruments (Fig. 5.9)

- Most of the instruments have single bevel that forms the primary cutting edge, e.g., gingival margin trimmer, enamel hatchet, and spoon excavator.
- These can be right or left bevel and mesial or distal bevel instruments.

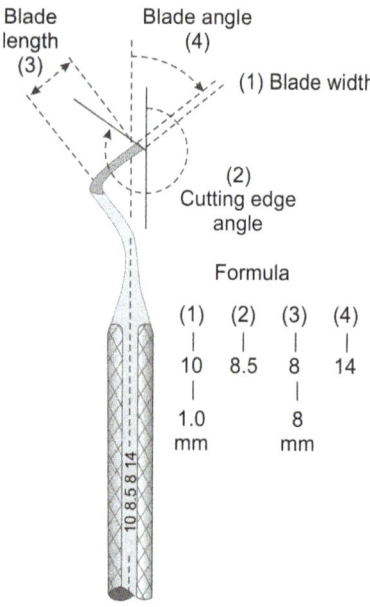

FIGURE 5.5: Schematic representation of four-number formula.

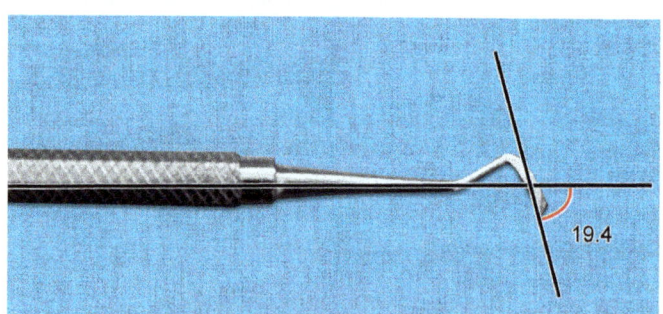

FIGURE 5.6: Schematic representation of measurement of primary cutting edge angle.

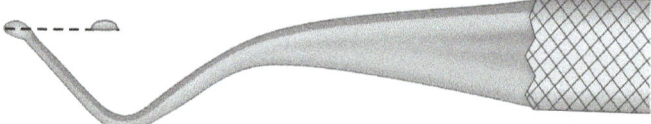

FIGURE 5.9: Single bevel instruments—Spoon excavator.

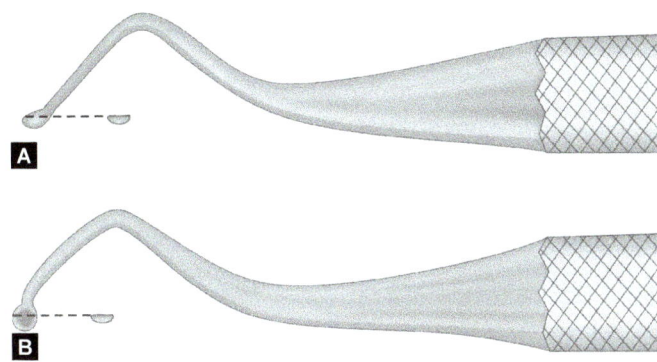

FIGURES 5.10A AND B: Schematic representation of circumferential bevel in a spoon excavator.

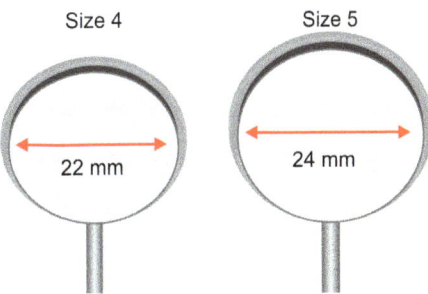

FIGURE 5.11: Different sizes of mouth mirror.

- **Right and left bevel instruments:** To determine right or left side of the bevel, primary cutting edge is held down pointing away. If bevel appears on right, it is the right instrument of the pair and if bevel appears on the left, it is left instrument of the pair. During use, move the instrument from right to left in right beveled instrument and from left to right in left beveled instrument.
- **Mesial and distal bevel instruments:** If we observe the inside of the blade curvature and the primary bevel is not visible then the instrument has a distal bevel and if the primary bevel can be seen from the similar view point the instrument has a mesial or reverse bevel.

Bibeveled Instruments

If two additional cutting edges extend from the primary cutting edges, then the instrument with secondary cutting edges is called bibeveled instrument. Only hatchets and hoes are bibeveled instruments.

Triple-beveled Instrument

If three additional cutting edges extend from the primary cutting edge, then the instrument is called triple-beveled instrument. It results in three distinct cutting edges and increases cutting efficiency of the instrument.

Circumferential Bevel

Here instrument blade is beveled at all its peripheries, e.g., spoon excavator **(Figs. 5.10A and B)**.

DESCRIPTION OF VARIOUS INSTRUMENTS

Mouth Mirrors

Mouth mirror is used as supplement to improve access to instrumentation. It has handle, shank and a mirror attached to a round metal disk at one end.

Sizes of Mouth Mirrors (Fig. 5.11)

Size 1	Size 2	Size 3	Size 4	Size 5
16 mm	18 mm	20 mm	22 mm	24 mm

Types

Mouth mirrors are of various types:
- **Front surface reflecting mirror:** Here the coating is present on front surface of the mirror to prevent image distortion. It is most commonly used due to good quality of image
- **Plane or flat surface:** It produces double image also called ghost image, therefore not recommended much, though it resists the scratch because reflecting surface is on back of the mirror lens
- **Concave surface:** It is used to provide different degrees of magnification, but it causes image distortion.

Uses

- Direct visualization of operating field
- Indirect visualization of oral structures that cannot be seen directly **(Fig. 5.12)**
- Illumination of operating area by reflecting light on to the tooth surface **(Fig. 5.13)**
- Refraction of soft tissues like the tongue, cheeks or lips for improved accessibility and visibility of the operating site **(Fig. 5.14)**.

Explorer

Explorer is commonly used as a diagnostic aid in evaluating condition of teeth especially pits and fissures.

Types of Explorer (Figs. 5.15A to D)

Tweezer (Fig. 5.16)

Tweezer has angled tip and is available in different sizes. It is used to place and remove cotton rolls and other small materials to and from the mouth.

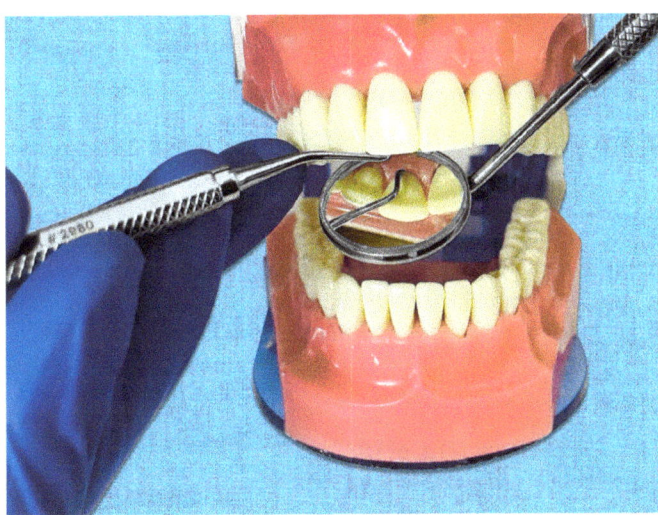

FIGURE 5.12: Indirect vision using mirror.

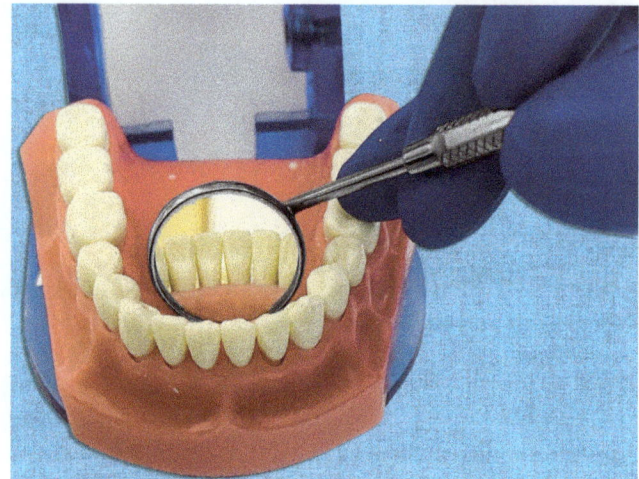

FIGURE 5.13: Illumination using mirror.

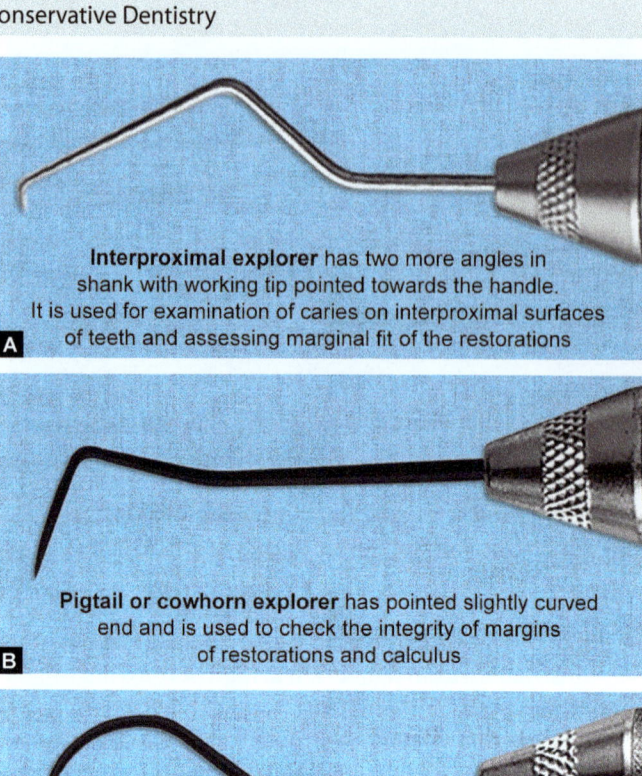

A. **Interproximal explorer** has two more angles in shank with working tip pointed towards the handle. It is used for examination of caries on interproximal surfaces of teeth and assessing marginal fit of the restorations

B. **Pigtail or cowhorn explorer** has pointed slightly curved end and is used to check the integrity of margins of restorations and calculus

C. **Shepherd's crook explorer** or **curved explorer** has got semilunar shaped working tip which is perpendicular to the handle. This is used for examining caries and irregular restoration margins

D. **Straight explorer** is used for examining occlusal surfaces of teeth for caries and margins of restorations

FIGURES 5.15A TO D: Different types of explorers: (A) Interproximal; Pigtail or cowhorn; (C) Shepherd's crook or curved; (D) Straight.

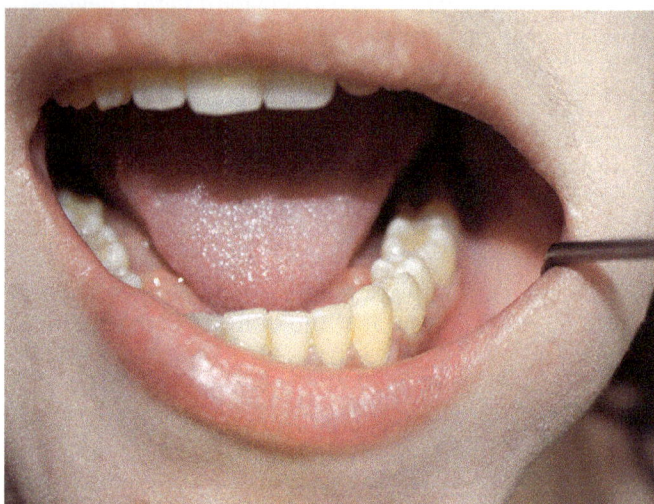

FIGURE 5.14: Refraction of cheek or lips for better accessibility and visibility.

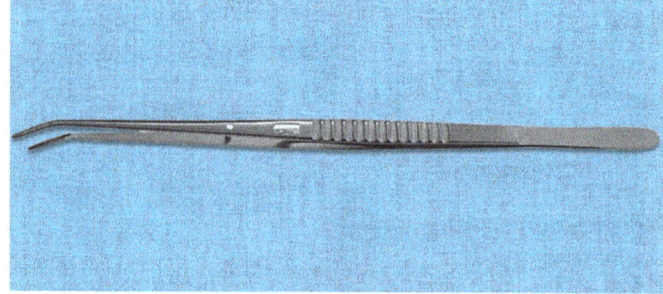

FIGURE 5.16: Tweezer.

Probe (Fig. 5.17)

Though probe almost looks like straight explorers, but it has blunt end which is marked with graduations. Probe is used for measuring pocket depth but in operative dentistry, it is used to check dimensions of tooth preparation.

HAND CUTTING INSTRUMENTS

Excavators

Ordinary Hatchet

- An ordinary hatchet excavator is a bibeveled instrument in which cutting edge of blade is directed in same plane as that of long axis of the handle
- It is used to prepare and sharpen the line angles
- It is also used for preparing retentive areas for direct filling gold in anterior teeth.

Hoe Excavators (Fig. 5.18)

- Primary cutting edge of blade is perpendicular to the long axis of handle
- It is a single-planed instrument which cuts in vertical, push and pull, right, and left motions
- It is used to shape and plane the tooth preparation walls and to form the line angles in class III and V restorations for direct filling gold.

Instruments Used in Operative Dentistry

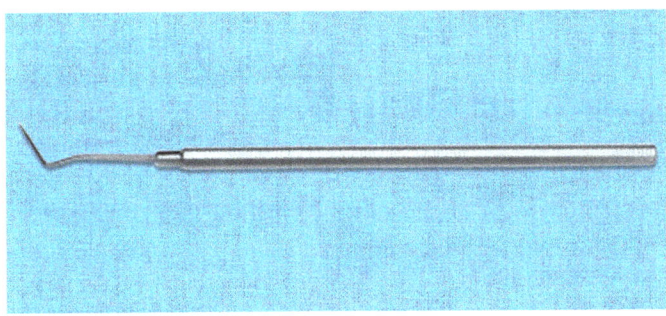

FIGURE 5.17: Probe.

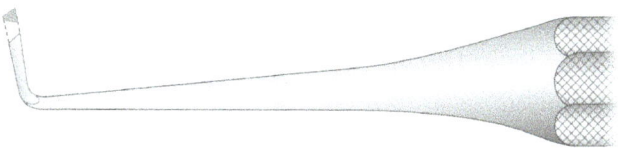

FIGURE 5.18: Hoe excavator.

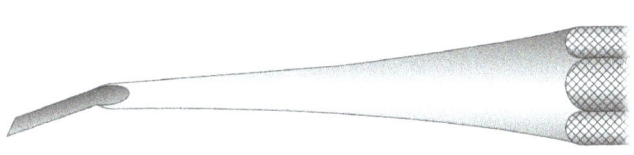

FIGURE 5.19: Angle former excavator.

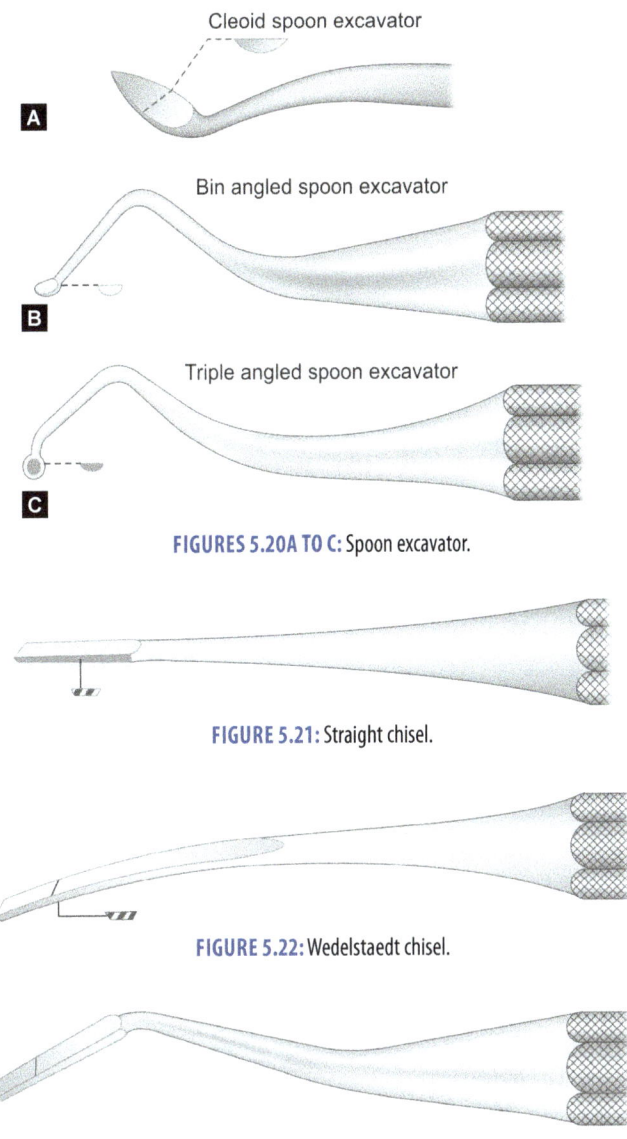

FIGURES 5.20A TO C: Spoon excavator.

FIGURE 5.21: Straight chisel.

FIGURE 5.22: Wedelstaedt chisel.

FIGURE 5.23: Binangled chisel.

Angle Former

- Angle former is a type of excavator which is monoangled with the cutting edge sharpened at an angle to long axis of the blade **(Fig. 5.19)**
- Blade of angle former is beveled on sides as well as at the end, this forms three cutting edges, thus resulting in a triple-beveled instrument
- It cuts in vertical push or pull motion for accentuating line and point angles, to establish retention form in direct filling gold restoration.

Spoon Excavator

- It is a double-ended instrument with a spoon, claw, or disk-shaped blade shank is bin- or triple-angled to facilitate accessibility **(Figs. 5.20A to C)**
- It is used to remove caries and debris in the scooping motion from the carious teeth and for carving amalgam restorations and wax patterns.

Chisels

Straight Chisel

- It has straight blade in line with shank and handle **(Fig. 5.21)**
- In this, primary cutting edge is in a plane perpendicular to long axis of the handle
- It is used with a push or pull motion
- It is used with straight thrust force in push motion for cutting enamel.

Curved/Wedelstaedt Chisel

- This instrument is almost similar to straight chisel except for slight vertical curvature in its shank **(Fig. 5.22)**
- It can be mesially or distally beveled
- It is mainly used for cleaving undermined enamel.

Binangle Chisel

- It has two different angles—one at the working end and other at the shank **(Fig. 5.23)**
- It is mesially or distally beveled and is used to cleave the undermined enamel.

Enamel Hatchet (Fig. 5.24)

- Hatchet is a paired instrument in which blades makes 45–90° angle to the shank
- In paired right and left hatchets, blades are beveled on opposite sides to form their cutting edges
- Hatchet is used for cleaving enamel and planing cavity dentinal walls so as to have sharp outline of the preparation.

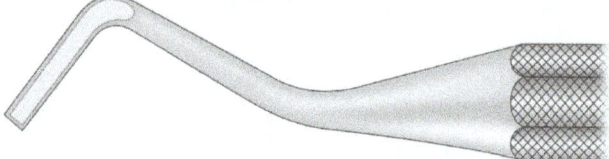

FIGURE 5.24: Enamel hatchet.

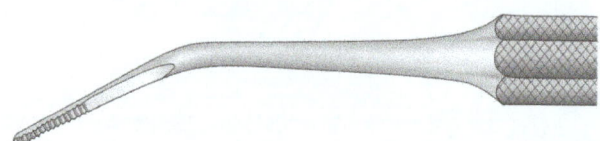

FIGURE 5.26: Files.

Files

Blades of files have serrations called teeth. These are used in push and pull motion to remove excess material especially at gingival margins **(Fig. 5.26)**.

Carvers: Cleoid-Discoid (Fig. 5.27)

- In cleoid, it is claw-like and in discoid it is disk-like. These instruments have sharp cutting edges as spoon excavators but blade to shaft relationship is similar to chisels
- It is used for removing caries, carving occlusal anatomy of amalgam restorations or wax patterns.

RESTORATIVE INSTRUMENTS

Following are the commonly used instruments when temporary or permanent restoration is being done.

Cement Spatulas (Fig. 5.28)

- Cement spatula is made up of stainless steel or plastic, having wide nib with blunt edges, straight shank, and handle

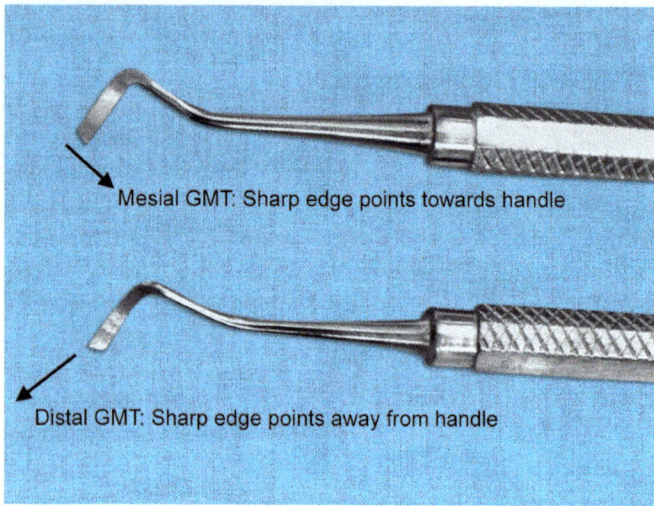

FIGURE 5.25: Mesial and distal gingival margin trimmer (GMT).

Gingival Margin Trimmer

- Gingival margin trimmer (GMT) is a modified hatchet which has working ends with opposite curvatures and bevels **(Fig. 5.25)**
- It is available in a set of two double-ended styles and is used in pairs
- **Mesial GMT:** In this, cutting edge of the instrument makes an acute angle with edge of the blade nearest to the handle
- **Distal GMT:** In this, cutting edge of instrument makes acute angle with edge of blade farthest from handle
- GMT is used in lateral scraping motion.

Uses of GMT

- Used in proximal box of class II preparation with horizontal strokes to scrape the gingival wall and margin
- Mesial GMT is used to bevel a mesial gingival margin or accentuate a distal axiogingival angle. Distal GMT is used to bevel a distal gingival margin or accentuate a mesial axiogingival angle
- It is used in proximal box of class II preparation with horizontal strokes to scrape the gingival floor and margin.

Other Cutting Instruments

Knives

- These are finishing knives having thin knife-like blade
- These are used in scrap and pull motion for removing excess restorative material on gingival, facial or lingual margins of a proximal restoration
- For contouring surface of class V restoration.

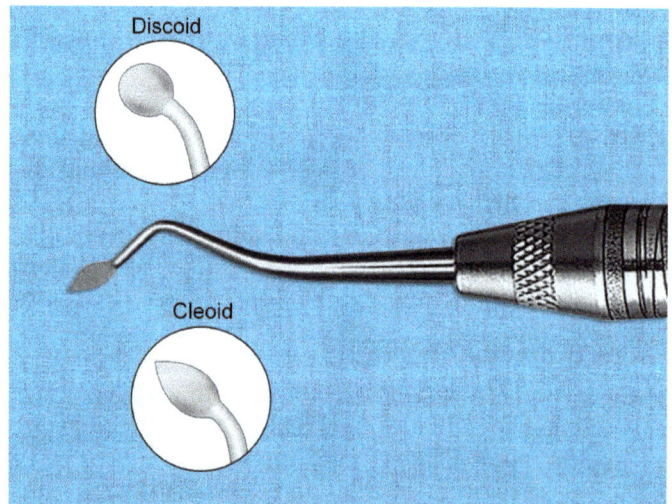

FIGURE 5.27: Cleoid discoid carver.

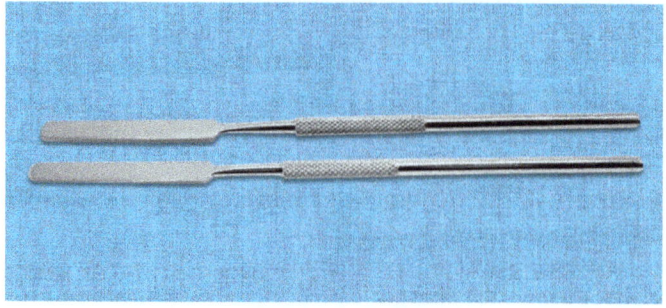

FIGURE 5.28: Cement spatulas.

- Blunt end is used for mixing impression materials and cements like zinc phosphate, glass ionomer cement, etc.

Plastic Filling Instrument (Fig. 5.29)
- It is a double-ended instrument with flat nib at one end and round condenser nib at other end
- It is used to carry and place cement into the cavity and to check convenience form of tooth preparation.

Condensers (Fig. 5.30)
- Condensers are used to pack material into prepared cavity
- Nibs can be round, elliptical, diamond, triangular, parallelogram, etc. Depending upon serrations they can be serrated (for spherical amalgam) and nonserrated (for admixed amalgam).

Amalgam Carrier
- Amalgam carrier carries the freshly prepared amalgam restorative material to the prepared tooth
- Amalgam carrier has hollow working end, called barrel, into which the amalgam is packed for transportation (**Fig. 5.31**). Lever of amalgam carrier is located on top of the carrier. When lever is depressed, the amalgam is expelled into the preparation
- After restoration is completed, any remaining amalgam alloy is expelled out from the carrier into the amalgam well, otherwise if the amalgam is allowed to harden in the carrier, it will no longer be serviceable.

Carvers (Fig. 5.32)
- Carvers have sharp cutting edges to shape and contour the surface of filling materials in their plastic state, waxes, molds, and patterns
- They have different designs and shapes, for example
    - Hollenback carver (knife edged elongated bibeveled)
    - Diamond (Frahm's carver)
    - Ward 'C' carver
    - Discoid cleoid carver
    - Interproximal carver.

Burnisher (Figs. 5.33A and B)
- Burnisher is a double ended instrument with smooth spherical working ends to produce surface of restoration shiny and lustrous
- Nibs can be egg shaped, ball shaped, beaver tail shaped, apple shaped, conical, bullet shaped, fish tail or hourglass shaped.

Burnishers are used for final condensation of amalgam and shaping of metal matrix bands.

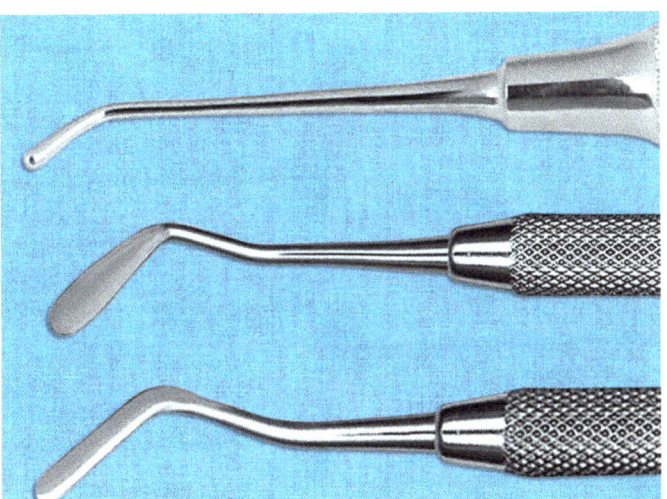

FIGURE 5.29: Plastic filling instrument.

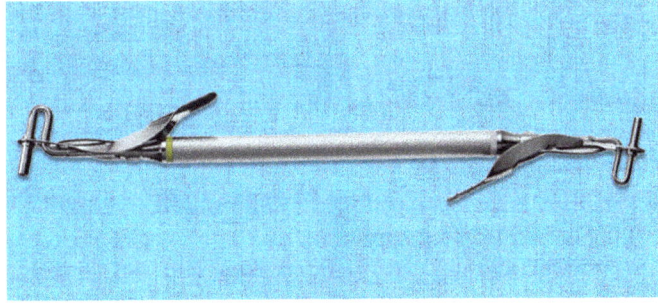

FIGURE 5.31: Amalgam carrier.
(*Courtesy*: Hu-Friedy).

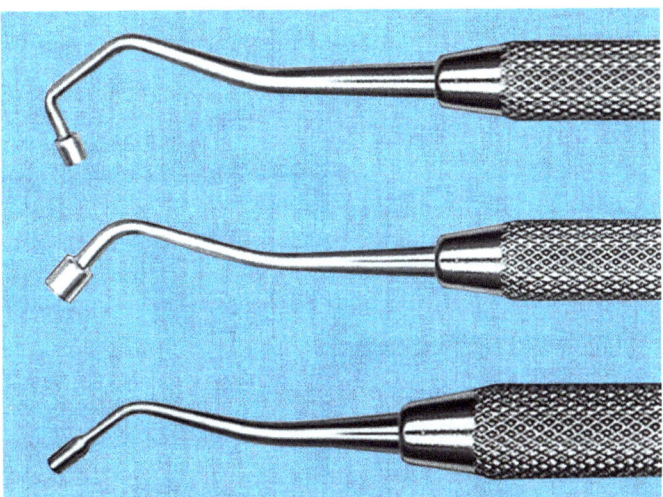

FIGURE 5.30: Different types of condensers.
(*Courtesy*: Hu-Friedy).

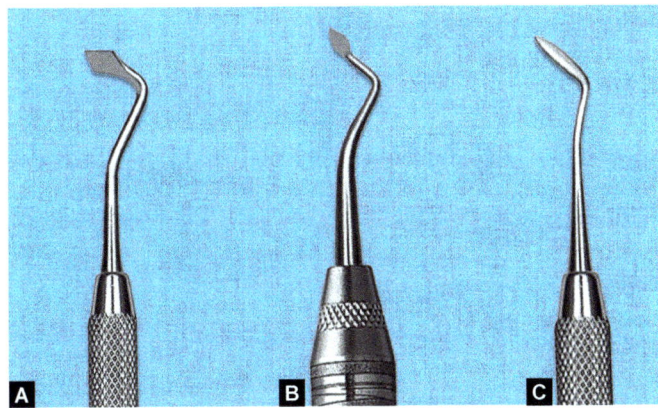

FIGURES 5.32A TO C: (A) Diamond carver; (B) Cleoid discoid carver; (C) Hollenback carver.
(*Courtesy*: Hu-Friedy).

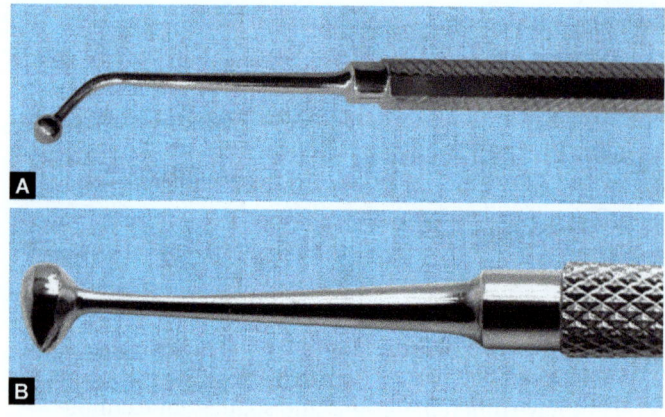

FIGURES 5.33A AND B: (A) Ball burnisher; (B) Egg shaped burnisher.

- This grasp is most commonly used for preparing a tooth in the lingual aspect of maxillary anterior and occlusal surface of maxillary posterior teeth.

Composite Resin Instruments (Fig. 5.34)

These are set of instruments with a coating of titanium nitride. Since Titanium nitride is 40% harder than stainless steel, it is not scratched by filler particles of composite resin. It also resists sticking of resin.

INSTRUMENT GRASPS

Modified Pen Grasp

- Modified pen grasp is similar to the pen grasp except the operator uses the pad of the middle finger on the handle of the instrument rather than going under the instrument **(Figs. 5.35A and B)**
- Positioning of the fingers in this manner creates a triangle of forces or tripod effect, which enhances the instrument control. Here palm of the operator faces away from the operator
- This position stabilizes the instrument and allows the middle finger to help push the instrument down.

Inverted Pen Grasp

- In inverted pen grasp, finger positions are the same as for the modified pen grasp except that hand is rotated so that palm faces toward the operator **(Fig. 5.36)**

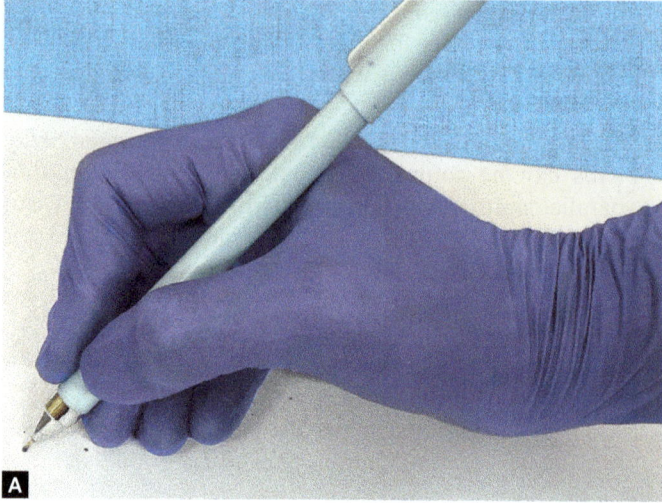

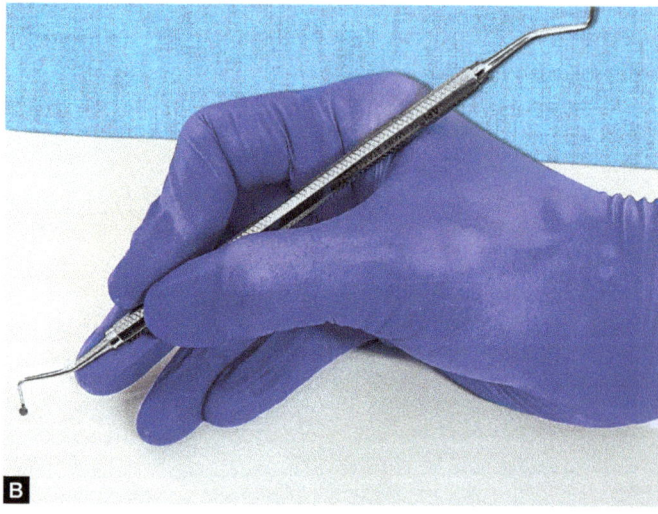

FIGURES 5.35A AND B: (A) Normal pen grasp; (B) Modified pen grasp.

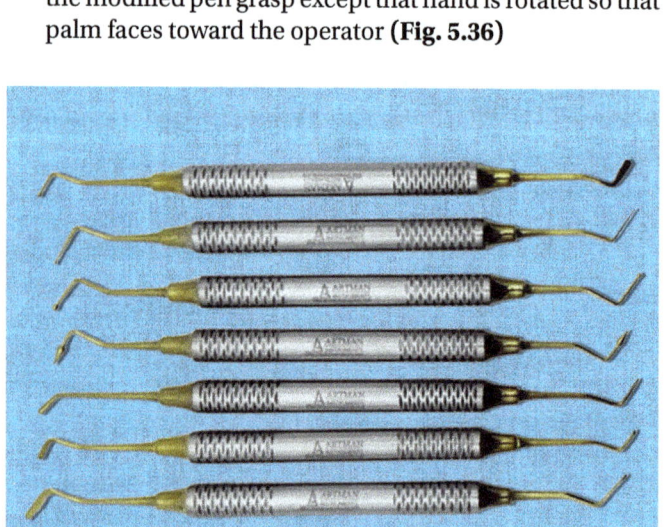

FIGURE 5.34: Instruments used for composite restorations.

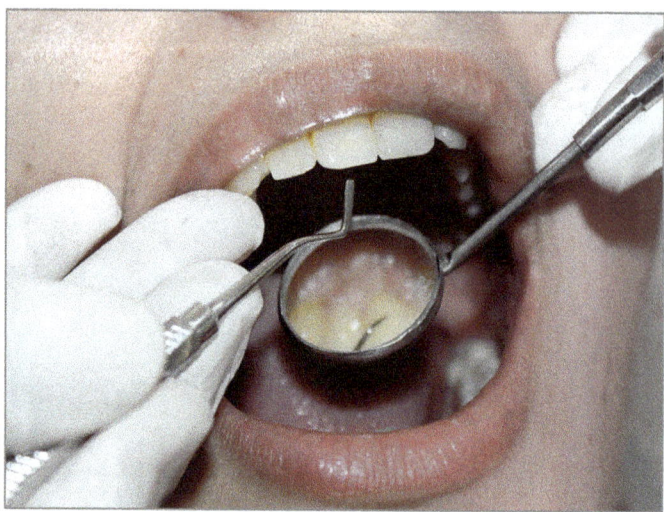

FIGURE 5.36: Inverted pen grasp.

Palm and Thumb Grasp

- This grasp is same as that for holding the knife for peeling the skin of an apple. Here, instrument is grasped very near to its working end so that thumb can be braced against the teeth so as to provide control during instrument movements **(Figs. 5.37A and B)**
- Shaft of the instrument is placed on the palm of the hand and grasped by the four fingers to provide firm control, while the thumb is free to control movements and provide rest on an adjacent tooth of the same arch
- To achieve the thrust action with the fingers and palm, instrument is forced away from the tip of the thumb which is at the rest position.

Modified Palm and Thumb Grasp (Figs. 5.38A and B)

- Instrument is held like the palm grasp but the pads of all the four fingers press the handle against the palm and pad and first joint of the thumb. Here tip of the thumb rests on the tooth being prepared or the adjacent tooth
- Modified palm and thumb grasp provides more control to avoid slipping of instrument. This grasp is commonly used in maxillary anterior teeth.

FINGER RESTS

The finger rest helps to stabilize the hand and the instrument by providing a firm rest to the hand during operative procedures. Finger rests can be:

Conventional (Fig. 5.39)

In this, the finger rest is just near or adjacent to the working tooth.

Cross-arch

In this, the finger rest is achieved from tooth of the opposite side but of the same arch.

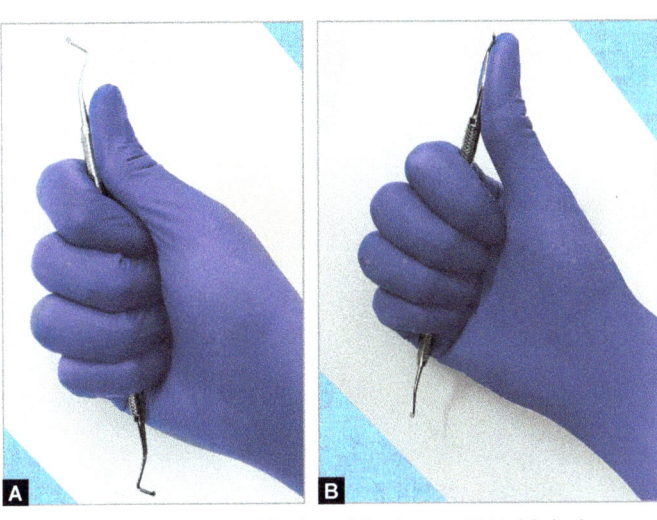

FIGURES 5.37A AND B: (A) Palm and thumb grasp; (B) Modified palm and thumb grasp.

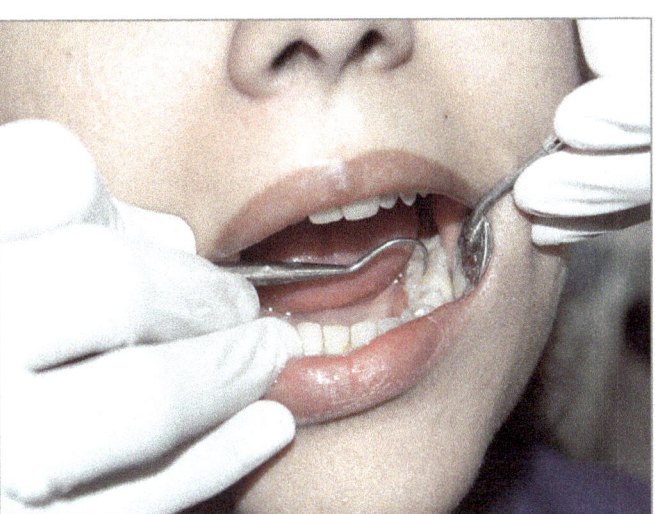

FIGURE 5.39: Cross-arch intraoral finger rest.

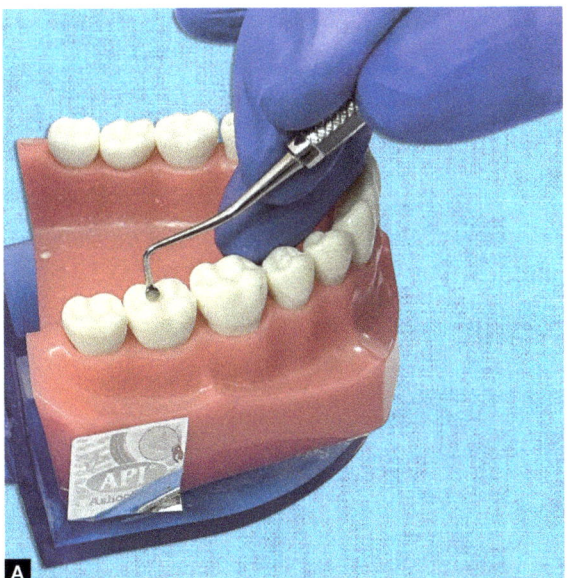
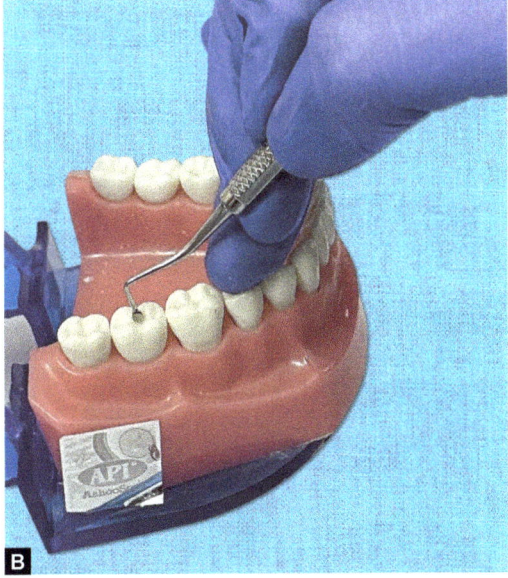

FIGURES 5.38A AND B: (A) Conventional finger rest on adjacent tooth; (B) Conventional finger on finger rest.

Opposite Arch

Here, the finger rest is achieved from tooth of the opposite arch.

METHODS OF USE OF INSTRUMENTS

- Instrument is effectively used when it is moved from bevel to nonbevel side
- Instrument should always be held parallel to the wall being worked upon. Holding an instrument at this angle may increase its cutting but it may also cause damage or fracture of the tooth
- For buccal wall, one side of instrument is used and for lingual wall, the other side of instrument should be used.

ROTARY CUTTING INSTRUMENTS

Rotary cutting instruments are those instruments which rotate on an axis to do the work of abrading and cutting on tooth structure.

Types of Rotary Cutting

- **Handpiece:** It is a power device
- **Bur:** It is a cutting tool.

HANDPIECES

Handpiece is a device for holding rotating instrument, transmitting power to it and positioning it intraorally.

Types of Handpiece

Contra-angle Handpiece

In this, head of handpiece is first angled away from and then back toward the long axis of the handle.

- **Air-rotor contra-angle handpiece (Fig. 5.40A):**
  - It gets power from the compressed air supplied by the compressor
  - Speed range is 100,000 to 300,000 rpm
  - Used for tooth preparation and removal of old restorations.
- **Micromotor (Fig. 5.40B):**
  - It gets power from electric micromotor or airmotor
  - Used for finishing and polishing procedures.

Straight Handpiece

- In straight handpiece, long axis of bur lies in same plane as long axis of handpiece
- Can be attached to micromotor or airmotor
- It is used in oral surgical and laboratory procedures **(Fig. 5.40C)**.

Table 5.1 summarizes rotary speed ranges in operative dentistry with their advantages and disadvantages.

DENTAL BURS (FIG. 5.41)

Bur is a rotary cutting instrument which has bladed cutting head. It removes tooth structure either by chipping it away or by grinding.

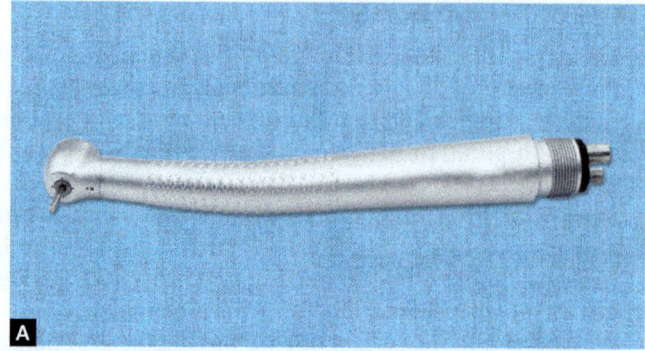

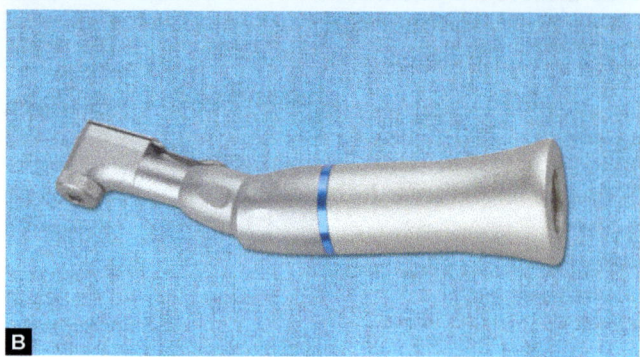

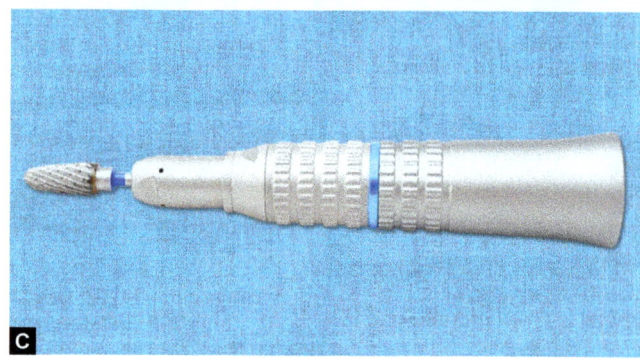

FIGURES 5.40A TO C: (A) Air-rotor contra-angled handpiece; (B) Micromotor contra-angle handpiece; (C) Straight handpiece.

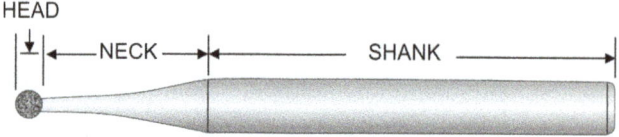

FIGURE 5.41: Parts of dental bur.

Classifications of Burs

- According to their **mode of attachment to the handpiece:**
  - Latch type
  - Friction grip type.
- According to the **length of their head:**
  - Long
  - Short
  - Regular.
- According to head **shape:**
  - Round bur
  - Inverted cone

Instruments Used in Operative Dentistry

TABLE 5.1: Rotary speed ranges in operative dentistry.

Speed	Range (rpm)	Commonly used bur (with this speed)	Uses	Advantages	Disadvantages
Low speed	Less than 12,000	Steel burs with or without lubricant	■ Polishing and finishing ■ Drilling holes for implants ■ Excavation of caries	■ Good tactile sense	■ Ineffective cutting ■ Time consuming ■ Operator fatigue ■ Produce patient discomfort
Medium speed	12,000 to 200,000	Diamond burs with lubricant	■ Tooth preparations ■ Making small tooth preparations ■ Refining tooth preparations ■ Refining occlusion	■ Fine tactile sense	■ More heat production ■ Not fit for larger preparations ■ Large preparations can cause operators fatigue
High speed	More than 200,000	Tungsten carbide burs with lubricant	■ Tooth preparations ■ Removal of old restorative materials ■ Crown preparations for fixed prosthesis	■ Ease for operator ■ Faster preparation takes less time ■ Less fatigue for patient and operator ■ Quadrant dentistry is possible ■ Bur life is enhanced ■ Less chances of apprehension and strain for patient	■ Overcutting is possible ■ Less tactile sense ■ Iatrogenic errors are more common ■ Impairment of visibility due to air-water spray

- Pear-shaped
- Wheel-shaped
- Tapering fissure
- Straight fissure
- End-cutting bur.

Parts of a Bur

Shank

- Shank is that part of the bur that fits into the handpiece, accepts the rotary movement from the handpiece and controls the alignment and concentricity of the instrument
- **Shank design:** Depending upon mode of attachment to handpiece, shanks of burs are of following types **(Figs. 5.42A to C)**:
- **Straight handpiece shank:**
  - In these burs, shank part is like a cylinder into which bur is held with a metal chuck which has different sizes of shank diameter
  - These are used for finishing and polishing of restorations.
- **Latch-type angle handpiece shank:**
  - Here, posterior portion of shank is made flat on one side so that end of bur fits into D-shaped socket at bottom of bur tube
  - Instrument is not retained in handpiece with chuck but with a latch which fits into the grooves made in bur shank
  - These instruments are commonly used in contra-angle handpiece for finishing and polishing procedures.
- **Friction-grip angle handpiece shank:**
  - Here, shank is simple cylinder which is held in handpiece by friction between shank and metal chuck

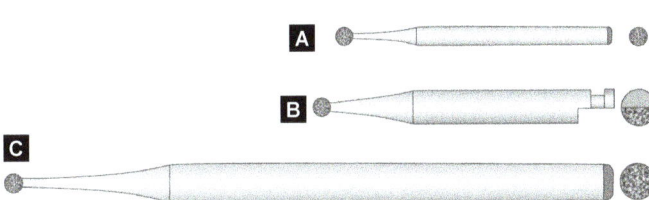

FIGURES 5.42A TO C: Different types of bur: (A) Straight bur; (B) Latch type; (C) Friction grip.

- In these, shank is much smaller than latch-type instruments
- This design is used for high-speed handpiece.

Neck

Neck connects head and shank. It is tapered from shank to the head.

Head

- The term "bur shape" refers to the contour or silhouette of the bur head. It is working part of the bur
- Bur head can be of different shapes and sizes. Depending upon shape of bur head, burs are named as round, inverted, pear, straight, tapered, etc.

Types of Bur (Fig. 5.43)

Round Bur

- Spherical in shape
- Used for initial entry into the tooth, removal of caries, extension of the preparation and for the placement of retentive grooves.

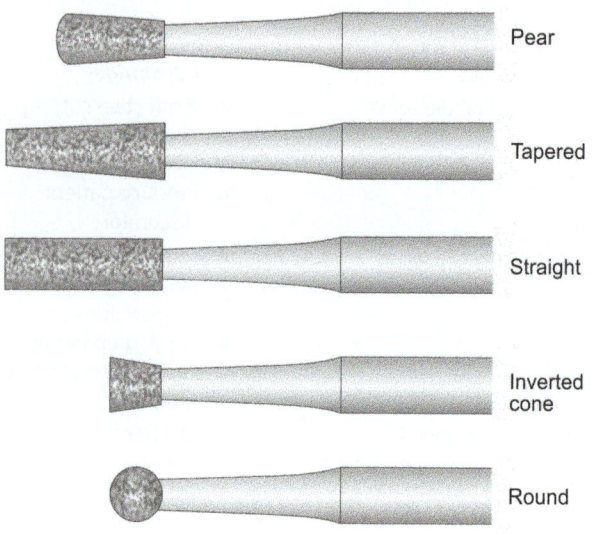

FIGURE 5.43: Schematic representation of designs of bur heads.

Inverted Cone Bur
- It has flat base and sides tapered toward shank
- Used for establishing wall angulations and providing undercuts in tooth preparations.

Pear-shaped Bur
- Head is shaped like tapered cone with small end of cone directed toward shank
- Used in class I tooth preparation for gold foil
- A long length pear bur is used for tooth preparation for amalgam.

Straight-fissure Bur
It is parallel-sided cylindrical bur of different lengths and is used for amalgam tooth preparations.

Tapering-fissure Bur
It is tapered-sided cylindrical but sides tapering toward tip and is used for inlay and crown preparations.

End-cutting Bur
It is used for carrying the preparation apically without axial reduction.

Bur Design
Bur head consists of uniformly spaced blades with concave areas in between them. These concave depressed areas are called chip or flute spaces. Bur tooth terminates in cutting edge or blade.

Blade has two surfaces (**Fig. 5.44**):
1. **Blade face/Rake face:** It is the surface of bur blade on the leading edge
2. **Clearance face:** It is the surface of bur blade on the trailing edge.

Rake Angle
This is angle that the face of bur tooth makes with the radial line from center of the bur to the blade (**Fig. 5.44**). Rake angle can be positive, negative or zero rake angle.

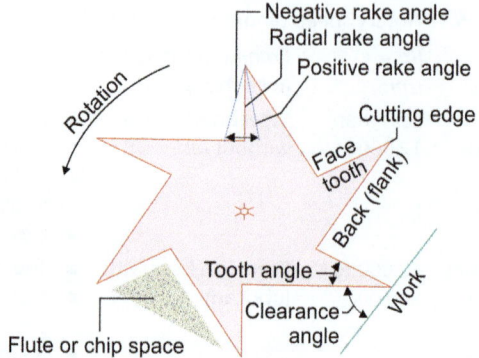

FIGURE 5.44: Bur design showing rake angle, clearance angle, and edge angle.

- **Positive rake angle:** When radial line leads the face
- **Negative rake angle:** When rake face is ahead of radial line
- **Zero rake angle:** When rake face and radial line coincide each other.

Clearance Angle
This is the angle between clearance face and the work (**Fig. 5.44**). It provides adequate chip space for clearing debris.

DIAMOND ABRASIVE INSTRUMENTS
Diamond instruments consist of three parts (**Fig. 5.45**):
1. A metal blank
2. Powdered diamond abrasive
3. Bonding agent to hold the abrasive particles together and binds the particles to metal blank.

Classification of Abrasives According to Abrasive Particle Size (Fig. 5.46)
- *Coarse grit diamond burs* (125–150 μ particle size)—*Green*
- *Medium grit diamond burs* (88–125 μ particle size)—*Blue*
- *Fine grit diamond burs* (60–80 μ particle size)—*Red*
- *Very fine grit diamond burs* (30–40 μ particle size)—*Yellow*.

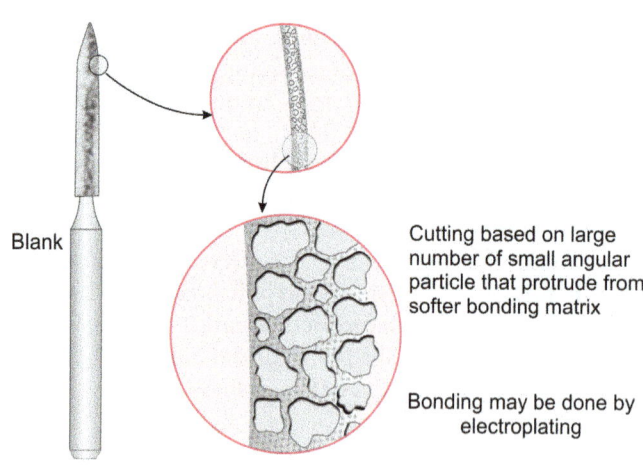

FIGURE 5.45: Powdered diamond abrasive.

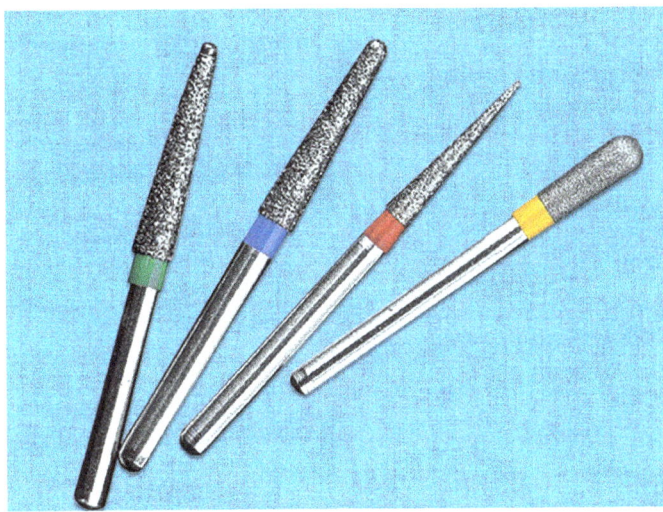

FIGURE 5.46: Coarse, medium, fine, superfine diamond points.

Abrasive stones are available as mounted and unmounted. The mounted stones have abrading head which is joined to the shank and the attachment part. In unmounted stones, the abrading head is supplied separately which can be attached to the mandrel when required.

MATRICING

It is the procedure by which a temporary wall is built opposite to the axial wall, surrounding the tooth structure which has been lost during the tooth preparation.

MATRIX

It is an instrument which is used to hold the restoration within the tooth while it is setting.

Parts of Matrix

Retainer

It holds the band in desired position and shape. Retainer can be a mechanical device, floss, metal ring or impression compound.

Band

It is a piece of metal or polymeric material used to give support and form to the restoration during its insertion and setting. Commonly used materials for bands are stainless steel and cellulose acetate

CLASSIFICATION

According to Method of Retention

- **Mechanically retained**, e.g., Ivory matrix retainers No. 1 and 8, Tofflemire universal dental matrix band retainer.
- **Self-retained**, e.g., copper or stainless-steel bands, automatrix.

According to the Tooth Preparation for which they are Used (Table 5.2)

TABLE 5.2: Enlists various matrices used according to the type of tooth preparation.

Types of preparation	Matrices and retainers
Class I with buccal or lingual extension	Double banded Tofflemire matrix (Bartons matrix)
Class II tooth preparation	<ul><li>Ivory matrix number 1</li><li>Nystrom's retainer</li><li>Ivory matrix number 8</li></ul>
Class II mesio-occlusodistal (MOD) tooth preparation	<ul><li>Tofflemire matrix</li><li>Steele's siqveland self-adjusting matrix, copper band matrix</li><li>Anatomical matrix band</li><li>"T" shaped matrix band</li><li>Retainerless automatrix</li></ul>
Class III tooth preparation	<ul><li>"S" shaped matrix band</li><li>Cellophane matrix strips</li><li>Mylar strips</li></ul>
Class IV tooth preparation	<ul><li>Cellophane strips</li><li>Aluminum foil</li><li>Transparent crown form</li></ul>
Class V tooth preparation	<ul><li>Custom made plastic matrix</li><li>Window matrix</li><li>Tin foil matrix</li><li>S-shaped matrix</li><li>Anatomic matrix</li><li>Aluminum or copper collars</li></ul>

Ivory Matrix Holder (Retainer) No. 1 (Fig. 5.47)

- Ivory matrix holder number 1 is most commonly used matrix band holder for unilateral class II tooth preparations
- Matrix holder has a claw at one end with two flat semicircle arms having a pointed projection at the end. On other end

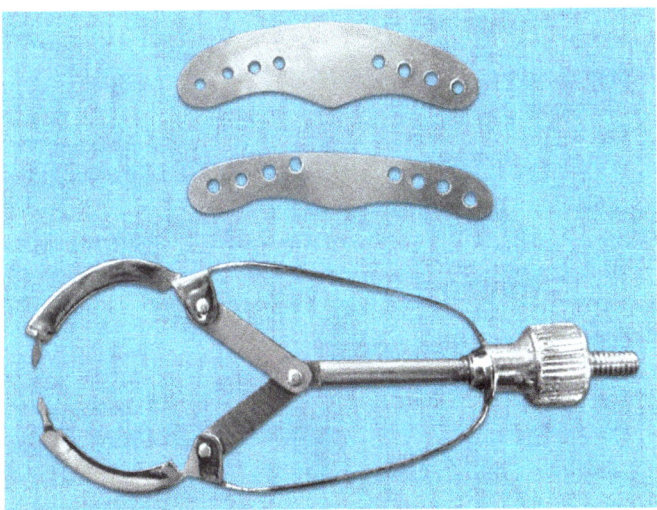

FIGURE 5.47: Ivory No. 1 matrix retainer and band.

of matrix band holder, there is a screw which on rotating clockwise brings ends of both claws closer to each other
- Keeping the matrix band around the tooth, the screw of the retainer is tightened so that the band perfectly fits around the tooth. After this, wedge is placed which also helps in further adaptation of the matrix band to the tooth.

Ivory Matrix Band Retainer No. 8 (Fig. 5.48)

- Ivory matrix band retainer holds the matrix band that encircles the tooth to provide missing walls on both proximal sides
- The matrix band is made up of thin sheet of metal so that it can pass through the contact area of the unprepared proximal side of the tooth.

TOFFLEMIRE UNIVERSAL MATRIX BAND RETAINER (DESIGNED BY DR BR TOFFLEMIRE)

It is also well known as "universal" matrix because it can be used in all types of tooth preparations of posterior teeth.

Parts of Tofflemire Retainer (Fig. 5.49)

Head (Fig. 5.50A)

It has slot for positioning of matrix. It is U-shaped with two slots in open side. Open side of the head should be held facing gingivally when the band is placed around the tooth.

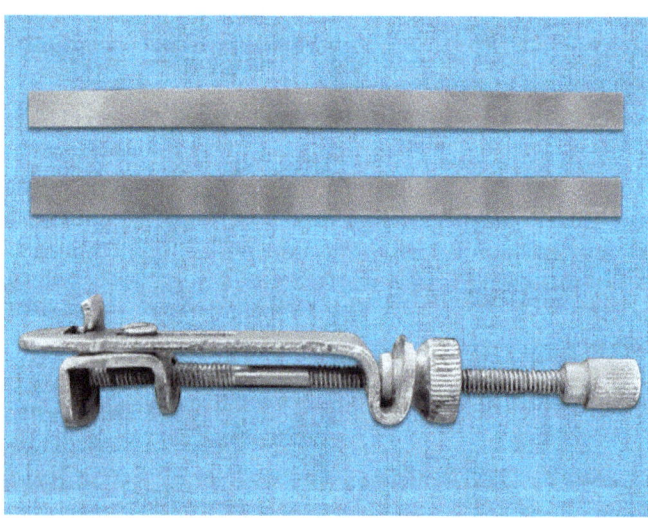

FIGURE 5.48: Ivory No. 8 matrix retainer and bands.

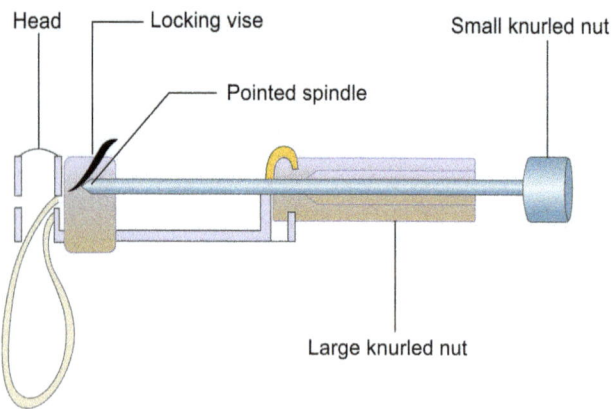

FIGURE 5.49: Parts of tofflemire retainer.

Locking Vise (Fig. 5.50B)

It has a diagonal slot. This portion is located near the head for placing band in the retainer and helps in positioning of band around the tooth.

Pointed Spindle (Fig. 5.50C)

Pointed spindle is used to adjust the distance between head and locking vise and to adjust the size of loop of matrix band.

Large Knurled Nut (Fig. 5.50D)

It is also known as rotating spindle. It helps in adjusting the size of loop of matrix band against the tooth.

Small Knurled Nut (Fig. 5.50E)

It helps in tightening the band to retainer by turning it clockwise.

Placement of Tofflemire Retainer and Band (Figs. 5.51A to E)

- First open the large knurled nut by turning it counter clockwise so that locking vise is at least ¼ inches from the head (**Fig. 5.51A**)
- Hold the knurled nut (large) with one hand, open the small knurled nut in opposite direction (counter clockwise) for clearance of diagonal slot for reception of matrix band (**Fig. 5.51B**)
- Bring the two ends of matrix band together to form loop. This loop can be projected straight, right or left side (**Fig. 5.51C**)
- Turn the small knurled nut clockwise to tighten the band to the retainer (**Fig. 5.51D**)
- After securing the band tightly to the retainer, position the band around the tooth to be restored
- For final adaptation of matrix band to the tooth, tighten the large knurled nut by turning it clockwise and finally place wedge to secure the band well adapted to the cavity walls (**Fig. 5.51E**).

Figures 5.51A to D shows common mistakes which are to be avoided while placing tofflemire retainer and band.

Indications of Tofflemire Matrix

- Class I tooth preparations with buccal or lingual extensions
- Unilateral or bilateral class II MOD tooth preparations
- Class II compound tooth preparations having more than two missing walls.

Advantages

- Easy to use
- Sturdy and stable in nature
- Provides good contact and contours
- Can be easily removed
- Can be sterilized
- Can be used both from facial as well as lingual side
- Economical.

Disadvantages

Cannot be used in badly broken teeth or extensive class II restorations.

Instruments Used in Operative Dentistry

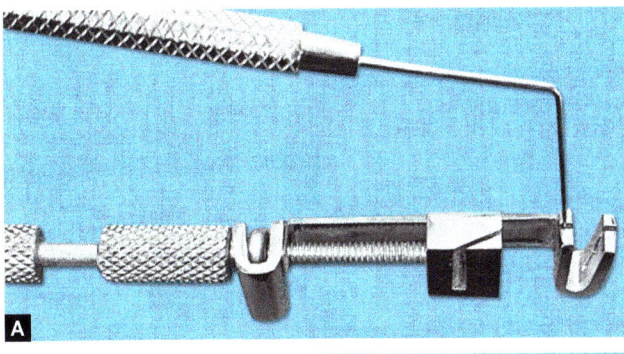
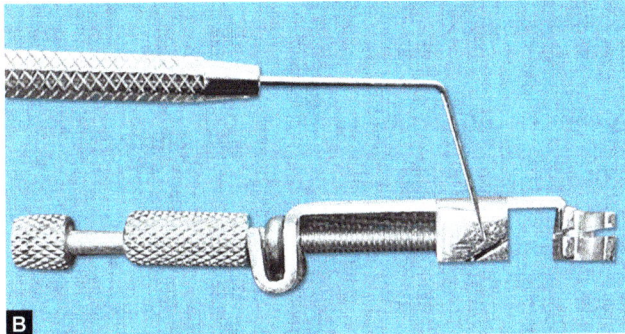
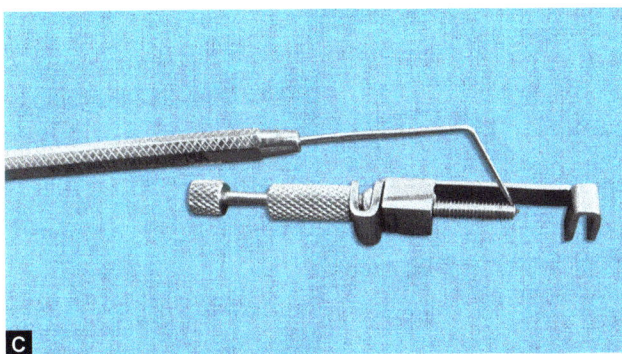
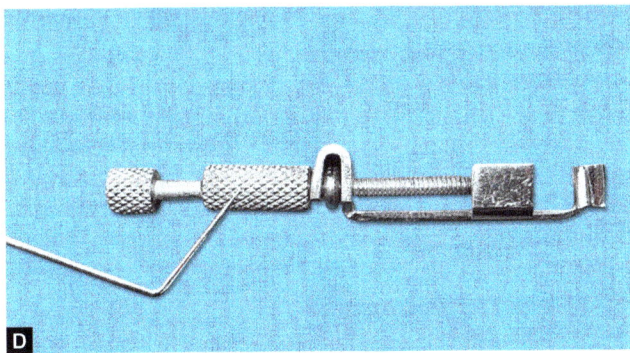
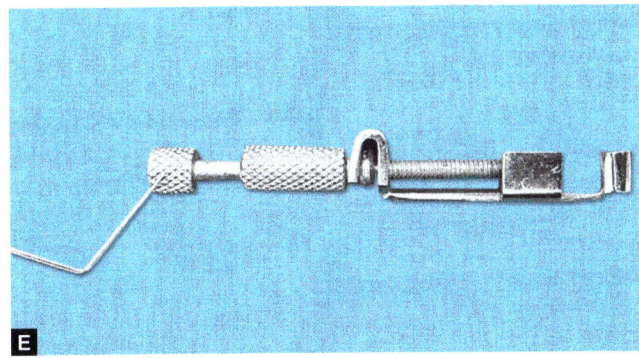

FIGURES 5.50 A TO E: Showing parts of tofflemire retainer; (A) Head; (B) Locking vise; (C) Pointed spindle; (D) Large knurled nut; (E) Small knurled nut.

T-shaped Matrix Band (Figs. 5.52A to D)

- This is preformed brass, copper or stainless-steel matrix bands without a retainer
- In this band, the long arm of the T surrounds the tooth and overlaps the short arm of the T
- Band is adapted according to tooth shape and size and stabilized using wedges and impression compound. may be used to provide further stability to the band.

Transparent Crown Forms Matrices

- These are plastic crowns which can be contoured according to tooth shape and size
- After selecting appropriate crown form, it is trimmed to fit 1 mm beyond the preparation margins
- These are indicated for bilateral class IV preparations.

Clear Plastic Matrix Strips (Fig. 5.53)

- These are transparent matrix strips used for tooth colored restorations because they allow light to be transmitted during polymerization of composite restorations
- These are used for class III and IV composite restorations.

SEPARATION OF TEETH

Definition

Separation of teeth is defined as the process of separating the involved teeth slightly away from each other or bringing them closer to each other and/or changing their position in one or more dimensions.

Methods of Tooth Separation

Two methods used for tooth separation are:
Rapid or immediate separation: Rapid separation is most frequently used method in which tooth separation can be achieved in very short span of time.

Principles Used in Rapid Separation

- **Wedge principle:** A pointed, wedge-shaped mechanical device is inserted beneath the contact area of teeth to produce the separation, e.g., Elliot separator and wedges. Wedges are used for rapid tooth separation during tooth preparation and restoration.

Advantages

- Provide space to compensate for thickness of matrix band
    - Help in retracting and depressing the interproximal gingival area, thus help in minimizing trauma to soft tissue.
- Help in stabilization of retainer and matrix during condensation of area
- Prevent gingival overhang of restoration.

Types of Wedges

- **Wooden wedges:** Wooden wedges are made from soft wood like pine or hard wood like oak (**Fig. 5.55**). These are most commonly used and preferred as they can be

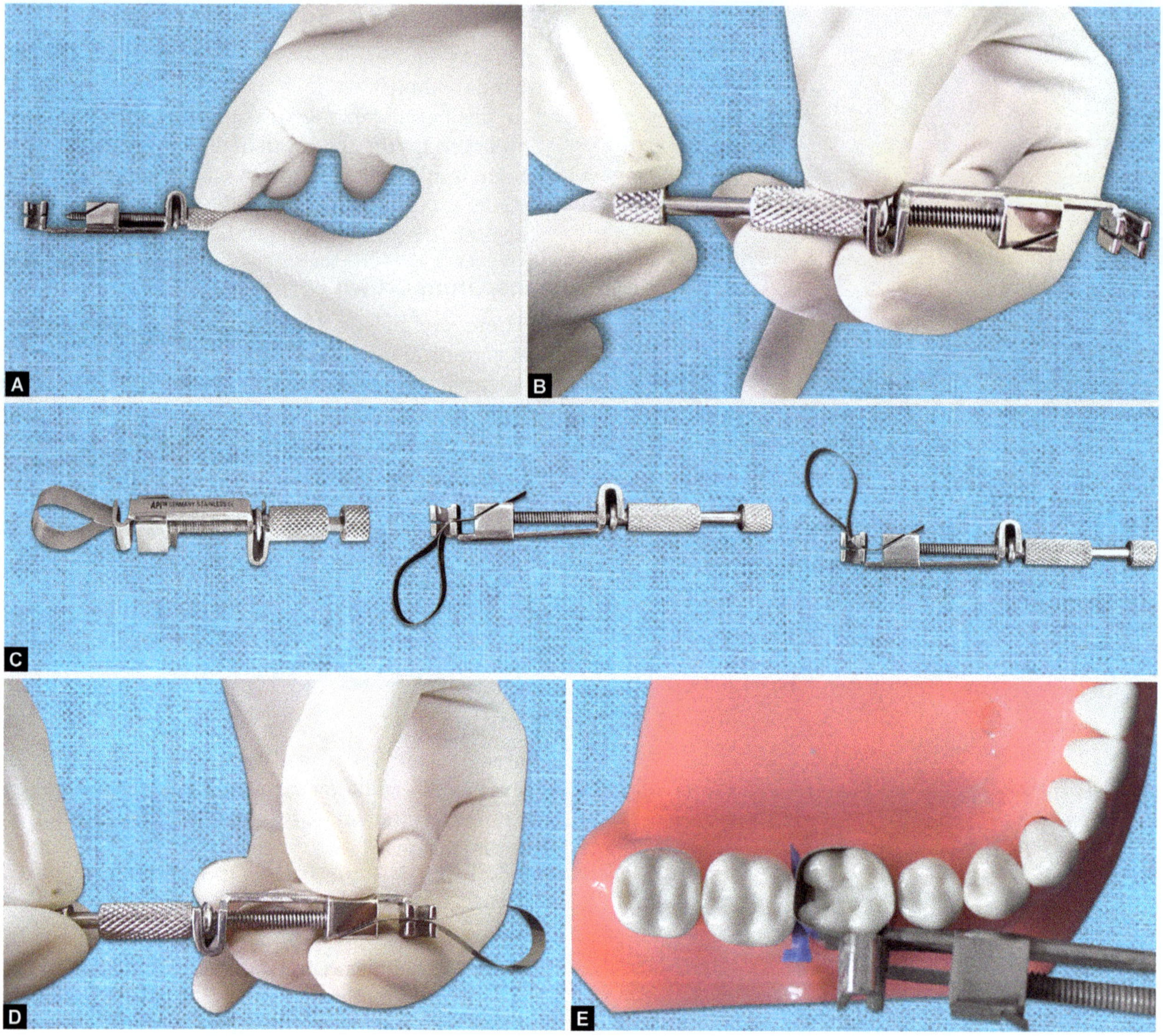

FIGURES 5.51A TO E: Placement of Tofflemire retainer: (A) Open the large knurled nut by turning it counter clockwise so that locking vise is at least ¼ inches from the head; (B) Hold large knurled nut with one hand, open the small knurled nut in opposite direction so as to receive matrix band; (C) Bring the two ends of matrix band together to form loop. This loop can project in straight, left or right; (D) Turn the small knurled nut clockwise to tighten the band to the retainer; (E) Position the band around the tooth to be restored.

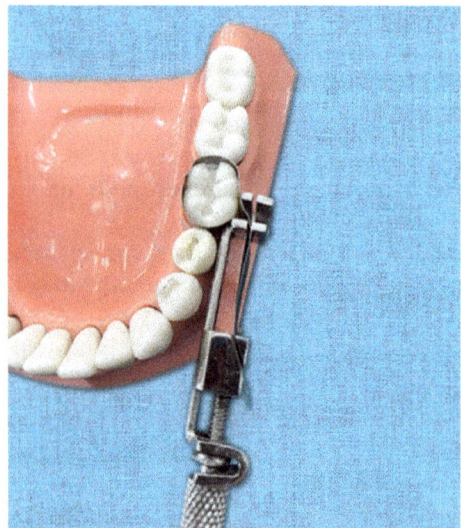

FIGURE 5.52A: Slot should not be directed occlusally, it should be directed gingivally.

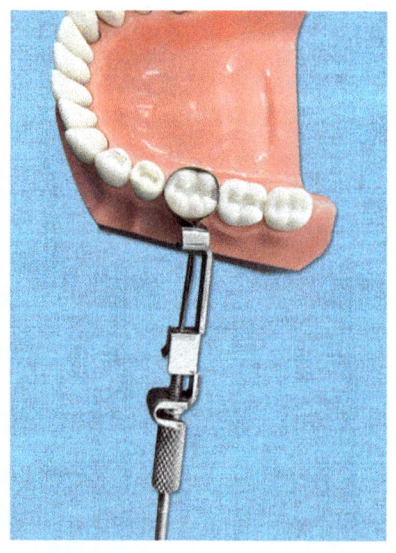

FIGURE 5.52B: Tofflemire retainer should be placed parallel to arch directed anteriorly.

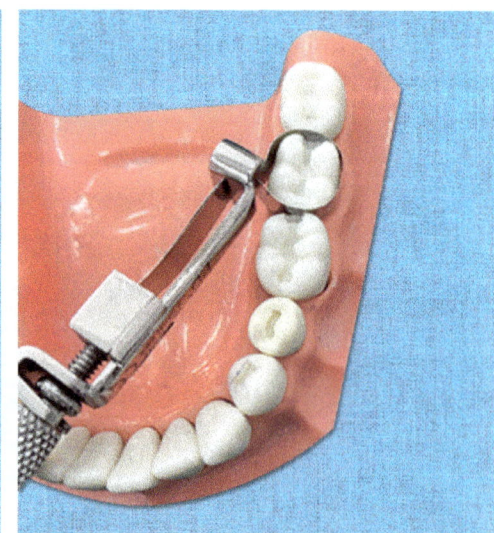

FIGURE 5.52C: Retainer should not be placed lingually as it interferes with tongue.

Instruments Used in Operative Dentistry

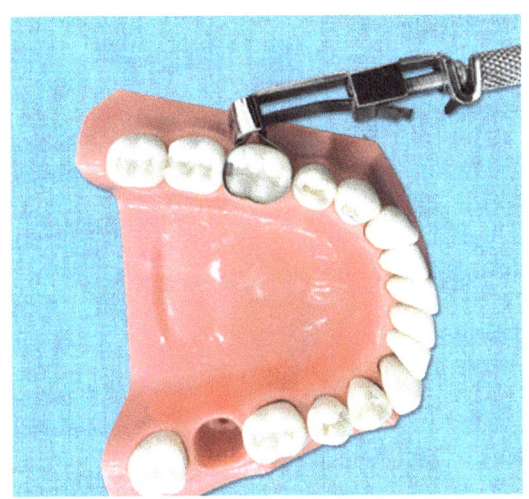

FIGURE 5.52D: Tofflemire band and retainer should be well adapted and fitted to the tooth, it should not be loosely placed.

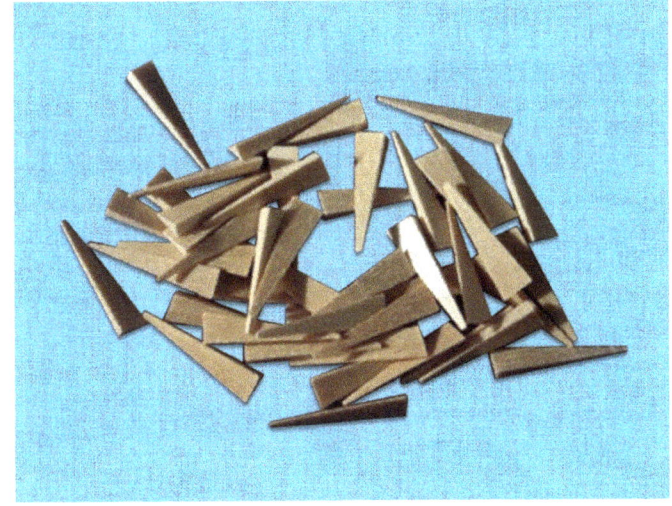

FIGURE 5.55: Wooden wedges.

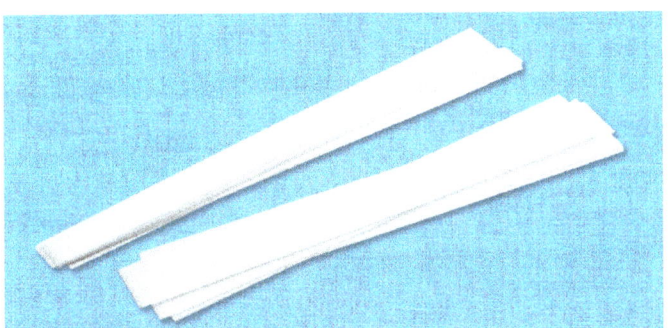

FIGURE 5.53: Mylar strips.

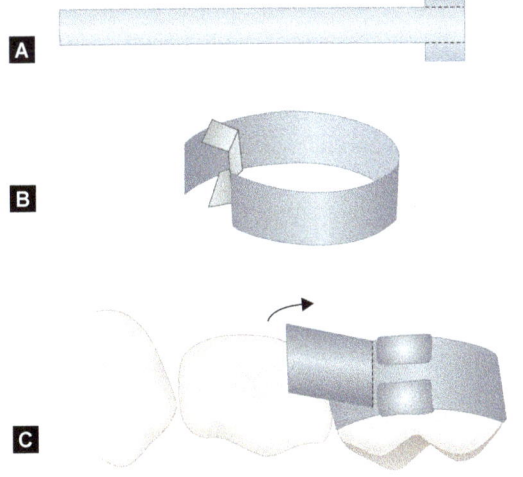

FIGURES 5.54A TO C: Procedure for placement of T-shaped matrix band.

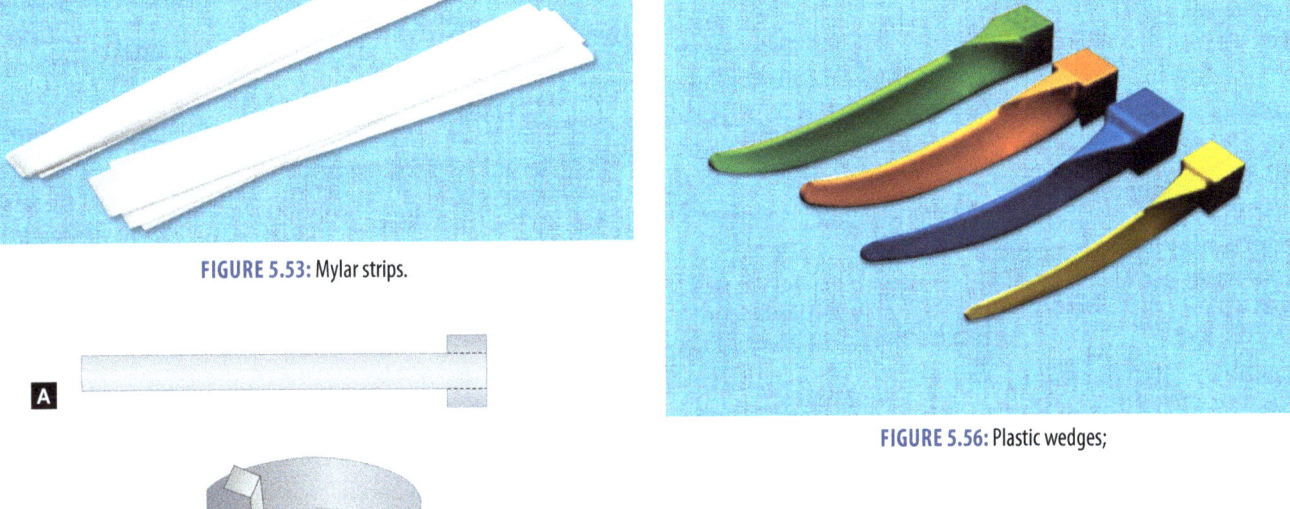

FIGURE 5.56: Plastic wedges;

easily trimmed and can adapt well in gingival embrasure. These are available in two shapes

- **Triangular wedge:** It is most commonly used type of wedge. It has two parts; apex and the base. Apex of the wedge usually lies towards contact area and base lies in contact with gingiva
- **Round wedge:** It is made from wooden tooth picks by trimming the apical portion.

- *Plastic wedges:* Though commercially available but they are not much preferred because trimming and adaptability is difficult in some cases **(Fig. 5.56)**.

Wedging Techniques
- Select the appropriate wedge as per requirement
- Wedge is placed beneath the contact area in the gingival embrasure.
- It is usually placed from lingual embrasure area since it is wider than buccal area. But, if irritates tongue; it can placed from buccal side.

Modified Wedging Techniques
Double Wedging (Fig. 5.57A)
In this technique, two wedges are used; one from buccal embrasure and another from lingual embrasure for better adaptation of matrix band at cervical area of tooth. This technique is used when there is spacing between adjacent teeth where single wedge is not sufficient.

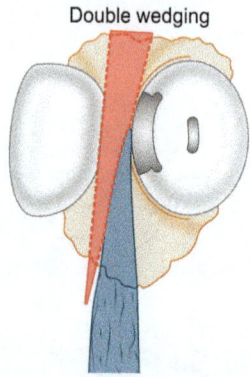

FIGURE 5.57A: In double wedging technique, two wedges are used, one for buccal embrasure and another from lingual embrasure.

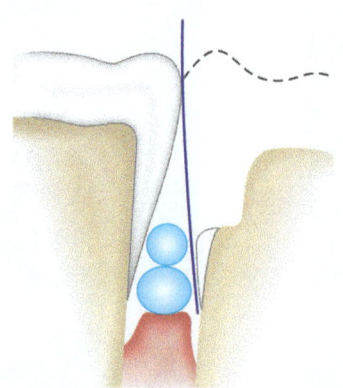

FIGURE 5.57B: In piggyback wedging technique, larger wedge is placed as normal, other smaller wedge is placed over the larger one.

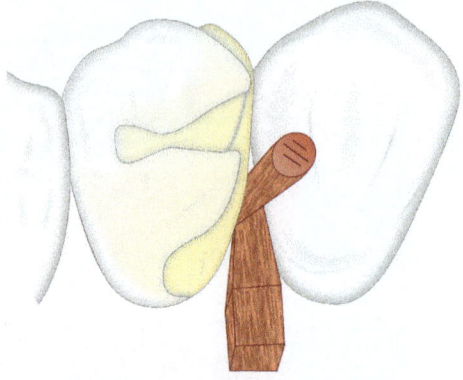

FIGURE 5.57C: In wedge wedging technique, one wedge is placed as normal, another wedge is placed between the wedge and matrix band at right angle to the first wedge.

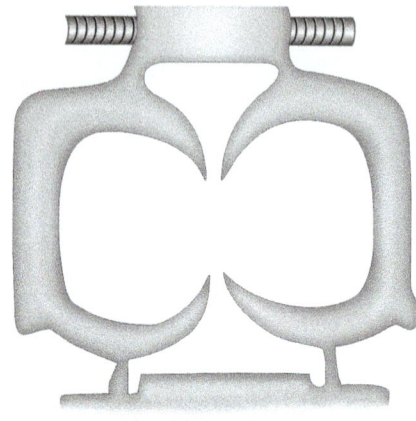

FIGURE 5.58: Ferrier double bow separator.

Piggyback Wedging (Fig. 5.57B)

In this technique two wedges are used; one (larger) wedge is placed as used normally, while the other smaller wedge is piggy backed over larger one. It is indicated in shallow proximal box with gingival recession where a single wedge lies much apically to the gingival margin.

Wedge Wedging (Fig. 5.57C)

In this technique, one wedge is placed as normal, and another wedge is placed between the wedge and matrix band at right angle to first wedge.

Traction Principle (Fig. 5.58)

This principle uses mechanical devices which engage the proximal area of the tooth with holding arms, separation of teeth occurs by moving the holding arms apart from each other. It uses Ferrier double bow separator and noninterfering true separator.

Slow or Delayed Separation

In this separation, teeth are slowly and gradually shifted apart by inserting material between the teeth. This separation usually takes long time, i.e., from several days to weeks. It uses rubber dam sheet, ligature wire, gutta percha stick for separation.

VIVA QUESTIONS

Q.1 What is Black's system of nomenclature for instruments?
Ans.
- **Order:** Function or purpose of the instrument, e.g., excavator, condenser
- **Suborder:** Position, mode or manner of use, e.g., push, pull
- **Class:** Design or form of the working end, e.g., hatchet, spoon excavator
- **Subclass:** Shape of the shank, e.g., binangle, contra-angle.

Q.2 What are different parts of hand instruments?
Ans.
- Handle or shaft
- Shank
- Blade or nib.

Q.3 What are different bevels of instruments?
Ans.
- Single bevel instruments
    - Right and left bevel instruments
    - Mesial and distal bevel instrument
- Bibeveled instrument
- Triple-beveled instrument.

Q.4 What is 3 number formula?
Ans.
- First number of the formula indicates width of the blade or primary cutting edge in tenths of a millimeter
- Second number indicates length of blade in millimeters
- Third number indicates the angle which blade forms with long axis of handle.

Q.5 What is 4 number formula?
Ans.
- First number of the formula indicates width of the blade or primary cutting edge in tenths of a millimeter
- Second number indicates angle formed by primary cutting edge and long axis of the instrument handle.
- Third number indicates length of blade in millimeters

- Fourth number indicates angle which the blade forms with the long axis of the handle or the plane of the instrument in clockwise centigrade.

Q.6 What are uses of mouth mirror?
Ans.
- Direct vision
- Indirect illumination
- Retraction
- Transillumination.

Q.7 What are uses of explorer?
Ans.
- For examining caries on occlusal and interproximal surfaces
- For examining restoration overhangs on proximal surfaces.

Q.8 What are the uses of tweezers?
Ans. Tweezers are used to place and remove cotton rolls and other small materials.

Q.9 What are single and double-planed instruments?
Ans. If the shank angle and blade are in single plane, it is a single-planed instrument. For example; hatchet.
If the shank angle and blade are not in same plane, it is a double-planed instrument. For example; GMT.

Q.10 What is spoon excavator?
Ans. It is a double-ended instrument which has spoon, claw, or disk-shaped blade.

Q.11 What are uses of spoon excavator?
Ans.
- Remove soft caries and debris
- For carving amalgam restorations and wax patterns.

Q.12 What is straight chisel?
Ans. In straight chisel, cutting edge of chisel is prependicular to plane of instrument.

Q.13 What are different bevels of instrument?
Ans.
- *Single-bevel instruments:* Here single bevel forms the primary cutting edge
- *Bibeveled instrument:* If two additional cutting edges extend from the primary cutting edges, then the instrument with secondary cutting edges is called bibeveled instrument
- *Triple-beveled instrument:* If three additional cutting edges extend from the primary cutting edge, then the instrument is called triple-beveled instrument.

Q.14 What is a GMT?
Ans. It is a modified hatchet which has working ends with opposite curvatures and bevels.

Q.15 Which instrument is used to break the proximal contact?
Ans. Enamel hatchet.

Q.16 How do you differentiate mesial and distal GMT?
Ans. GMT is mesial if cutting edge tip forms an acute angle to shaft. It is distal if angle is obtuse.

Q.17 What is angle former?
Ans. It is a type of excavator in which cutting edge sharpened at an angle to the long axis of the blade.

Q.18 What is amalgam carrier?
Ans. Amalgam carrier carries the freshly prepared amalgam to the prepared tooth.

Q.19 What is burnisher and its use?
Ans. Burnisher is a single- or double-ended instrument with smooth rounded working end.
It is used to smoothen and polish the restorations.

Q.20 What are uses of plastic instrument?
Ans.
- To mix, carry and place cements
- To check the convenience form of tooth preparation.

Q.21 How many types of carvers are there?
Ans.
- *Hollenback carver/wards C carver:*
  - Double ended, binangled instrument
  - Used to carve amalgam and inlay wax patterns.
- *Diamond carver/Frahm's carver:* Has bibeveled cutting edge
- *Interproximal carver:* It has very thin blade and is used for carving proximal surfaces
- *Discoid–cleoid carver:* Is used for carving occlusal surface.

Q.22 What do you mean by rotary instruments?
Ans. Rotary cutting instruments are those instruments which rotate on an axis to do the work of abrading and cutting on tooth structure.

Q.23 What are different parts of a dental bur?
Ans.
- "Bur is a rotary cutting instrument which has bladed cutting head"
- *Parts:* Shank, neck and head.

Q.24 What are different types of bur shanks?
Ans.
- Straight handpiece shank
- Latch-type handpiece shank
- Friction-grip handpiece shank.

Q.25 What are the uses of round bur?
Ans. Used for removal of caries, extension of the preparation and for the placement of retentive grooves.

Q.26 What is use of inverted cone bur?
Ans. Used for establishing wall angulations and providing undercuts in tooth preparations.

Q.27 What is use of straight fissure bur?
Ans. Used for tooth preparation.

Q.28 What is rake angle?
Ans. It is the angle between the rake face and the radial line.

Q.29 What is clearance angle?
Ans. It is the angle between the clearance face and the work.

Q.30 What is significance of clearance angle?
Ans. Clearance angle provides a stop to prevent the bur edge from digging into the tooth and provides adequate chip space for clearing debris.

Q.31 Define concentricity.
Ans. It is a direct measurement of symmetry of the bur head.

Q.32 What do you mean by run-out?
Ans. It measures the accuracy with which all the tip of blades pass through a single point when bur is moving.

Q.33 What is tooth separation?
Ans. It is the process of separating the involved teeth slightly away from each other or bringing them closer to each other and/or changing their spatial position in one or more dimensions.

Q.34 What is purpose of tooth separation?
Ans.
- For examination of initial proximal caries
- For providing accessibility to proximal area during preparation of class II and class III tooth preparations
- Matrix can be placed easily during restoration of class II restoration
- It helps in repositioning of shifted teeth.

Q.35 What are different methods of tooth separation?
Ans.
- Slow or delayed separation
- Rapid or immediate separation.

Q.36 What are different ways of slow separation?
Ans.
- Separating rubber ring/bands
- Rubber dam sheet
- Ligature wire/copper wire
- Gutta-percha stick
- Oversized temporary crowns
- Fixed orthodontic appliances.

Q.37 What are different ways of rapid separation?
Ans.
- Ferrier double bow separator
- Non-interfering true separator
  - Elliot separator
  - Wedges.

Q.38 What is Elliot separator?
Ans. Elliot separator is used for rapid separation of teeth which works on wedge principle. It is also known as "crab claw" separator because of its design.

Q.39 What is ferrier separator?
Ans.
- It is used for rapid separation of teeth and works on the traction principle
- It has 2 bows, each bow engages the proximal contact area of tooth just gingival to contact area of tooth
- A "wrench" system is used for turning the threaded bars, this helps in causing separation.

Q.40 What are wedges?
Ans. Wedges are used for rapid tooth separation. They can be made up of wood or plastic.

Q.41 What are different types of wedges?
Ans.
- Wooden wedges
- Plastic wedges
- Available in two shapes:
  - Triangular
  - Round.

Q.42 Why are advantages of wooden wedges?
Ans.
- Adapt well in the gingival embrasure
- Easy to use
- Wooden wedges absorb water, thus increase the interproximal retention
- Provide stabilization to matrix band.

Q.43 What are functions of wedges?
Ans.
- Help in rapid separation of teeth
- Prevent gingival overhang of restoration
- Help in stabilization of retainer and matrix during restorative procedures
- Help in retracting and depressing the interproximal gingival area, thus help in minimizing trauma to soft tissue.

Q.44 What are different techniques of wedging?
Ans.
- Double wedging
- Wedge wedging
- Piggyback wedging.

Q.45 Define matricing?
Ans. It is the procedure by which a temporary wall is built opposite to the axial wall, surrounding the tooth structure which has been lost during the tooth preparation.

Q.46 What are requirements of a matrix band?
Ans.
- Rigidity
- Adaptability
- Easy to use
- Nonreactive
- Height and contour
- Application
- Sterilization
- Inexpensive.

Q.47 What are different materials used for matricing?
Ans.
- Stainless steel
- Polyacetate
- Cellulose acetate
- Cellulose nitrate.

Q.48 What are functions of matrix band?
Ans.
- To confine the restoration during setting
- To provide proper proximal contact and contour
- To provide optimal surface texture for restoration
- To prevent gingival overhangs.

Q.49 What are matrix retainers?
Ans. It holds a band in desired position and shape.

Instruments Used in Operative Dentistry

Q.50 What is ivory No. 1 retainer? What are its advantages and disadvantages?

Ans. Here the matrix holder has a claw at one end with two flat semicircle arms having a pointed projection at the end. Band used with this matrix has one margin slightly projected in its middle part. Keeping the matrix band around the tooth, the screw of the retainer is tightened so that the band perfectly fits around the tooth.

Indication

For unilateral class II tooth preparations.

Q.51 Describe Ivory No. 8 retainer?

Ans. Ivory matrix band retainer holds the matrix band that encircles the tooth to provide missing walls on both proximal sides. It is indicated in unilateral or bilateral class II preparations (MOD).

Q.52 What are advantages and disadvantages of Tofflemire retainer?

Ans. **Advantages:**
- Can be used from both facial and lingual sides
- Economical
- Sturdy and stable in nature
- Provides good contact and contours
- Can be easily removed
- Can be sterilized.

Disadvantages
- Cannot be used in badly broken teeth
- Does not offer optimal results with resin restorations.

Q.53 What are indications of Toffeimire retainers?

Ans.
- Class I tooth preparations with buccal or lingual extensions
- Unilateral or bilateral class II (MOD) tooth preparations
- Class II compound tooth preparations having more than two missing walls.

Q.54 What are different types of Tofflemire bands?

Ans.
- Flat bands
- Precontoured bands.

Q.55 What is T-band matrix?

Ans. In T-shaped matrix long arm of the T surrounds the tooth and overlaps the short arm of the T. It is indicated in unilateral or bilateral class II (MOD) tooth preparations.

Q.56 What is 'S' Shaped matrix?

Ans. In this, stainless steel matrix band is taken and twisted like "S" with the help of a mouth mirror handle. The contoured strip is placed interproximally over the facial surface of tooth and lingual surface of bicuspid.

Q.57 What are the consequences of not restoring proximal area?

Ans.
- Food impaction leading to recurrent caries
- Change in occlusion and intercuspal relations
- Rotation and drifting of teeth
- Trauma to the periodontium.

Q.58 What is mylar strip?

Ans. Mylar strip is a transparent matrix strip used for tooth-colored restoration. It is burnished over the end of a steel instrument to produce a convexity. This convex contoured surface is positioned facing the proximal surface of the tooth to be restored.

Q.59 Name different types of wedging techniques?

Ans.
- Single wedging technique
- Double wedging
- Wedge wedging
- Piggyback wedging.

Q.60 What is double wedging technique?

Ans.
- Here two wedges are used; one is inserted from buccal embrasure and another from lingual.
- It is used when single wedge is not sufficient due to interproximal spacing and widening of proximal box is there in buccolingual dimension.

Q.61 What is wedge wedging technique?

Ans.
- Here two wedges are used, one wedge is inserted from lingual embrasure area while another is inserted between the wedge and matrix band at right angle to first wedge
- It is indicated specially for mesial aspect of maxillary first premolar because of presence of flutes in root near the gingival area.

Q.62 What is Piggyback wedging technique?

Ans.
- Here two wedges are used, larger wedge is inserted as used normally, and then smaller wedge (Piggyback) is inserted above the larger one
- It is indicated when there is shallow proximal box with gingival recession.

Q.63 What is double matricing technique (Balter's technique).

Ans. In case of buccal or lingual preparations, it is difficult to form cervico-occlusal contour of buccal and lingual surface because of the convexity of occlusal two-third. In these cases, second band is inserted to cover the occlusal part of buccal or lingual surface between the tooth and the band which is already applied. Both bands can be stabilized using a softened compound between the bands.

Q.64 How can you identify mesial and distal GMT?

Ans. If sharp edge of blade points toward the handle, it is a mesial GMT. If sharp edge of blade points away from the handle, it is a distal GMT.

Q.65 Why are some instruments made double ended?

Ans. Some instruments are made double ended so that one end can cut from left to right and other end from right to left. For example, spoon excavator.

Chapter 6: Chair Position and Dental Operatory

Chapter Outline
- Operating stool
- Considerations for dentists while treating patients
- Dental chair positions
- Antisepsis in clinics
- Definitions
- Universal precautions
- Sterilization of dental handpiece
- COVID-19 and dentistry

INTRODUCTION

The patient and operator positions are important for the benefits of both individuals. A patient, who is comfortably seated in dental chair with right posture is going to experience less muscular strain, less fatigue and is more cooperative during the treatment. The same is the case with operator. If operator maintains proper position and posture during treatment, the operator is less likely to get strained, fatigued, and be more efficient and has less chances of getting musculoskeletal disorders. Most of the restorative dental procedures can be completed while sitting.

Following points should be kept in mind in relation to dental chair:
- It should be able to provide comfort to the patient and total body support during working
- Headrest of chair should be attached for supporting patient's chin and reducing strain on chin muscles
- It should be able to provide maximum working area to the operator
- It should be placed at the convenient location with adjustable control switches
- Foot switches are preferred to improve infection control.

OPERATING STOOL

Many types of operating stools are commercially available **(Fig. 6.1)**. An operating stool should have following features like it should:
- Have casters for mobility and easy movement
- Be sturdy and well balanced
- Have a seat which is well padded with cushion
- Have adjustable backrest to provide full support to the dentist.

CONSIDERATIONS FOR DENTISTS WHILE TREATING PATIENTS

- Dentist should sit on the middle of the chair cushion rather than edges
- Back should be straight. Head should be erect and should not be bent or drooping **(Figs. 6.2A and B)**
- Hip should sit at an angle of 90° with the thighs parallel to the floor
- Heels of the feet should touch the floor. When working in 11 O'clock or 12 O'clock position, feet should be spread apart so that legs and the chair base form a tripod which creates the stable position. Avoid placing legs behind patient's chair
- Elbow should be close to the sides and at the level of patient's mouth
- Forearm while working should be parallel to the floor
- Maintain proper working distance during dental procedure. This will result in increased cooperation and confidence from the patient. When the patient is properly positioned, the dentist's eyes should be 14–16 inches from the treatment site **(Fig. 6.3)**
- Avoid/minimize body contact with patient. Operator should not rest forearms on the patient's shoulders and hands on the face of the patient

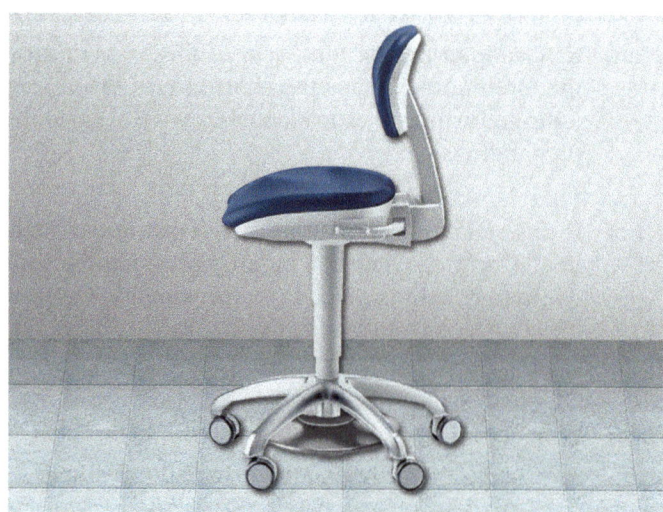

FIGURE 6.1: Operating stool.

Chair Position and Dental Operatory

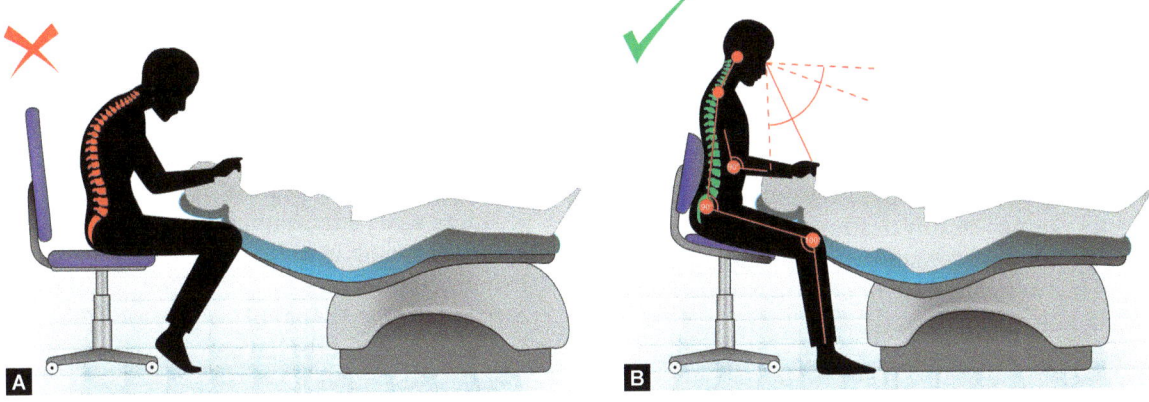

FIGURES 6.2A AND B: Incorrect and correct operator posture while performing dental procedures.

- Patient's head can be rotated backward or forward or from side to side for operator's ease and visibility while doing work
- While working on maxillary arch:
  - Back of chair should be slightly 45° to the floor
  - Maxillary occlusal surfaces should be perpendicular to the floor
- While working on mandibular arch:
  - Back of chair should be almost parallel to the floor
  - Mandibular occlusal surface should be oriented 45° to the floor.

DENTAL CHAIR POSITIONS

There are four general chair positions, viz; upright, reclined at 45°, supine and Trendelenburg.

Upright Position

This is the initial position of chair from which further adjustments are made **(Fig. 6.4A)**. This position is mainly used for initial patient seating, consultation and conclusion of treatment.

Reclined at 45°

Here, the chair is reclined at 45° **(Fig. 6.4B)**. This position is preferred while working for mandibular teeth. Patient should have chin down position and mandibular occlusal surfaces, almost at 45° to the floor for optimal working on mandibular teeth.

Supine

In this, chair position is such that patient's head, knees and feet are approximately at the same level **(Fig. 6.4C)**. This position is preferred while working for maxillary teeth. Patient should have chin up position for optimal access of maxillary teeth.

ANTISEPSIS IN CLINICS

Goal of infection control is to eliminate or reduce the number of microbes from being transferred from one person to another.

Microorganisms can spread from one person to another via direct contact (by touching soft tissues or teeth of patients), indirect contact (injuries with contaminated

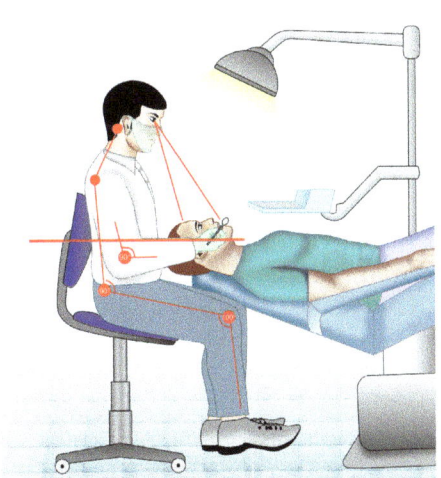

FIGURE 6.3: Distance considerations while working on a patient.

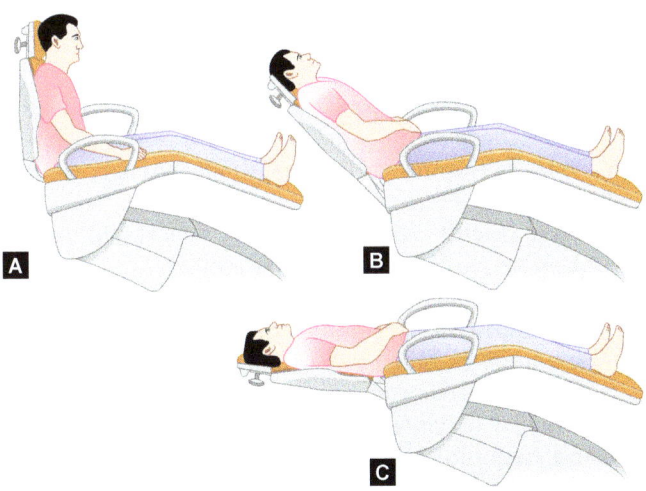

FIGURES 6.4A TO C: (A) Upright position; (B) Reclined at 45°; (C) Supine.

sharp instruments, needlestick injuries, or contact with contaminated equipment and surfaces), and droplet infection (by large particle droplets spatter which is transmitted by close contact).

DEFINITIONS

Cleaning: It is the process that physically removes contamination but does not necessarily destroy microorganisms. It is a prerequisite before decontamination by disinfection or sterilization of instruments since organic material prevents contact with microbes, inactivates disinfectants.

Disinfection: It is the process of using an agent that destroys germs or other harmful microbes or inactivates them, usually referred to chemicals that kill the growing forms (vegetative forms) but not the resistant spores of bacteria.

Antisepsis: It is the destruction of pathogenic microorganisms existing in their vegetative state on living tissue.

Sterilization: Sterilization involves any process, physical, or chemical that will destroy all forms of life, including bacterial, fungi, spores, and viruses.

Aseptic technique: It is the method that prevents contamination of wounds and other sites by ensuring that only sterile objects and fluids come into contact with them, and that the risks of airborne contamination are minimized.

UNIVERSAL PRECAUTIONS

- **Personal hygiene:** Follow the proper hygiene protocol to avoid cross infection
- **Personal protection equipment (PPE)/barrier technique:** Use of barrier technique includes gown, face mask, protective eye wear, and gloves
  - *Protective gown:* Protective gown should be worn to prevent contamination of normal clothing and protect the skin of the clinician from exposure to blood and body substances
  - *Face mask:* A surgical mask that covers both the nose and mouth should be worn by the clinician during procedures. Mask prevents the splatter from contaminating the face
  - *Head cap:* Hairs should be properly tied and covered with a head cap
  - *Protective eyewear:* Eyewear should be clear, antifog, distortion free, close fitting and shielded
  - *Face shield:* Chin length plastic face shield can be worn as alternate to protective eyewear
  - *Gloves:* Gloves should be worn to prevent contamination of hands when touching mucous membranes, blood, saliva, and to reduce the chances of transmission of infected microorganisms from clinician to patient.
- **Hand hygiene:** Hand hygiene significantly reduces potential pathogens on the hands and is considered the single most critical measure for reducing the risk of transmitting organisms to patients and dentists. Handwashing instructions
  - Wet hands with warm water
  - Apply adequate amount of soap to achieve lather
  - Rub vigorously for a minimum of 15 seconds, covering all surfaces of hands and fingers. Pay particular attention to finger tips, between fingers, backs of hands, and base of thumbs, which are the most commonly missed areas
  - Rinse well with running water
  - Dry thoroughly with a disposable paper towel.
- **Immunization:** All members of the dental team (who are exposed to blood or blood-contaminated articles) should be vaccinated against hepatitis B, tuberculosis, varicella, measles, rubella, etc.

STERILIZATION OF DENTAL HANDPIECE

According to Centres for Disease Control (CDC), the following guidelines represent a general approach to handpiece sterilization and maintenance.
- Clean the surface of handpiece using mild detergent for 30 seconds to remove contaminants. Alcohol or any chemical solution should never be used as a cleaning agent as it can dehydrate spores and increase resistance to sterilization
- Dry off the handpiece to prevent the corrosion
- Lubricate the handpiece using lubricating spray oil into the drive airline. Run the handpiece to expel excess oil to evenly distribute the oil through the bearings, and to expel excess oil to prevent coagulation during autoclaving. Sterilize the handpiece by autoclave and chemical method.

Sterilization of Dental Burs

After use, place the burs in 0.2% glutaraldehyde and sodium phenate (sporicidin) for at least 10 minutes. Then clean the burs using bur brush or ultrasonic cleaner and sterilize by autoclaving. Burs should be protected from rust by submerging them in 2% sodium nitrite solution.

COVID-19 AND DENTISTRY

The present outbreak of a coronavirus-associated with acute respiratory disease called coronavirus disease-19 (COVID-19) is the documented spillover of an animal coronavirus to humans.

According to the WHO, a pandemic is defined as the "worldwide spread of a new disease. The first transmission to humans was in Wuhan, China. It was initially reported to WHO on 31st December, 2019. On 30th January, 2020, the WHO declared the COVID-19 outbreak a global health emergency.

Transmission (Fig. 6.5)

The novel coronavirus has four stages of transmission.

Stage 1 is the first appearance of the disease through people with a travel history, with everyone contained, their sources traced, and no local spread from those affected. The number of those infected would be quite low at this stage.

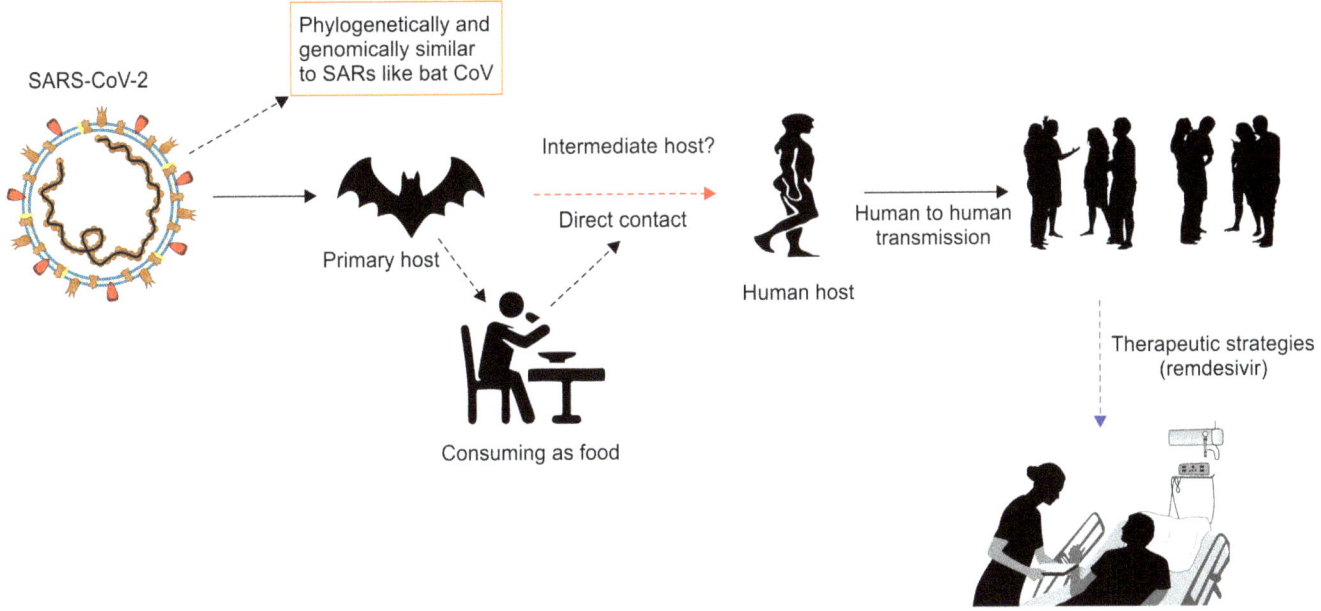

FIGURE 6.5: Schematic representation showing transmission of SARS-CoV-2.

Stage 2 is local transmission, when those who were infected and have a travel history spread the virus to close friends or family. At this stage, every person who came in contact with the infected can be traced and isolated.

Stage 3 is community transmission, when infections happen in public and a source for the virus cannot be traced. At this stage, large geographical lockdowns become important as random members of the community start developing the disease.

Stage 4 is when the disease actually becomes an epidemic in a country, such as it was in China, with large numbers of infections and a growing number of deaths with no end in sight. It is then considered to be endemic or now prevalent in the region.

Post-COVID Dentistry

A dentist's life is not same post-COVID-19. The serious implications on cross infection ensure that the use of the indispensable air turbine drills and ultrasonic devices that induce aerosol are restricted.

Few precautions to be taken:
- Telephonic prescreening should be done prior to giving appointment to patients
- Ask patient to wear mask and preferably come alone without any attender
- Take the history and consent of patients arriving at the facility
- Recommended guidelines for dental professionals
- Recommended treatment protocols.

Guidelines for Preparation of Dental Operatory

Waiting Area
- It needs to be spacious and arrangements of chairs to be made following physical distancing norms.
- Fomite bearing articles like magazine to be removed from waiting area.
- Only patient should be allowed in the waiting areas and should be advised to visit alone.
- Commonly touched surfaces like door handles, reception tables, chair handles need to be sprayed regularly by the auxiliary staff with sodium hypochlorite
- An arrangement of hand hygiene practice (sensor based sanitizer dispenser (**Fig. 6.6**), foot controlled sanitizer dispenser or hand washing area) to be kept at entry of waiting area.
- Staff with infrared thermal scanner at the entry of waiting area for thermal scanning of the patients must be present
- Respiratory/ coughing etiquettes, with disposable tissues and foot-controlled waste disposal unit in the waiting room should be present.

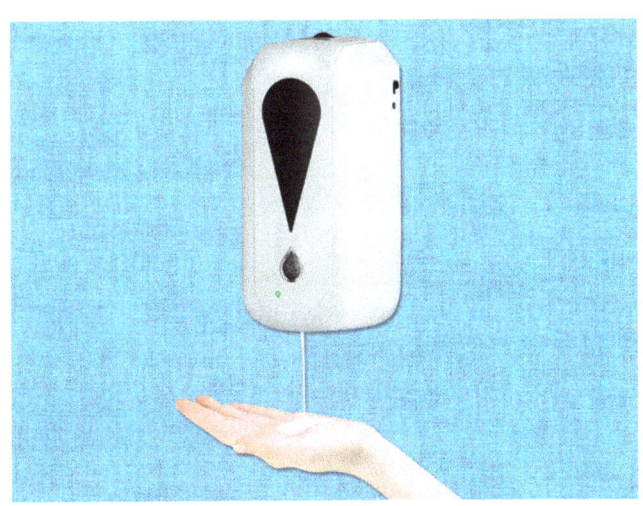

FIGURE 6.6: Sensor based sanitizer dispenser.

- Washroom etiquettes to be followed rigidly. All contact areas need to be sanitized, and the washroom needs to be fumigated frequently.

Operating Area
- It should be spacious with windows/vents for air circulation
- Air must flow from less contaminated zone to more/potentially more contaminated zone (Patient area)
- Air must be exhausted from the contaminated zone to the external environment or recirculated through HEPA filters
- Cover all the fomite bearing surfaces like the X-ray machine, viewer, computers, micromotors, scalers, chair handles, overhead light handles with disposable plastic sheets which need to be replaced after every day and after major procedures
- All the stationary items must be removed from the operatory.

Additional Armamentarium Recommended to Reduce the Aerosol Transmission in an Operatory
- *HEPA filters (Fig. 6.7A):* High-efficiency particulate air (HEPA), also known as high-efficiency particulate absorbing and high efficiency particulate arrestance, is an efficiency standard of air filter.
- *Plasma air sterilizer (Fig. 6.7B):* Plasma air sterilizers can be used and continuously run for air disinfection in an environment with human activity. So, these can be used in office rooms and waiting rooms.
- *Fogger machine (Fig. 6.7C):* Fogger machine with sodium hypochlorite can be used efficiently in sterilizing the contacting surfaces like dental chairs, door handles, table tops. These must be repeated 2–3 times a day in a clinic to minimize the transmission of COVID-19.

Personal Protective Equipment (Fig. 6.8)
Personal protective equipment's (PPEs) are protective gears designed to safeguard the health of workers by minimizing the exposure to a biological agent.

Components of PPE are goggles, face-shield, mask, gloves, coverall/gowns (with or without aprons), head cover and shoe cover.

Face Shield and Goggles
Protection of the mucous membranes of the eyes/nose/mouth by using face shields/goggles is an integral part of standard and contact precautions.

Masks
A triple layer medical mask is a disposable mask, fluid resistant, provide protection to the wearer from droplets of infectious material emitted during coughing/sneezing/talking. An N-95 respirator mask is a respiratory protective device with high filtration efficiency to airborne particles.

If mask is damaged or soiled, or if breathing through the mask becomes difficult, one should remove the face mask, discard it safely, and replace it with a new one.

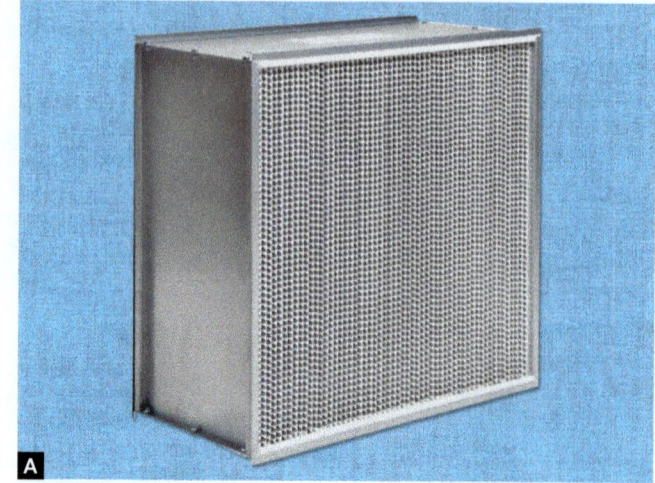
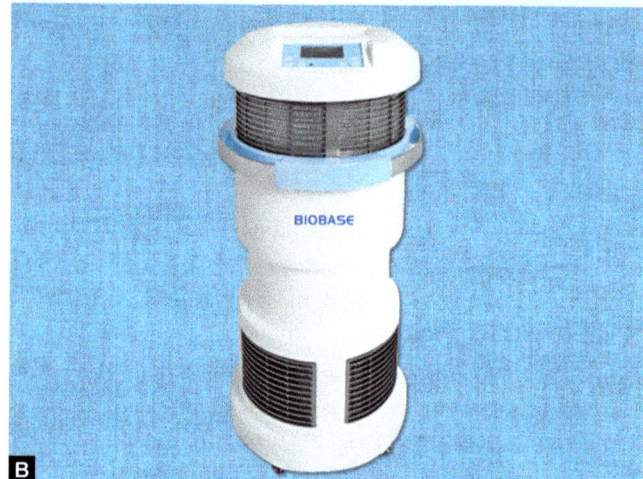
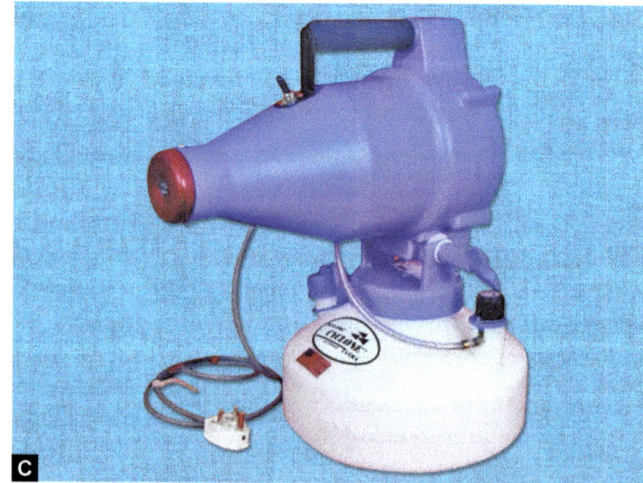

FIGURES 6.7A TO C: (A) HEPA filter; (B) Plasma air sterilizer; (C) Fogger machine.

Gloves
When a person touches an object/surface contaminated by COVID-19 infected person, and then touches his own eyes, nose, or mouth, he may get exposed to the virus. Care should be exercised while handling objects/surface potentially contaminated by suspect/confirmed cases of COVID-19.

Coverall/Gowns
Coverall/gowns are designed to provide 360µ° protection because they are designed to cover the whole body,

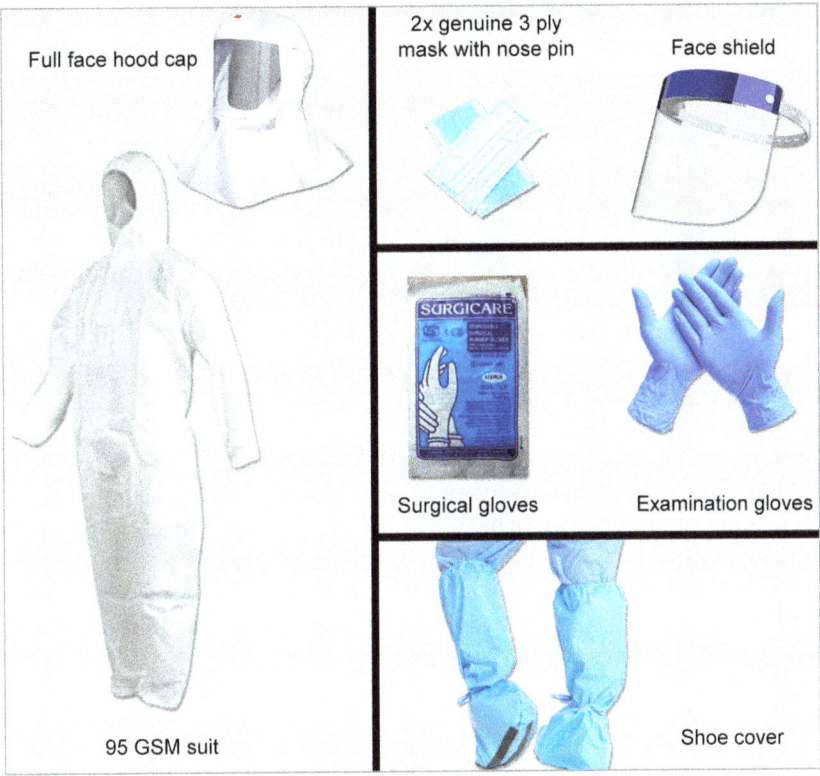

FIGURE 6.8: Personal protective equipment's.

including back and lower legs. Gowns are considerably easier to put on and for removal. An apron can also be worn over the gown for the entire time the health worker is in the treatment area.

Shoe Covers

Shoe covers should be made up of impermeable fabric to be used over shoes to facilitate personal protection and decontamination.

Head Covers

One should use a head cover that covers the head and neck while providing clinical care for patients. Hair and hair extensions should fit inside the head cover.

If basic PPE, including surgical facemasks are not available, do not proceed with any dental procedure, regardless of emergency/urgent patients.

If a patient with a confirmed diagnosis for COVID-19 within the last 14 days, who presents with respiratory symptoms, is treated in the dental office, or if any patient is treated without the appropriate PPE, these are considered high-risk scenarios. Dentist and members of the dental team should proceed to 14 days quarantine.

Preparing the Operatory for Each Patient

- Flush all water lines for 30 seconds before attaching handpieces to the lines.
- If an ultrasonic scaler is to be used, flush the scaler line for 30 seconds before attaching the tip.
- Cover the following items with plastic bags of appropriate size (large, small) if they will be touched at any time during treatment.
- Cover the following items with plastic wrap (cover all strips) if they will be touched at any time during treatment.
  - Light handle(s)
  - Light switch(es)
  - Ultrasonic scaler hose (if used) (2 feet from coupling)
  - X-ray viewer box light switch
  - Computer mouse
- Set up all items to be used in the planned procedure. Instruments and items that may or will contact the patient's mucous membranes must be disposable or sterilized prior to use. Inspect the integrity of each package containing sterile instruments/equipment. Open each package aseptically.
  - Ultrasonic scalers must be covered with a large bag and the scaler handle covered with plastic wrap or a small bag.

The aim of the treatment should be to:
- Minimize the creation of aerosol by eliminating the usage of aerosol producing devices like the air turbine drills and ultrasonic instruments in practice.
- Reduce chair side time and minimize 'doctor to patient' contact.
- Perform procedures that will work well in the medium term and allow for future improvement or upgradations.
- Have a balanced approach towards satisfying patient's dental needs and looking after the well-being of the patient, doctor and support staff.

Additional Measures

- Use dental hand-piece with anti-retraction valves (it decreases the backflow of oral bacteria and viruses into

non-sterilizable dental unit hoses), 4-handed technique, high-volume saliva ejectors, and a rubber dam when appropriate to decrease possible exposure to infectious agents.
- For pediatric patients who cannot rinse, always have a rubber dam placed for all aerosol generating emergency procedures.
- When appropriate, use NSAIDs in combination with acetaminophen to manage dental pain.
- Clean and disinfect public areas frequently, including waiting rooms, door handles, chairs, and bathrooms. Patient companions should wait outside clinic or in car.
- Office manager and/or other staff should maintain a list of patients who will not be coming in for in person visits in charts or find another mechanism that fits dental office's workflow. It is critical that a list of dental patients that have been referred to other settings due to suspected COVID-19 infection be maintained.

After Patient Treatment

Following patient treatment, use the following protocol, in the order given, for cleaning-up:
- Complete all entries in the computer.
- Remove gloves.
- Wash your hands immediately.
- Dismiss the patient.
- Put on heavy-duty, nitrile rubber gloves.
- *Nitrile rubber is more puncture resistant than latex. Nitrile gloves may not prevent a puncture in your skin but they may prevent blood or other contamination on the instrument from entering the wound.*
- Discard needles and any disposable sharp instruments (e.g. scalpel blades, suture needles, broken instruments, endodontic instruments, used burs, orthodontic wires, and any item that could puncture skin) into the rigid biohazard (sharps) container at your unit. Use forceps to pick up these items.
- Hold the high-speed handpiece over the high-speed evacuator and activate the handpiece water line and air line (bur in) for 30 seconds before removing the handpiece.
- Place handpieces into the transportation cassette and place them to the side.
- Place all the dental instruments back into their cassettes in the correct order, removing all composite, amalgam, other non-biologic waste and biologic waste.
- Disinfect all portable equipment and supplies with Cavicide disinfectant, spray with Cavicide disinfectant and wipe clean the visible debris using paper towel. Then spray again with Cavicide and keep moist for at least 5 minutes.
- Return the dental instruments, handpieces and bur cassettes to sterilization.
- Remove all barriers, one at a time, from the unit and any portable equipment and discard into the plastic waste bag. When all barriers are removed, place the waste bag in a rigid waste receptacle. Avoid touching the contaminated side (outside) of the barriers against any clean surfaces.
- Any surface which is visibly contaminated with blood and all surfaces within 3 feet radius of the patient's mouth that were not covered during patient treatment, must be Sprayed with Cavicide disinfectant, wiped clean of visible debris, and then Sprayed with Cavicide and kept moist for at least 5 minutes.
- All surfaces within a 3 feet radius of the patient's mouth are considered contaminated and are treated as clinical contact surfaces. All disinfectants take time to act—often 5 minutes or more.
- Paper towels and napkins must be discarded.
- Flush all vacuum lines with tap water to prevent drying of blood and debris in the lines.

In Between Patients
- Clean PPE with soap and water, or if visibly soiled, clean and disinfect reusable facial protective equipment
- Non-dedicated and non-disposable equipment (e.g., handpieces, dental X-ray equipment, dental chair and light) should be disinfected according to manufacturer's instructions
- Handpieces should be cleaned to remove debris, followed by heat-sterilization after each patient.

Cleanup at the End of the Day
- Using heavy-duty, nitrile rubber gloves and Cavicide disinfectant, clean all operatory items and surfaces
- Disinfect all surfaces by liberally spraying them with Cavicide disinfectant
- Make sure the handpieces have been removed from the tubing, hold the handpiece tubings, operate the dental unit's handpiece flush valve and syringe until all of the water has been purged from the unit
- Before removing the nitrile utility gloves, wash them just as you would wash your hands and then dry them with paper towels. They can then be removed in a normal manner
- Broken equipment that has been contaminated with blood or other body fluids must be decontaminated and cleaned before being repaired in the laboratory or transported to the manufacturer for repair
- Storage and transport of contaminated items: If items such as models, dies, and bite registrations become contaminated, they are to be sprayed with Cavicide disinfectant, left wet for 3 minutes, rinsed, and placed into a clean container.

Disinfection of Hard Surfaces

Surface disinfection is done using the Cavicide/ Sodium hypochlorite disinfectant.

Glutaraldehyde based compounds should not be used for surface disinfection due to their potential toxicity.
- Clean the surface using the Cavicide/sodium hypochlorite and paper towels
- Spray the surface liberally with the Cavicide/sodium hypochlorite and make sure it remains moist for at least 5 minutes
- Dry the surface with paper towels or allow it to air dry.

Chair Position and Dental Operatory

Step 1: Telephonic prescreening protocol
- Fix appointments through phone only and discourage walk-in patients
- Hot spot matching and medical symptoms assessment
- Dental needs assessment
- Disclosure/consent form to be sent to patient electronically (if possible)
- Ask patient to wear mask and preferably come alone without any attender

Step 2: Reception/waiting area protocol
- Receptionist/staff: One Person
- Discourage footwear within clinic interiors/provide foot cover
- Record patient temperature using digital non-contact infrared thermometer
- Mandatory use of alcohol based hand rub (ABHR) and provide mask for everyone
- Seating arrangement with minimum 3 feet physical distancing
- Display patient education material on hand & cough hygiene
- Patient to submit signed disclosure/consent form

Step 3: Dental operatory protocol
- Keep the clinical operatory clutter-free
- Improve air circulation and avoid air-conditioners
- 0.01% NaOCl for disinfection of dental water lines
- Donning of appropriate PPE for dental surgeon and one dental assistant

Step 4: Patient assessment and treatment protocol
- Pre-procedural mouth rinse: 1% hydrogen peroxide or 0.2% povidone-iodine: 1 min
- Extra oral scrubbing of face with antiseptic wipe
- Diagnose and treatment plan into aerosol generating procedures (AGP) and non-aerosol generating procedures (Non-AGP)
- Four-handed dentistry and rubber dam application for AGP
- High volume suction and minimize IOPA usage

Aerosol generating procedures
Should be ideally done in designated isolation rooms which should be quipped with HEPA filters/augmented ventilation

Non-aerosol producing procedure

Step 5: Discharging patient
- Patient advised to re-mask and proceed to reception area
- Hand hygiene
- Electronic treatment records only
- Cashless payment preferred

Step 6A: Treatment borne contaminant removal protocol
Room should be well ventilated with a minimum 6 air changes per hour

Aerosol generating procedures

Non-aerosol generating procedures

HEPA air filter
(Min. 12 Air changes)

20 minutes
Air filtration with HEPA 13/14 filters

UVGI (Ultraviolet germicidal irradiation) + ventilation (min.6 air changes)

15 minutes
UV-c Irradiation of 245 nm, 40W per 100sq.ft.

Disinfectant defogging

30–45 minutes
Hydrogen peroxide (HPV) or chlorine dioxide

Only natural ventilation (min.6 air changes)

60 minutes
Cross ventilation and additional ventilators (fans)

Step 6B: Chairside disinfection protocol (min. 20 minutes)
- Instrument change
- Flushing of suction and spittoon drainage with 1% NaOCl
- Disinfect 3 feet area around chair and mop the clinical area

Step 7: Protocol at the end of the day
- Repeat step 6B and 6A
- Doffing of PPE in a separate area
- Bio-medical waste in double lined color-coded bags only

The basics of infection control will be same and should be incorporated into our daily practice for the welfare of both the patients as well as the doctor.

Disinfection of Equipment

- Put on a pair of heavy-duty, nitrile rubber gloves and protective eyewear
- Clean and dry all instruments to be disinfected
- Immerse them for at least 5 minutes in the glutaraldehyde or Cavicide solution.

For a dental healthcare personnel following steps need to be followed for a safe dental practice:

VIVA QUESTIONS

Q.1 What points should be kept in mind in relation to dental chair?

Ans.
- It should be able to provide comfort to the patient and total body support during working.
- Headrest of chair should be attached for supporting patient's chin and reducing strain on chin muscles
- It should be placed at the convenient location with adjustable control switches
- Foot switches are preferred to improve infection control.

Q.2 What should be the chair and patient position while working on maxillary and mandibular arch?

Ans. While working on maxillary arch:
- Back of chair should be slightly 45° to the floor
- Maxillary occlusal surfaces should be perpendicular to the floor

While working on mandibular arch:
- Back of chair should be almost parallel to the floor
- Mandibular occlusal surface should be oriented 45° to the floor.

Q.3 What are different dental chair positions?

Ans.
- Upright position
- Reclined at 45°
- Supine.

Q.4 How do you sterilize dental handpiece?

Ans.
- Clean the surface of handpiece using mild detergent for 30 seconds to remove contaminants.
- Dry off the handpiece to prevent the corrosion.
- Lubricate the handpiece using lubricating spray oil into the drive airline.
- Run the handpiece to expel excess oil to evenly distribute the oil through the bearings.
- Sterilize the handpiece by autoclave and chemical method.

Q.5 How do you sterilize the dental burs?

Ans. After use, place the burs in 0.2% glutaraldehyde and sodium phenate (sporicidin) for at least 10 minutes. Then clean the burs using bur brush or ultrasonic cleaner and sterilize by autoclaving.

Q.6 How do you protect the burs from rusting?

Ans. Burs should be protected from rust by submerging them in 2% sodium nitrite solution.

Q.7 How does COVID-19 spread?

Ans. The novel coronavirus has four stages of transmission
- **Stage 1** is the first appearance of the disease through people with a travel history, with everyone contained.
- **Stage 2** is local transmission, when those who were infected and have a travel history spread the virus to close friends or family.
- **Stage 3** is community transmission, when infections happen in public and a source for the virus cannot be traced.
- **Stage 4** is when the disease actually becomes an epidemic in a country.

Q.8 How do you do surface disinfection?

Ans. Disinfect all portable equipment and supplies with Cavicide disinfectant, spray with Cavicide disinfectant and wipe clean the visible debris using paper towel. Then spray again with Cavicide and keep moist for at least 5 minutes.

Q.9 What are components of PPE?

Ans.
- Face shield and goggles
- Masks
- Gloves
- Coverall/Gowns
- Shoe covers
- Head covers.

Q.10 Looking at COVID scenario, what should be the design of dental operatory?

Ans.
- Keep the clinical operatory clutter-free
- Improve air circulation and avoid air-conditioners
- 0.01% NaOCl for disinfection of dental water line
- Disinfect all portable equipment and supplies with Cavicide disinfectant.

Chapter 7: Principles of Tooth Preparation

Chapter Outline

- Terminology
- Number of line and point angles in different tooth preparations
- GV Black's classification of tooth preparation
- Stages of cavity preparation
- Initial cavity preparation stage
- Final stages of tooth preparation

INTRODUCTION

The most important procedure of operative dentistry is the tooth preparation so as to receive a restoration that can fulfill all its requirements. Therefore, it is a must for every operative clinician to be well aware of all the fundamentals of tooth preparation.

DEFINITION

Tooth preparation is the mechanical alteration of a defective, injured or diseased tooth in order to best receive a restorative material which will re-establish the healthy state of the tooth including esthetics correction when indicated along with normal form and function.

—*Sturdevant*

TERMINOLOGY

Simple Tooth Preparation

A tooth preparation involving only one tooth surface is termed simple preparation (**Fig. 7.1**), for example, occlusal preparation.

Compound Tooth Preparation

A tooth preparation involving two surfaces is termed as compound tooth preparation (**Fig. 7.2**), for example, mesio-occlusal or disto-occlusal preparation.

Complex Tooth Preparation

A tooth preparation involving more than two surfaces is called as complex tooth preparation (**Fig. 7.3**), for example, MOD preparation.

For communication and records purpose, the surface of tooth preparation is abbreviated by capitalizing the first letter.

For example,
- Preparation on the occlusal surface as "O".
- Preparation on the distal and occlusal surfaces as "DO".
- Preparation on mesial, occlusal and distal surfaces as "MOD".

Walls

Internal Wall

It is a wall in the preparation, which is not extended to the external tooth surface (**Fig. 7.4**).

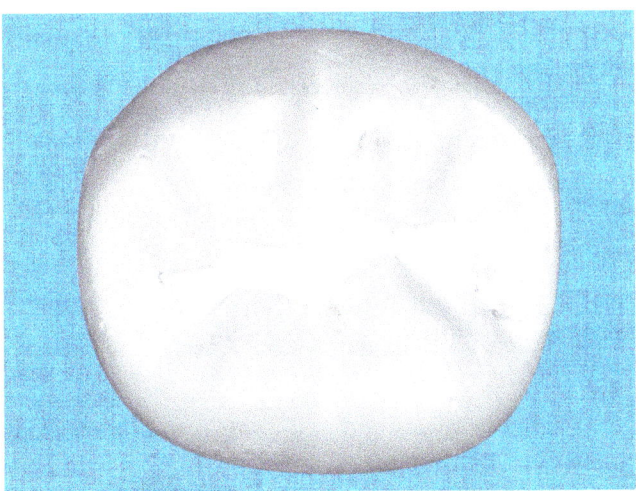

FIGURE 7.1: Simple tooth preparation involves only one tooth surface.

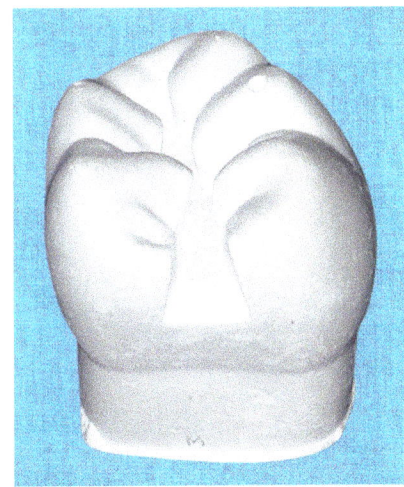

FIGURE 7.2: Compound tooth preparation involves two surfaces.

External Wall (Fig. 7.4)

An external wall is a wall in the prepared tooth that extends to the external tooth surface. External wall takes the name of the tooth surface toward, which it is situated.

Pulpal Wall

A pulpal wall is an internal wall that is toward the pulp and covering the pulp **(Fig. 7.5)**. It may be both vertical and perpendicular to the long axis of the tooth.

Axial Wall

It is an internal wall which is parallel to the long axis of the tooth **(Fig. 7.5)**.

Floor

Floor is a prepared wall which is usually flat and perpendicular to the occlusal forces directed occluso-gingivally, for example, pulpal and gingival floor **(Fig. 7.6)**.

Cavosurface Angle Margin

Cavosurface angle is formed by the junction of a prepared tooth surface wall and external surface of the tooth **(Fig. 7.7)**.

Line Angle (Fig. 7.8)

It is a junction of two surfaces of different orientations along the line. Its name is derived from the involved surfaces.

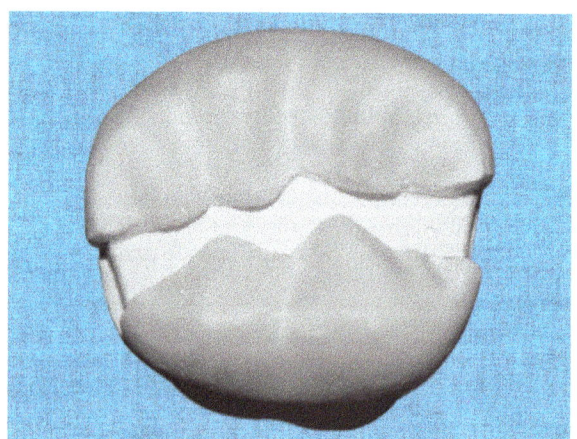

FIGURE 7.3: Complex tooth preparation involves more than two surfaces.

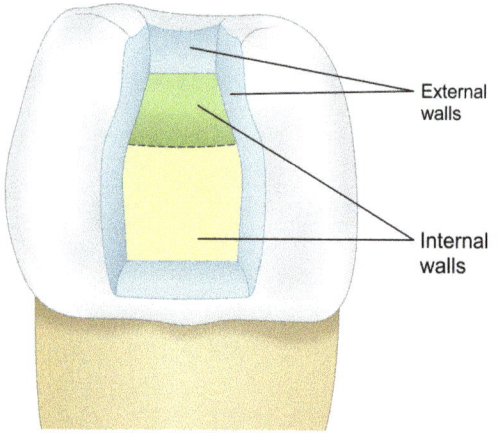

FIGURE 7.4: Schematic representation showing internal and external walls of tooth preparation.

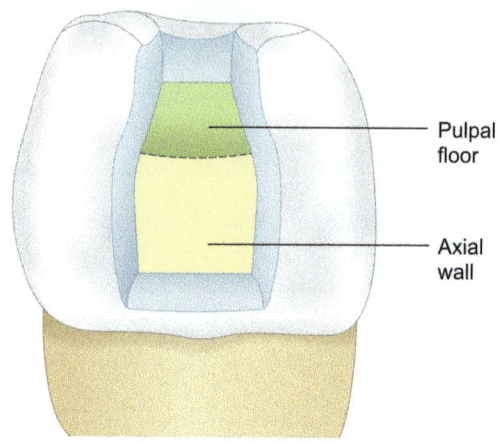

FIGURE 7.5: Schematic representation showing pulpal floor and axial wall.

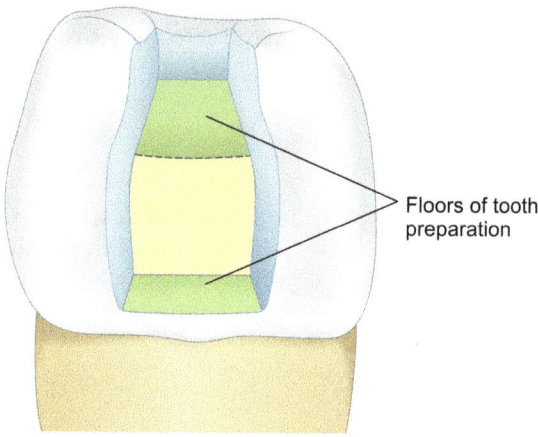

FIGURE 7.6: Schematic representation of gingival and pulpal floor.

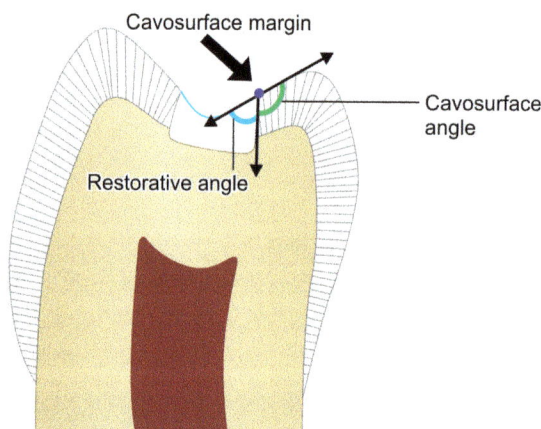

FIGURE 7.7: Schematic representation showing the cavosurface angle.

Point Angle (Fig. 7.8)

It is a junction of three plane surfaces or three line angles of different orientations. Its name is derived from its involved surfaces or line angles.

NUMBER OF LINE AND POINT ANGLES IN DIFFERENT TOOTH PREPARATIONS (FIGS. 7.9 TO 7.13)

Number of line angles and point angles in different tooth preparations are enumerated in **Table 7.1**.

Line and point angles of class I to class V tooth preparations are enlisted as following:

Principles of Tooth Preparation

TABLE 7.1: Number of line angles and point angles in different tooth preparation designs.

Type of tooth preparation	Line angles	Point angles
Class I	8	4
Class II	11	6
Class III	6	3
Class IV	11	6
Class V	8	4

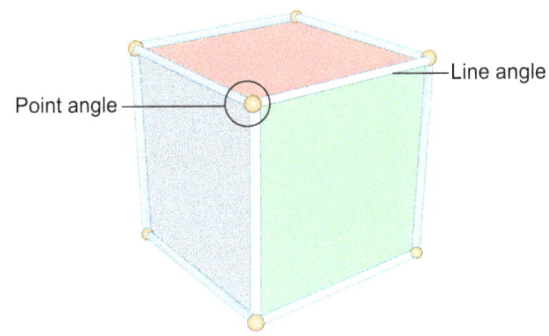

FIGURE 7.8: Schematic representation showing line and point angle. Line angle is a junction of two surfaces of different orientations along the line. Point angle is a junction of three plane surfaces or three line angles of different orientations.

Box 7.1: Facts

Earlier when the affected tooth was prepared because of caries, cutting of the tooth was referred to as cavity preparation. But nowadays many indications other than caries lead to preparation of the tooth. Hence, the term cavity preparation has been replaced by tooth preparation.

GV BLACK'S CLASSIFICATION OF TOOTH PREPARATION

- **Class I**: Preparation required to treat pit and fissure caries of the occlusal surfaces of premolars and molars, the occlusal two-third of buccal and lingual surface of molars, and palatal surface of maxillary incisors **(Fig. 7.9)**.
- **Class II**: Preparation required to treat caries on proximal surface of posterior teeth **(Fig. 7.10)**.
- **Class III**: Preparation required to treat lesions present on proximal surface of anterior teeth, not involving the incisal angles **(Fig. 7.11)**.

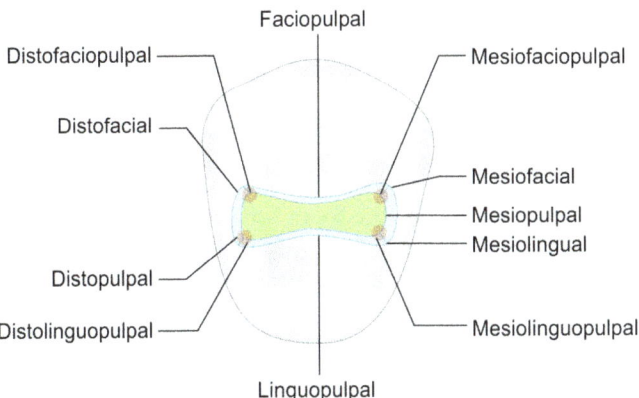

FIGURE 7.9: Class I tooth preparation showing line angles and point angles.

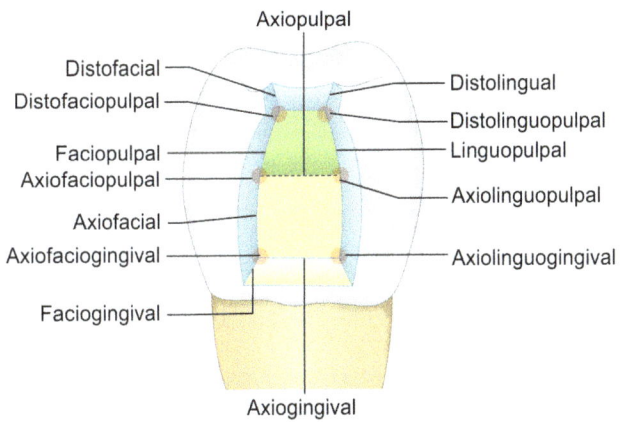

FIGURE 7.10: Class II tooth preparation showing line and point angles.

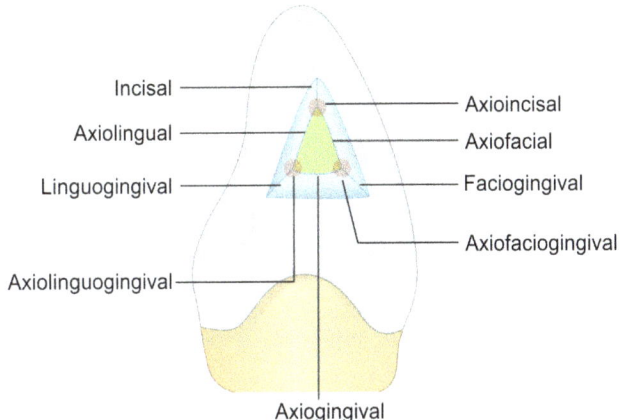

FIGURE 7.11: Class III tooth preparation showing line and point angles.

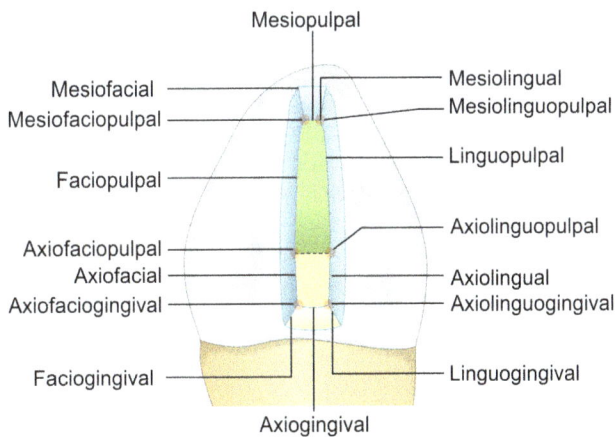

FIGURE 7.12: Class IV tooth preparation showing line and point angles.

- **Class IV**: Preparation required to treat lesions present on proximal surface of anterior teeth involving the incisal angle **(Fig. 7.12)**.
- **Class V**: Preparation required to treat caries present on gingival third of facial and lingual or palatal surfaces of all teeth **(Fig. 7.13)**
- **Class VI**: Preparation required to treat defects present on incisal edges of anterior and cusp tips of posterior teeth without involving any other surface.

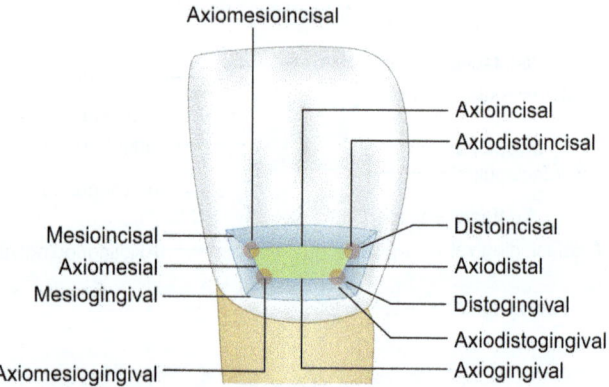

FIGURE 7.13: Class V tooth preparation showing line and point angles.

STAGES OF CAVITY PREPARATION

Box 7.2: Steps of tooth preparation

Stage I: Initial cavity preparation stage:
- Cutline form and initial depth
- Primary resistance form
- Primary retention form
- Convenience form

Stage II: Final cavity preparation stage:
- Removal of any remaining enamel pit or fissure, infected dentin and/or old restorative material, if indicated
- Pulp protection, if indicated
- Secondary resistance and retention form
- Procedures for finishing the external walls of the tooth preparation
- **Final procedures:** Cleaning, inspecting and sealing.

INITIAL CAVITY PREPARATION STAGE

Outline form and Initial Depth

Definition

Outline form is defined as "placing the preparation margins in the position they will occupy in the final tooth preparation except for finishing enamel walls and margins". It also includes preparing the initial depth of 0.2–0.8 mm into the dentin.

Principles

- Removal of all weakened and friable tooth structure.
- Removal of all undermined enamel.
- Incorporate all faults in preparation.
- Place all margins of preparation in a position to afford good finishing of the restoration.

Features for Establishing a Proper Outline Form (Fig. 7.14)

- Preserving cuspal strength.
- Preserving strength of marginal ridge.
- Minimizing the buccolingual extensions.
- If distance between two faults is less than 0.5 mm, connect them.
- Limiting the depth of preparation 0.2–0.8 mm into dentin.
- Using enameloplasty wherever indicated.

Outline form for Pit and Fissure Lesions

- Remove all defective portion and extend the preparation margins to healthy tooth structure. Rather than being

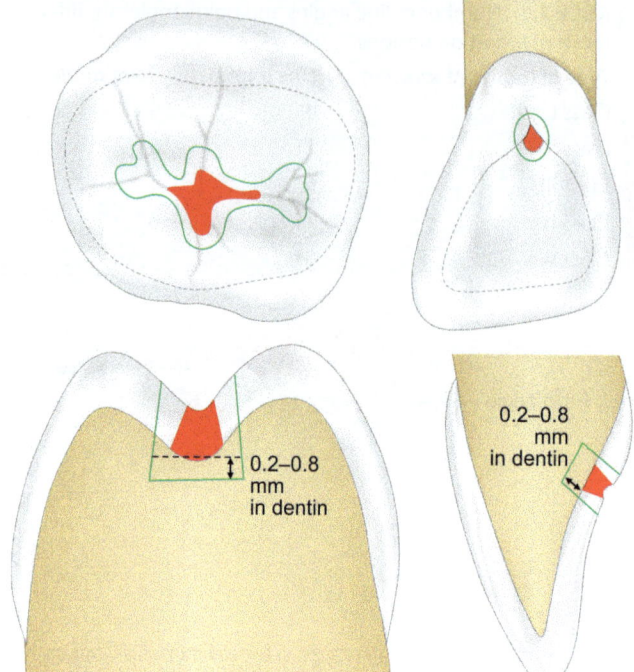

Initial depth of preparation should be 0.2–0.8 mm into dentin

FIGURE 7.14: Outline form for pit and fissure lesions.

straight, the outline form should form the smooth curves so as to preserve as much strong cusps as possible. This is called circumventing the cusps.
- Remove all unsupported enamel rods or weakened enamel margins.
- Limit the depth of preparation to 0.2 mm into dentin, though the actual depth of preparation may vary from 1.5–2 mm depending on the steepness of cuspal slopes and the thickness of the enamel
- Circumventing of cusps should be followed to have smooth free flowing outline form.
- If the thickness of enamel between two preparation sites is less than 0.5 mm, connect them to make one preparation, otherwise prepare as separate cavity preparations.
- Avoid ending the preparation margins in high stress areas, such as cusp eminences.
- Extend the preparation margins to include all pits and fissures which cannot be managed by enameloplasty.
- Isthmus width should be 1/4th of the intercuspal distance **(Fig. 7.15)**.
- Extend the outline form to facilitate the convenience for preparation and restoration.

Outline Form for Smooth Surface Lesions—Outline Form of Proximal Caries (Class II, III and IV Lesions)

Rules for Making Outline form for Proximal Preparation (Fig. 7.16)

- Extend the preparation margins until sound tooth structure is reached.
- Restrict the depth of axial wall 0.2–0.8 mm into dentin.
- Axial wall should be parallel to external surface of the tooth.
- Avoid terminating the margins on extreme eminences like cusp tips and marginal ridges.

Principles of Tooth Preparation

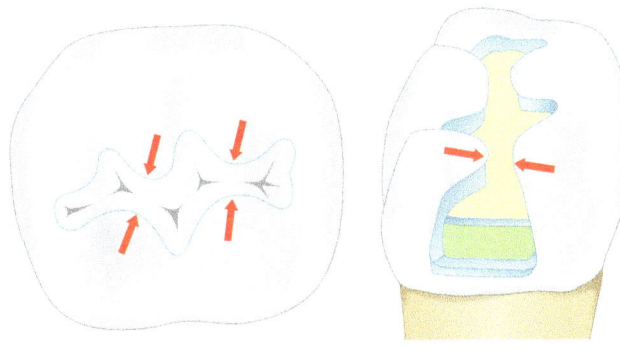

FIGURE 7.15: Isthmus width should be 1/4th of the intercuspal distance. Arrows showing isthmus of the cavity.

- In class II tooth preparation, place gingival seat apical to the contact but occlusal to gingival margin and have a clearance of 0.5 mm from the adjacent tooth. This clearance provides space for proper accessibility, visibility, instrumentation, and restoration **(Fig. 7.17)**.
- Facial and lingual margins of proximal box should extend in their respective embrasure areas so as to have clearance between prepared margins and adjacent tooth structure.

Rules for Class V Cavities
- Outline form is limited by extent of the lesion.
- Extensions are made mesially, distally, occlusally and gingivally till sound tooth structure is reached.
- Axial depth is limited to 0.8–1.25 mm pulpally.

Factors Affecting the Outline form of Proximal Preparations
- Extent of the caries on the proximal side.
- Contact relationship with adjacent tooth.
- Alignment of teeth and masticatory forces likely to fall on restorative material **(Figs. 7.18A and B)**.
- Esthetic requirement of the patient.

Enameloplasty
Enameloplasty is removal of sharp and irregular enamel margins of the enamel surface by "rounding" or "saucering" it and converting it into a smooth groove making it a self cleansable area **(Figs. 7.19A and B)**.

Indications
- It is done when caries is present in less than one-third thickness of the enamel.
- Presence of a shallow fissure crossing facial or lingual ridge.

Significance
Enameloplasty does not extend the outline form. This procedure should not be used unless a fissure can be made into saucer shaped area with mild removal of enamel.

Primary Resistance Form

Definition
Primary resistance form is that shape and placement of preparation walls to best enable both the tooth and restoration to withstand, without fracture, the stresses of masticatory forces delivered principally along the long axis of the tooth.

Factors Affecting Resistance Form
- Amount of occlusal contact
- Type of restoration used
- Amount of remaining tooth structure.

Features of Resistance Form
- *Box-shape or mortise form* of preparation with *flat pulpal and gingival floor* **(Fig. 7.20)**. Flat gingival and

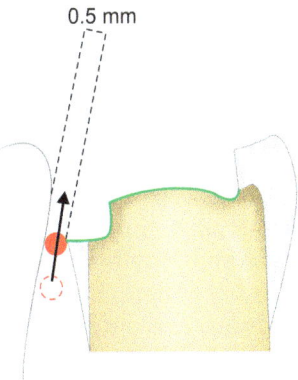

FIGURE 7.17: In proximal tooth preparation, gingival margin should clear adjacent tooth by 0.5 mm.

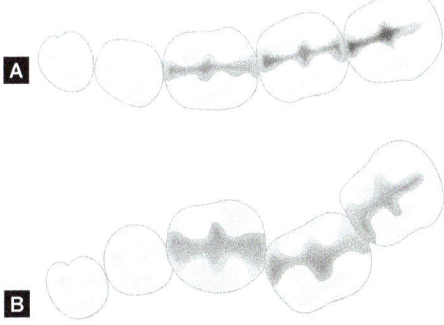

FIGURES 7.18A AND B: (A) Proper alignment of teeth requires less faciolingual extensions as compared to malaligned teeth; (B) Mal-alignment of teeth necessitates increase in faciolingual extensions.

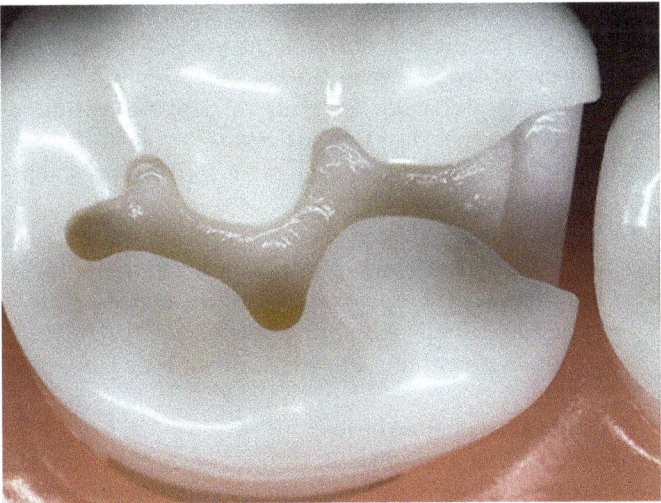

FIGURE 7.16: Ideal class II cavity preparation of mandibular 1st molar.

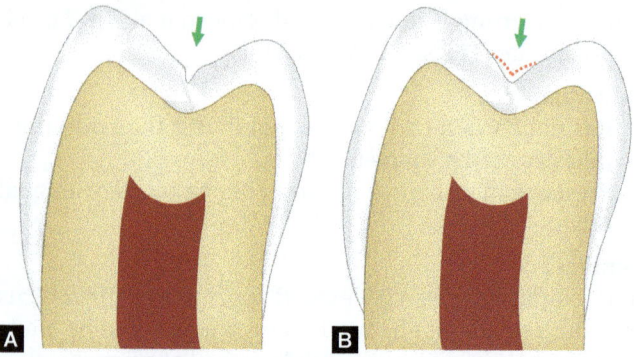

FIGURES 7.19A AND B: Enameloplasty: (A) Tooth with deep pit and fissure; (B) Removal of superficial enamel resulting in rounding of deep pit and fissure caries making it self-cleansable.

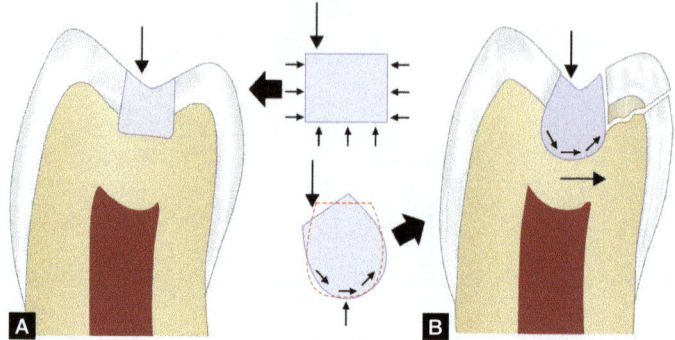

FIGURES 7.21A AND B: (A) Resistance form of tooth preparation provided by flat pulpal and gingival floor; (B) In case of rounded pulpal floor, the rocking motion of restoration results in wedging force which may result in failure of restoration.

pulpal floors help in resisting masticatory forces directed along the long axis of the tooth, thereby prevent the tooth fracture from wedging forces resulting from opposing cusps **(Figs. 7.21A and B)**
- *Adequate thickness of restorative material* depending on its respective compressive and tensile strengths to prevent the fracture of both the remaining tooth structure and the restoration **(Fig. 7.22)**.

Type of restoration	Minimum occlusal thickness
Cast metal	1–2 mm
Amalgam restorations	1.5 mm
Ceramics	2 mm
Composite	1–2 mm

- *Restrict the extension of external walls* to allow strong marginal ridge areas with sufficient dentin support.
- *Inclusion of weakened tooth structure* to avoid fracture under masticatory forces.
- *Rounding of internal line angles* to reduce the stress concentration points in tooth preparation **(Fig. 7.22)**.
- Consideration to *cusp capping* depending upon the amount of remaining tooth structure. Cusp capping is considered when outline form has involved half the distance from primary groove to cusp tip. Cusp capping becomes mandatory when outline form has involved two-thirds the distance from primary groove to cusp tip.

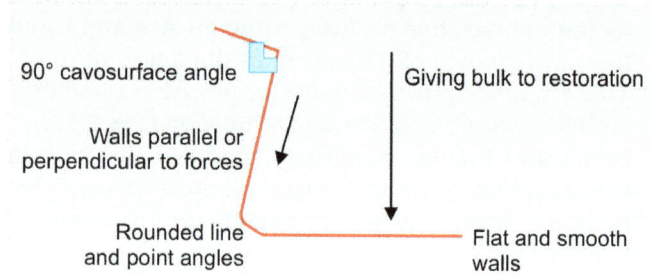

FIGURE 7.22: Features of resistance and retention form for amalgam.

Primary Retention Form

Definition
Primary retention form is that form, shape and configuration of the tooth preparation that resists the displacement or removal of restoration from the preparation under lifting and tipping masticatory forces.

Retention Form for Different Restorations
- **Amalgam:** Retention is increased in amalgam restoration by the following:
  - Providing occlusal convergence (about 2-5°) of the dentinal walls toward the tooth surface **(Fig. 7.22)**.
  - Giving slight undercut in dentin near the pulpal wall.
  - Providing occlusal dovetail **(Figs. 7.23A and B)**.
- **Cast metals:** Retention is increased in cast restorations by the following:
  - Close parallelism of the opposing walls with slight occlusal divergence of 2-5°.
  - Making occlusal dovetail to prevent tilting of restoration in class II preparations.
  - Use of secondary retention in the form of coves, skirts and dentin slot.
  - Give reverse bevel in class I compound, class II, and MOD preparations to prevent tipping movements.
- **Composites:** In composites, retention is increased by:
  - Micromechanical bonding between the etched and primed prepared tooth structure and the composite resin.
  - Providing enamel bevels.
- **Direct filling gold:** Elastic compression of dentin and starting point in dentin provide retention in direct gold fillings by proper condensation.

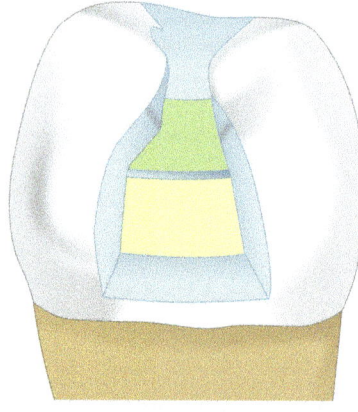

FIGURE 7.20: Box-shape or mortise form of preparation with flat pulpal and gingival floor.

Principles of Tooth Preparation

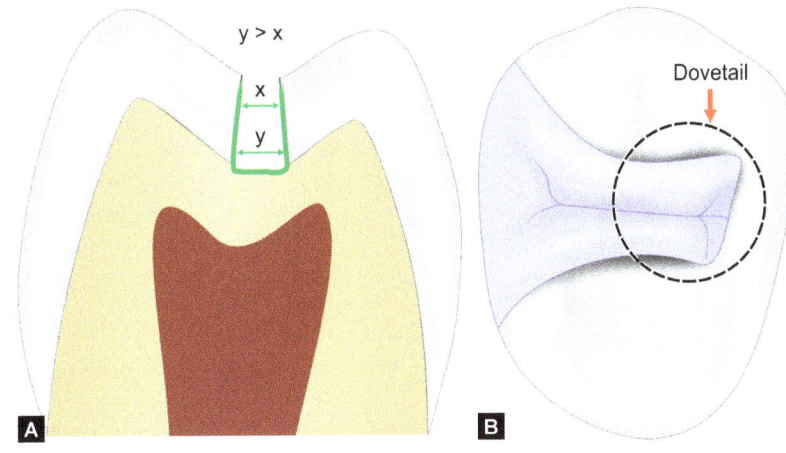

FIGURES 7.23A AND B: Retention to amalgam retention is provided by: (A) Convergence of walls; (B) Dovetail.

Convenience Form

Definition

The convenience form is that form which facilitates and provides adequate visibility, accessibility, and ease of operation during preparation and restoration of the tooth.

Features of Convenience Form

- To have adequate width and lateral extensions for restorative material.
- To provide proximal clearance from the adjacent tooth during class II preparation.
- Refining of line and point angles for starting points of direct filling gold.
- To provide occlusal divergence for cast gold inlays.

FINAL STAGES OF TOOTH PREPARATION

Removal of any Remaining Enamel Pit or Fissure, Infected Dentin and/or Old Restorative Material, if Indicated

Definition

It is defined as removal of any infected carious tooth structure or faulty restorative material which is left in the tooth after initial preparation. While removing the carious dentin, one should remove only infected dentin not the affected dentin. This is done by using:

- **Large sized round steel bur at slow speed** with light force in wiping motion. Large sized instrument minimizes the force per square millimeter applied to affected area, reducing the chances of mechanical pulp exposure.
- **Large spoon excavator** in lateral wiping motion, forces removal of infected dentin should be directed laterally and not towards the center of carious lesion. Caries are removed in a spiraling fashion, beginning with the most superficial caries at the outer lateral wall. As hard dentin is reached laterally, it is followed to the central area.

Table 7.2 shows the difference between infected dentin and affected dentin.

Removal of old restorative material is indicated, if:

- It affects esthetics of new restoration
- Tooth has secondary caries
- Tooth is symptomatic
- It compromises the placement of new restoration
- There is marginal deterioration of old restoration.

Pulp Protection

When remaining dentin thickness is less, pulpal injury can occur because of:

- Heat production by using high speed burs with less effective coolants
- Irritating restorative materials
- Galvanic currents due to restoration of dissimilar metals
- Excessive masticatory forces transmitted through restorative materials to the dentin and ingress of microorganisms and their noxious products through microleakage

Pulp protection is achieved using liners, varnishes and bases depending upon amount of remaining dentin thickness and type of restorative material used.

Varnish (Fig. 7.24)

Varnish is a natural gum like copal or a synthetic resin dissolved in an organic solvent like alcohol, acetone or ether. When applied on the tooth surface the organic solvent evaporates leaving behind a protective film which seals the dentinal tubules and reduces leakage around the restoration.

In case of amalgam restoration, varnish improves the sealing ability of the amalgam, until corrosion products are formed and reduces postoperative sensitivity by preventing microleakage. Use of varnish is contraindicated under glass ionomers because it interferes with bonding of tooth to glass ionomer cement. With composite resins varnish is not used because it interferes with polymerization of resins.

TABLE 7.2: Difference between infected and affected dentin.

Infected dentin	Affected dentin
It is a superficial layer of demineralized dentin	It is a deeper layer
Cannot be remineralized	Can be remineralized
Lacks sensation	It is sensitive
In this, intertubular layer is demineralized with irregularly scattered crystals	In this, intertubular layer is only partly demineralized

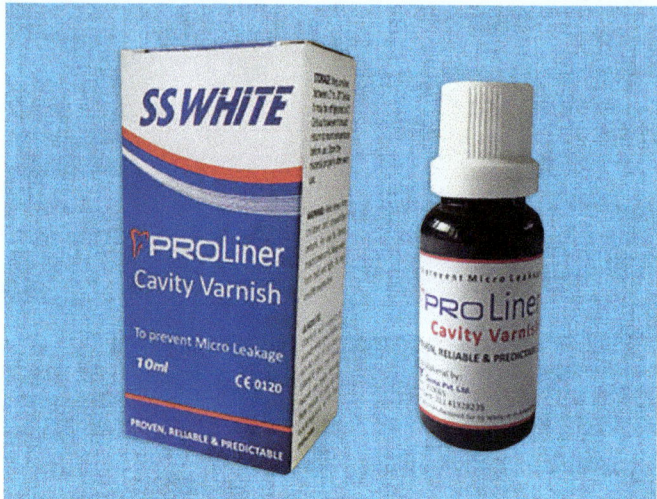

FIGURE 7.24: Varnish.

Cavity Liners

- Liner provides a thin barrier of 0.5 mm which protects the pulp tissue along with providing therapeutic benefit.
- Commonly used materials as liner are calcium hydroxide, glass ionomer cement, MTA and biodentine.
- Calcium hydroxide is most commonly used material as liner. It protects pulp from chemical irritation by its sealing ability, stimulating production of reparative and secondary dentin. It is compatible with all types of restorative materials. It is placed directly over the deepest part of preparation. It is then covered with resin modified glass ionomer cement.

Bases

Base is applied in thicker layers to provide thermal and mechanical protection for the pulp.

Mode of Application

After having optimal consistency, a small sesame seed size of base is attached to tip of explorer and carried in the prepared cavity, and applied on pulpal floor and axial wall. With the help of plastic carrier or ultra small cotton pellet held with cotton plier, pat the material and adapt it to the floor of the cavity.

Materials Used as Base

- **Zinc phosphate cement:** It is fast setting, has satisfactory mechanical properties, low solubility with excellent thermal insulation. But it does not adhere to dentin and has high acidity which irritates the pulp tissue
- **Polycarboxylate cement:** It chemically bonds to tooth structure, biocompatible and has moderate strength
- **Glass ionomer cement:** It is most commonly used liner and base because of its anticariogenic property, adhesion to tooth structure and biocompatible nature
- **Resin modified glass ionomer cements:** Resin modified glass ionomer cement was introduced to overcome problem of water sensitivity of conventional glass ionomer cements.

Guidelines of using liners, bases and varnishes for different restorative materials according to remaining dentin thickness is described in **Table 7.3**.

TABLE 7.3: Pulp protection with different restorative materials according to remaining dentin thickness.

Types of restoration	Shallow (RDT > 2.0 mm)	Moderately deep (RDT > 0.5–2 mm)	Deep (RDT < 0.5 mm)
Silver amalgam	Varnish, dentin bonding agent (DBA)	Base	Calcium hydroxide as liner and base
Glass ionomer cement	Not required	Not required	Calcium hydroxide as liner
Composite resins	Dentin bonding agent	Dentin bonding agent	Calcium hydroxide as liner followed by glass ionomer as base
Cast gold restorations	Luting cement	Base and luting cement	Calcium hydroxide liner, base and luting cement
Ceramic inlays and onlays	DBA and resin cement	DBA and resin cement	Calcium hydroxide liner, GIC base, DBA and resin cement

Secondary Resistance and Retention Forms

This step is needed in complex and compound tooth preparations where added preparation features are used to improve the resistance and retention form of the prepared tooth. These can be done by adding:
- Mechanical features.
- Conditioning procedures.

Mechanical Features (Fig. 7.25)

Many mechanical features are added in the tooth preparation to provide additional retention and resistance form.

These can be:
- **Retention grooves:** Retention grooves are placed on axiofacial and axiolingual line angles from gingival floor to occlusal surface.
- **Coves:** Coves are small conical depressions prepared in the proximal walls of class II preparations at axiofacial and axiolingual line angles thus resisting the proximal displacement of restoration.

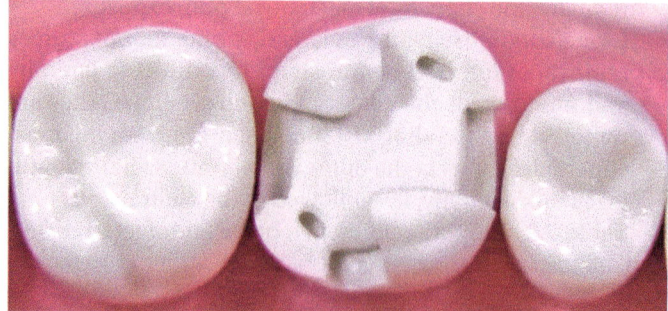

FIGURE 7.25: Photograph showing complex tooth preparation in mandibular 1st molar. Note the placement of internal box, and retention grooves for secondary retention form.

- **Slots or internal boxes:** These are 1.0–1.5 mm deep box-like grooves prepared in dentin to increase the surface area.
- **Locks:** Locks are usually prepared for class II amalgam restorations for increasing resistance and retention form.
- **Pins:** Different types of pins of various shapes and sizes are used to provide additional retention in amalgam, composite and cast restorations.
- **Amalgam pins:** Amalgam pins are vertical posts of amalgam anchored in dentin. Dentin chamber is prepared by using inverted cone bur on the gingival floor 0.5 mm into dentin with 1–2 mm depth and 0.5–1 mm width **(Fig. 7.26)**.

Conditioning Procedures

Treatment of the preparation walls by conditioning procedures, etching, and bonding increases the adhesive property of tooth preparation. These procedures are done for glass ionomer cements, composites or ceramic restorations.

Procedures for Finishing the External Walls of the Tooth Preparation

Definition

Finishing of tooth preparation walls is further development of a specific cavosurface design and degree of smoothness which produces maximum effectiveness of the restorative material being used.

Objectives

- To have smooth marginal junction between restoration and tooth surface.
- To provide maximum strength for both tooth and restorative material at and near the margins.
- To have smooth blending of restoration and tooth surface at the margins.

Factors Affecting Type of Finishing Necessary for External Walls

- Direction of enamel rods.
- Choice of restorative material.

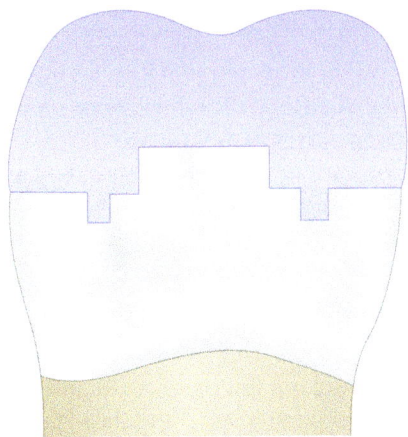

FIGURE 7.26: Secondary retention in the form of amalgam pins to increase the retention of the restoration.

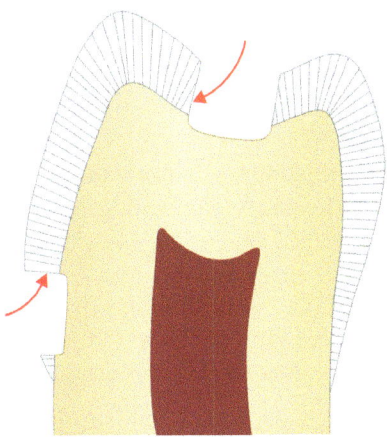

FIGURE 7.27: At the margins, all the enamel walls should have full length rods supported by dentin.

- Location of the margins.

To avoid fracture of the tooth structure at the margins, all enamel walls should have full length of enamel rods supported by sound dentin **(Fig. 7.27)**.

Features

Degree of Smoothness or Roughness of the Walls

This varies according to type of restorative material used. Smooth surface is indicated for cast metal restorations whereas roughness of the walls can be given in case of amalgam, direct filling gold, and composite resin restorations.

Design of Cavosurface Angle

This also varies according to type of restorative material used. For amalgam, 90° cavosurface angle or butt joint is recommended due to low edge strength of the material. For composite and cast metal restorations, bevel is indicated for better marginal sealing and better bonding.

Final Procedures: Cleaning, Inspecting and Sealing

Final step in tooth preparation is cleansing of the preparation. This includes the removal of debris, drying of the preparation, and final inspection before placing restorative materials.

- Cleaning of tooth preparation using warm water.
- Drying the tooth preparation using air, dry cotton pellets.
- Sterilization of preparation walls using very mild alcohol free disinfectant: Use of mild disinfectant in tooth preparation serves the purpose of disinfection.

■ VIVA QUESTIONS

Q.1 What is tooth preparation?

Ans. It is a mechanical alteration of a defective, injured or diseased tooth in order to best receive a restorative material which will re-establish the healthy state of the tooth including esthetic correction when indicated along with normal form and function.

Q.2 What are different causes of loss of tooth structure?

Ans. Most common cause is dental caries. Other causes can be trauma resulting in tooth fracture, attrition, abrasion, erosion, tooth malformation, hypoplasia, tooth resorption, etc.

Q.3 What is simple, compound and complex tooth preparations?

Ans. A tooth preparation involving only one tooth surface is termed as simple preparation. For example, mesial, distal, occlusal, buccal, lingual tooth preparation.

A tooth preparation involving two surfaces is termed as compound tooth preparation. For example, mesio-occlusal (MO), disto-occlusal (DO), mesiolingual (ML), or distobuccal (DB) tooth preparation.

A tooth preparation involving more than two surfaces is called as complex tooth preparation. For example, mesio-occlusodistal (MOD), facio-occlusolingual (FOL) or mesioincisodistal (MID) tooth preparation.

Q.4 Define class I tooth preparation.

Ans. Class I preparations occur on the occlusal surfaces of premolars and molars, the occlusal two-third of buccal and lingual surface of molars and lingual surface of incisors.

Q.5 Define class II tooth preparation.

Ans. Preparations on the proximal surface of premolars and molars are class II.

Q.6 Define class III tooth preparation.

Ans. Preparations on the proximal surface of anterior teeth and not involving the incisal angles are class III.

Q.7 Define class IV tooth preparation.

Ans. Preparations on the proximal surface of anterior teeth also involving the incisal angle falls under class IV.

Q.8 Define class V tooth preparation.

Ans. Preparations on gingival third of facial and lingual or palatal surfaces of all teeth came under class V.

Q.9 Define class VI tooth preparation.

Ans. Preparations on incisal edges of anterior and cusp tips of posterior teeth without involving any other surface come under Class VI.

Q.10 What are different walls and floors of a tooth preparation?

Ans.
- Buccal
- Lingual/palatal
- Mesial
- Distal
- Axial wall
- Occlusal/incisal
- Pupal floor
- Gingival seat.

Q.11 Who is father of modern operative dentistry?

Ans. GV Black.

Q.12 What is floor of the cavity?

Ans. Floor is the flat surface of prepared cavity which is perpendicular to the occlusal forces which are directed occlusogingivally.

For example, pulpal and gingival floors.

Q.13 Define a line angle.

Ans. It is a junction of two surfaces of different orientations along the line. Its name is derived from the involved surfaces.

Q.14 What is a point angle?

Ans. It is a junction of three plane surfaces or three line angles of different orientations. Its name is derived from its involved surfaces or line angles.

Q.15 Do we have line angle at cavosurface margin?

Ans. No, because line angle is the junction between two prepared parts of tooth preparation. Cavosurface margin is the junction of prepared tooth with unprepared tooth surface.

Q.16 If class II tooth preparation involves only proximal surface, why do we make occlusal preparation also?

Ans. Occlusal preparation is done for convenience form. Since directly reaching the affected area with bur is difficult because of close proximity of the adjacent tooth therefore an occlusal preparation is made through which proximal surface is reached.

Q.17 Why is class VI added to Black's classification?

Ans. Black classified the cavities according to some order and pattern of caries in affected teeth. But he did not include the areas which he assumed might not be attacked by caries, though in reality they might be affected. Simon later modified Black's classification and added class VI. The class VI are the tooth preparations which occur in the areas not covered by any of the other five classes like cusp tips, incisal two-third of anterior teeth, etc.

Q.18 What is enamel and dentinal wall?

Ans. Enamel wall is portion of prepared external wall consisting of enamel.

Dentinal wall is portion of prepared external wall consisting of dentin.

Q.19 What will be the treatment if caries involve proximal surface of anterior tooth without involving incisal edge and caries at palatal pit?

Ans. If lesions are not interconnected they are treated as separate preparations.

But if they are connected, the preparation is class III with lingual extension.

Q.20 What is treatment for caries present on buccal surface and proximal surface of a molar?

Ans. If lesions are not interconnected and small, they are treated as separate class II and class I preparations. But

Principles of Tooth Preparation

if lesions are large and interconnected, it is treated as proximo-occlusobuccal preparation.

Q.21 What is similarity between class II, III, IV and V preparations?
Ans. All occur on smooth surfaces.

Q.22 What is common between class II, III, IV preparations?
Ans. All these occur on proximal surfaces.

Q.23 How is tooth preparation done?
Ans. It is done by use of hand and rotary instruments.

Q.24 What are different steps of tooth preparation?
Ans.
- Stage I—Initial tooth preparation steps:
  - Outline form and initial depth.
  - Primary resistance form.
  - Primary retention form.
  - Convenience form.
- Stage II—Final tooth preparation steps:
  - Removal of any remaining caries, infected dentin and/or old restorative material, if indicated.
  - Pulp protection, if indicated.
  - Secondary resistance and retention form.
  - Procedures for finishing the external walls of the tooth preparation.
  - Cleaning, inspecting and sealing.

Q.25 Define outline form. List the factors influencing the outline form?
Ans. *The outline form means:*
- Placing the preparation margins to the place they will occupy in the final tooth preparation except for finishing enamel walls and margins
- Maintaining the initial depth of 0.2–0.8 mm into the dentin.

Factors affecting outline form:
- Extension of carious lesion
- Proximity of the lesion to other deep structural surface defects
- Relationship with adjacent and opposing teeth
- Caries index of the patient
- Need for esthetics
- Restorative material to be used.

Q.26 What is extension for prevention?
Ans. This concept was given by GV Black which advocated involvement of all pits and fissures even if they are unaffected by caries.

Q.27 What do you mean by breaking the contact?
Ans. In case of class II, III and IV caries, there is always a contact with the adjacent tooth. In these cases, whether caries are below or above the contact, the contact has to be broken so as to bring preparation margins into the embrasures for easy cleansability. If preparation margins end in non-cleansable areas, food stagnation in those areas may result in secondary caries.

Q.28 What should be ideal depth of the preparation?
Ans. Ideal depth should be 0.5 mm below DEJ, especially for non-adhesive materials. Since enamel is inelastic, it cannot be used for providing retentive and resistance form. So depth of preparation should be increased till elastic dentin is reached. Preparation should not end at dentinoenamel junction. This area is sensitive because of lateral branching of dentinal tubules and cytoplasmic extensions of odontoblasts.

Q.29 How does convenience form affects outline from?
Ans. This is specially seen in case of class II, III and IV preparations where adjacent tooth is present. In these cases it is impossible to reach the proximal area without cutting occlusal surface, otherwise adjacent tooth is cut.

But if adjacent tooth is missing, one can gain entry to proximal box without cutting the occlusal surface.

Q.30 What is meant by cuspal contour?
Ans. Cuspal contour means making preparation at uniform depth providing equal dentin thickness between pulp and the preparation. Since cusps are conical in shape, if pulpal floor is made straight it may result in uneven dentin thickness. The areas where less of dentin is present, preparation will be closer to pulp, resulting in its damage.

Q.31 Why should not preparation have sharp angles?
Ans. If preparation has sharp angles, it leads to concentration of stresses at those areas which may fracture the restoration. So to avoid stress concentration, preparation should have gentle curves and smooth walls.

Q.32 What is significance of stress bearing areas?
Ans. When opposing teeth come in contact, they contact only some areas of occlusal surfaces. These areas where they contact are stress bearing areas.
Significance: Preparation margins should not end at stress bearing areas otherwise stresses are met partially by the tooth and partially by restoration resulting in separation between the two. This can fracture the restoration or may result in marginal leakage. So preparation margin should be avoided at stress bearing areas. They should be kept entirely either on tooth surface or on restorative material.

Q.33 How is outline form affected by direction of enamel rods?
Ans. Enamel rods extend perpendicular from DEJ to enamel in a slightly wavy course. In vertical direction, they appear to converge towards a pit from DEJ, whereas they diverge as they move towards cusp tip from the DEJ.

In horizontal section, enamel rods flare out from DEJ towards outer surface.

Because of the direction of enamel rods, following walls are flared externally:
- Buccal and lingual walls of proximal box.
- Mesial and distal walls of buccal and lingual boxes of class I extensions.
- All walls of class V preparation.

If these walls are made to converge towards each other, this will result in unsupported enamel rods which may fracture later on.

Q.34 How does esthetics affect outline form?
Ans.
- For class III preparation, labial enamel is kept intact
- Preparation margins should be kept into embrasures for better esthetics
- Reverse curve is given in maxillary premolars.

Q.35 How does age affect outline form?
Ans. Because of presence of deep pits and fissures, young teeth are more caries prone, therefore for a young patient, a conventional preparation is indicated.

For older patients, a conservative preparation is indicated. In these patients teeth become less susceptible to caries because of following reasons:
- Attrition of teeth.
- Cumulative effect of fluoride from food, water supply, dentifrices, etc.
- Older patient may follow oral instructions better.

Q.36 Define resistance form.
Ans. It is that shape and placement of preparation walls to best enable both the tooth and restoration to withstand, without fracture the stresses of masticatory forces delivered principally along long axis of the tooth.

Q.37 What are factors affecting resistance form?
Ans.
- Amount of occlusal stresses
- Type of restoration used
- Amount of remaining tooth structure.

Q.38 What is extension for resistance?
Ans. When outline is extended for reinforcing the weakened tooth structure, it is referred as extension for resistance. For example, when preparation involves more than one-half of the cusp, outline is extended in which cusp is reduced and cuspal coverage is done.

Q.39 Why is floor of preparation made perpendicular to occlusal forces?
Ans. When masticatory forces are applied perpendicular to floor, there is equal and opposite force offered by preparation floor to resist the masticatory forces.
If pulpal floor is made at an angle, it will split occlusal forces into two components:
1. Perpendicular component which is resisted by occlusal forces, this helps in seating of the restoration.
2. Lateral component of force along the surface of floor.

Q.40 Is pulpal floor always horizontal?
Ans. No the mandibular premolar has a lingual tilt, so the pulpal floor is also made with lingual tilt.

Q.41 Why should a restorative material have bulk?
Ans. To have resistance form a restorative material should have sufficient bulk, for example for amalgam, at least 1.5–2 mm of depth is required.

Q.42 Why should be unsupported enamel removed from the preparation?
Ans. If enamel is not supported by dentin, it can fracture by masticatory forces because of its brittle nature.

Q.43 What is as isthmus and its significance?
Ans. Isthmus is the narrow connection between two portions of a preparation (occlusal and proximal). Most of the restoration failures occur at isthmus area. If it is very narrow, restoration will be very weak at that area. If isthmus is very wide, the remaining tooth structure will become very weak.

Q.44 When should two adjacent preparation be connected??
Ans. If healthy tooth structure between two preparations is less then 0.5 mm, the two adjacent preparations are joined to form one large preparation. For example, mesial and distal pits of maxillary first molar.

Q.45 What is retention form?
Ans. It is that form, shape and configuration of the tooth preparation that resists the displacement or removal of restoration from the preparation under lifting and tipping masticatory forces.

Q.46 What are factors affecting retention form?
Ans.
- Proximity between tooth and restoration
- Parallelism of opposing walls
- Total surface area of contact.

Q.47 What area different modes of retention?
Ans.
- Providing occlusal convergence
- Providing occlusal dovetail
- Close parallelism of the opposing walls
- Use of secondary retention in the form of coves, skirts and dentin slot
- Use of bevels.

Q.48 How is retention achieved in amalgam restoration?
Ans.
- Occlusal convergence—inverted truncated shape
- Occlusal dovetail
- Undercuts.

Q.49 What is meant by inverted truncated shape of the cavity?
Ans.
- It means internal outline form is greater than external outline form with pulpoocclusal convergence of the preparation walls
- It is indicated for incrementally added direct restoration material like amalgam.

Principles of Tooth Preparation

Q.50 How does dentin help in retention?
Ans. Due to elastic nature of dentin, there is microscopic movement of dentinal walls (away from each other) when a restorative material is being condensed in the preparation. Once the restorative material sets, dentin comes back to its original position resulting in better retention and more gripping action.

Q.51 What is significance of dovetail?
Ans. It helps in retention in proximal direction. In other words, dovetail holds the proximal restoration from dislodging proximally.

Q.52 What is undercut?
Ans. Undercut is a mode of retention which is prepared with an inverted cone bur in line angles of the preparation. While preparing undercut, one should take care to make the cut in the wall and not into the floor. While restoration, one should take care that only the restorative material should be filled in the undercut area, and not the base.

Q.53 What are secondary means of retention?
Ans.
- Grooves and coves
- Slots, locks and pins
- Internal box
- Skirts
- Amalgam pins
- Beveled enamel margins.

Q.54 What is convenience form?
Ans. The convenience form is that form which facilitates and provides adequate visibility, accessibility and ease of operation during preparation and restoration of the tooth.

Q.55 What is meant by convenience for access?
Ans. In case of class II and III preparations, due to presence of adjacent tooth, one has to cut the occlusal or labial surface. This outline for gaining access to carious lesion is called as convenience for access.

Q.56 What do you mean by removal of remaining caries?
Ans. In some teeth, if any caries remain on the deeper part of preparation after gaining resistance and retention form, these are removed carefully without causing any harm to pulp. If attempts are made for complete caries removal at the initial stages only, one might end up for over cutting so it is always advised to incorporate retentive and resistance features before complete caries removal is done.

Q.57 Which instrument is used for removal of remaining caries?
Ans.
- Low-speed handpiece with the round bur
- Spoon excavator.

Q.58 Difference between affected and infected dentin?
Ans. *Infected dentin:*
- It is a superficial layer of demineralized dentin
- Cannot be remineralized
- Lacks sensation
- In this, intertubular layer is demineralized with irregularly scattered crystals
- Collagen fibers are broken down, appear as only indistinct cross bands
- It can be stained with:
  - 0.2% propylene glycol
  - 10% acid red solution
  - 0.5% basic fuschin.

Affected dentin:
- It is a deeper layer
- Intermediate demineralized dentin
- Can be remineralized
- It is sensitive
- In this, intertubular layer is only partly demineralized
- Distinct cross bands are present
- It cannot be stained with any solution.

Q.59 What precautions should be taken while removing deep carious lesion?
Ans. Use slow-speed handpiece with the round bur or spoon excavator that will fit in the carious lesion used with light force and a wiping motion.
Forces for removal of infective dentin should be directed laterally and not towards the center of the carious lesion.

Q.60 Which instrument is used for removal of unsupported enamel rods?
Ans. Chisel, hoe or hatchet is used for removal of unsupported rods.

Q.61 For smoothening the gingival seat which instrument is used?
Ans. GMT is used for making gingival seat.

Q.62 How do you check convenience form?
Ans. After tooth preparation, insert the small amalgam condenser into all parts of preparation. If even the small instrument does not enter some parts of tooth preparation, tooth preparation is widened.

Q.63 Is breaking of contact also required for insertion of matrix band?
Ans. No, the main reason for breaking a contact is to bring the preparation margins in self cleansable area. For matrix band insertion, teeth can be separated using separators rather than cutting natural teeth structure.

Q.64 For preparations near gingival margins, where should be gingival seat located?
Ans. As we know gingival area is a delicate area, any irritant present at tooth–gingival interface can cause inflammation of soft tissue and epithelial attachment. One should always try to keep the gingival margins supragingivally for easy cleansability. Subgingival margins are given only when:
- Decay extends subgingivally.
- Old restoration is present subgingivally.
- A biocompatible restorative material is used for esthetic concerns.

Q.65 Where is gingival seat prepared for class II preparation?
Ans. Just beyond the caries or contact point whichever is more.

Q.66 Why are marginal ridge/transverse or oblique ridges preserved during tooth preparation?
Ans. Since ridges are the strongest areas with high density of dentin as compared to others, these act as stress bearing areas and thus, need to be preserved.

Q.67 What is minimal gingival clearance between teeth in class II tooth preparation?
Ans. 0.5 mm.

Q.68 What is minimal facial and lingual clearance between teeth in class II tooth preparation?
Ans. 0.2–0.3 mm.

Q.69 Why should be the contact point broken in class II preparation?
Ans. Contact has to be broken so as to bring cavity margins outside the contact area into the embrasure both occlusogingivally and buccolingually for easy cleansability. If contact area is not broken, it can lead to debris accumulation and therby secondary caries.

Q.70 What are stress bearing areas in cavity preparation?
Ans. During occlusion, some areas of occlusal surface come in contact either in centic or eccentric position, these are stress bearing areas.
Significance: Cavity margins should not be placed on stress bearing areas as this may lead to stress distribution both to tooth and restoration resulting in their separation.

Q.71 Why should not the pulpal floor be placed on DEJ?
Ans. Because of branching of dentinal tubules and cytoplasmic branches, this area is very sensitive, so pulpal floor should be avoided on DEJ.

Q.72 What should be the width of gingival seat?
Ans. 0.8 mm. 0.3 mm in enamel and 0.5 mm in dentin.

Q.73 What is ideal width of marginal ridge?
Ans. 1.5 mm for premolars 2 mm for molars. Marginal ridge width less than 1.6 mm results in undermining of the marginal ridge and reduced resistance form.

Q.74 Where should be the gingival seat placed in class II tooth preparation?
Ans. It is placed cervical to the contact point so as to break contact with the adjacent tooth and to have restoration with self-cleansable margins.

Q.75 What will happen if gingival seat is placed very shallow at the same level with pulpal floor?
Ans. Inadequate removal of the proximal carious lesion and inadequate retention form.

Q.76 What should be the clearance from adjacent tooth in class II tooth preparation?
Ans. 0.5 mm. Clearance >0.5 mm: excessive loss of tooth structure, unesthetic display of amalgam facially and chances of damaging interdental gingival clearance <0.5 mm: inadequate caries removal and difficulty in placement of matrix band.

Q.77 Why should the floor of cavity preparation be placed in dentin not enamel?
Ans.
- Since enamel is inelastic and brittle in nature, it cannot be used for providing resistance form. However, dentin being softer than enamel acts as cushion support to enamel and prevents its fracture.
- If enamel margin is left unsupported during cavity preparation, it may undergo fracture under forces of mastication.
- Preparation should not end at dentinoenamel junction because this area is sensitive because of lateral branching of dentinal tubules and cytoplasmic extensions of odontoblasts.
- Due to elastic nature of dentin, there is microscopic movement of dentinal walls (away from each other) when a restorative material is being condensed in the preparation. Once the restorative material sets, dentin comes back to its original position resulting in better retention and more gripping action.

Principles of Tooth Preparation

COLOR PLATE 1

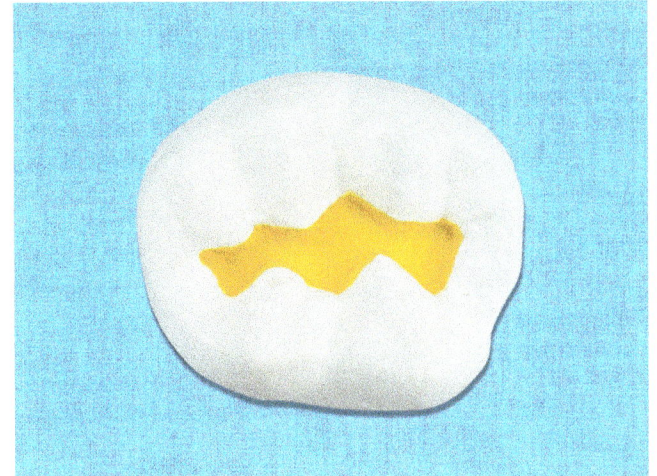

Class I tooth preparation in mandibular first molar.

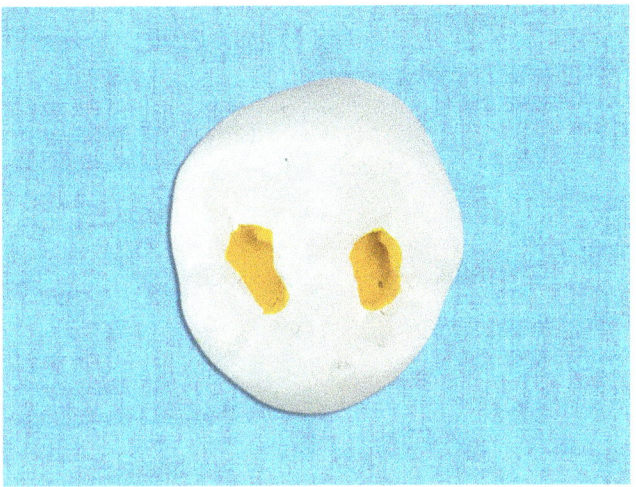

Conservative class I cavity preparation in mandibular premolar.

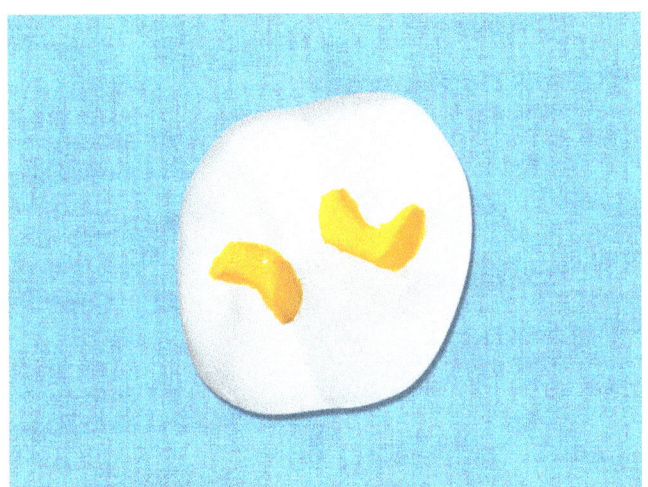

Conservative class I cavity preparation in maxillary first molar.

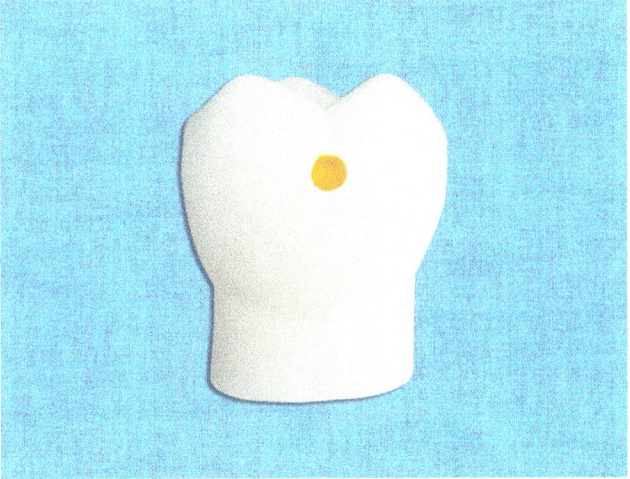

Conservative class I cavity (buccal pit) preparation in mandibular first molar.

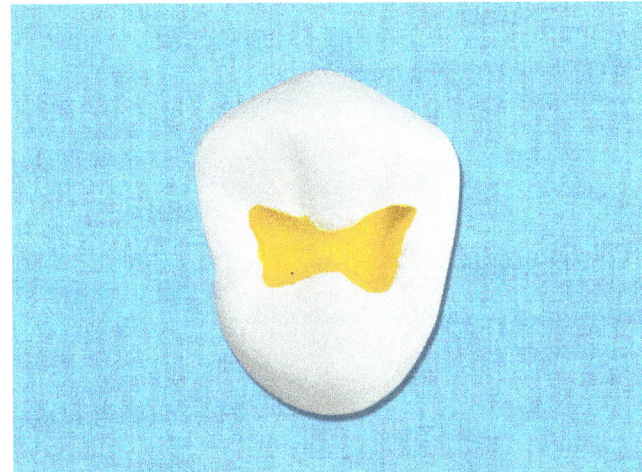

Class I cavity preparation in maxillary premolar.

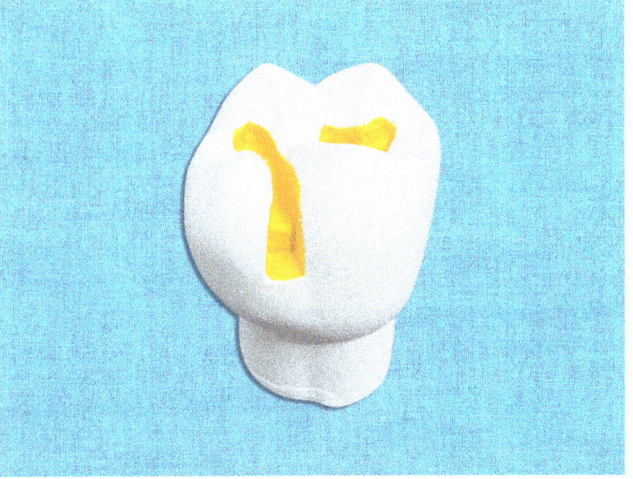

Palatal extension (class I cavity) preparation in maxillary first molar.

COLOR PLATE 2

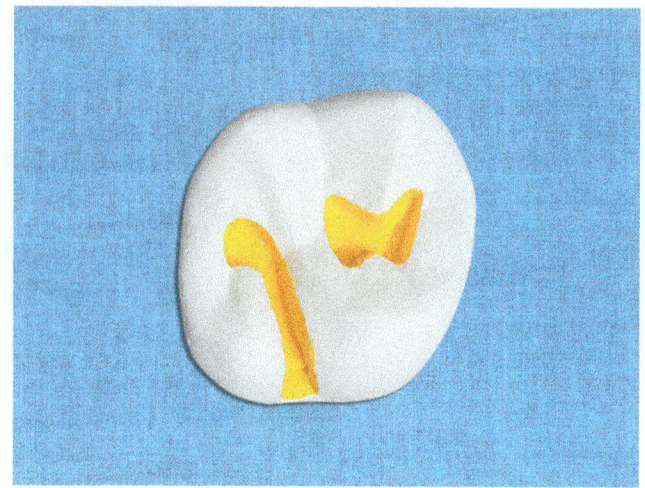

Palatal extension and mesial pit preparation in maxillary first molar.

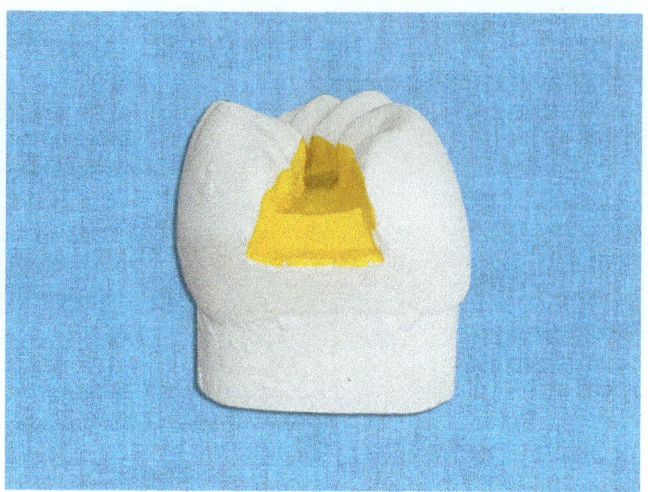

Class II cavity preparation in mandibular first molar.

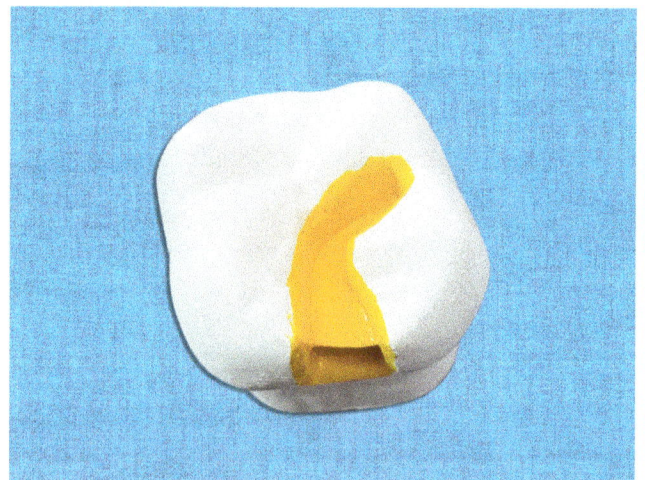

Class II cavity preparation in maxillary first molar.

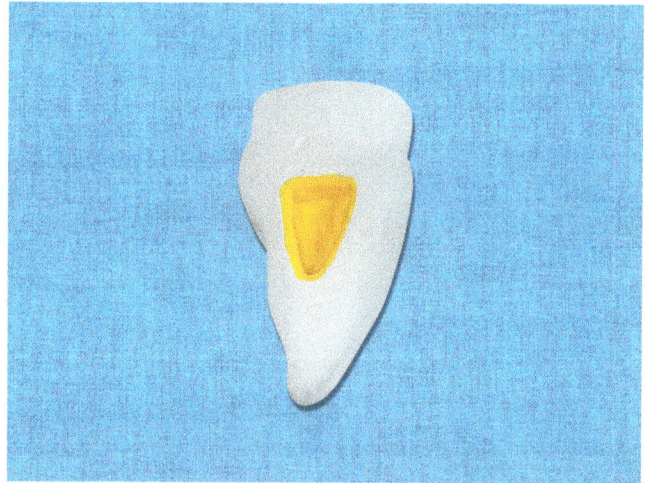

Class III cavity preparation in maxillary incisor.

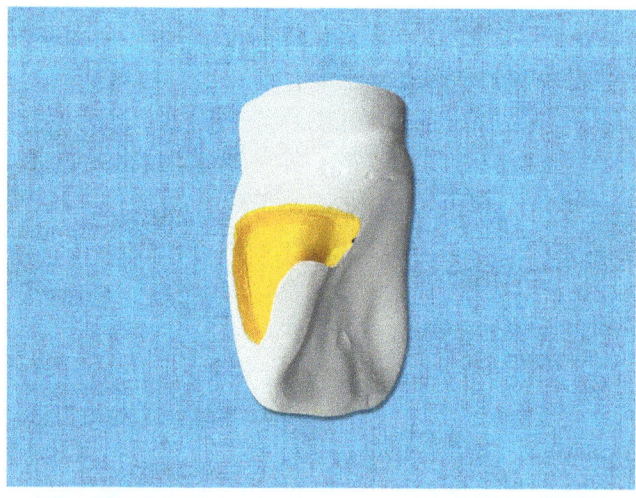

Class III cavity preparation with dovetail in maxillary incisor.

COLOR PLATE 3

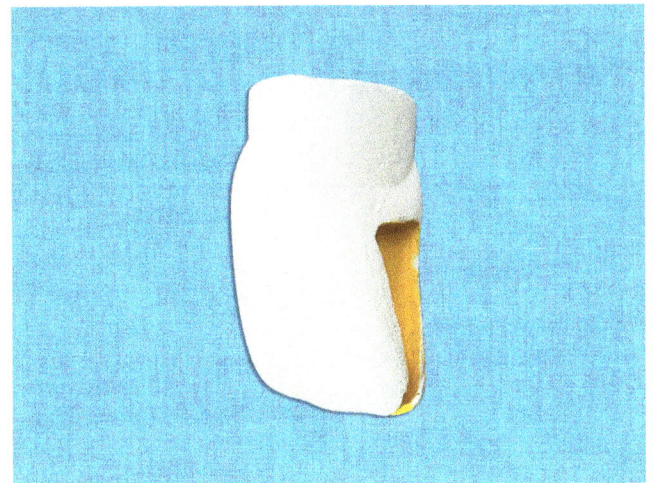
Class IV cavity preparation in maxillary incisor.

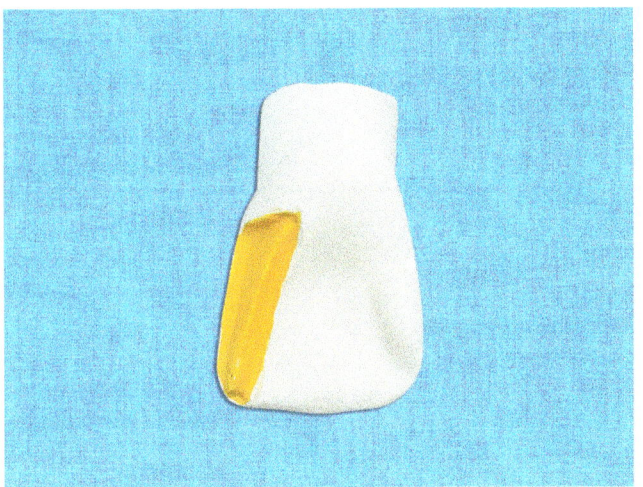
Class IV cavity preparation in maxillary incisor.

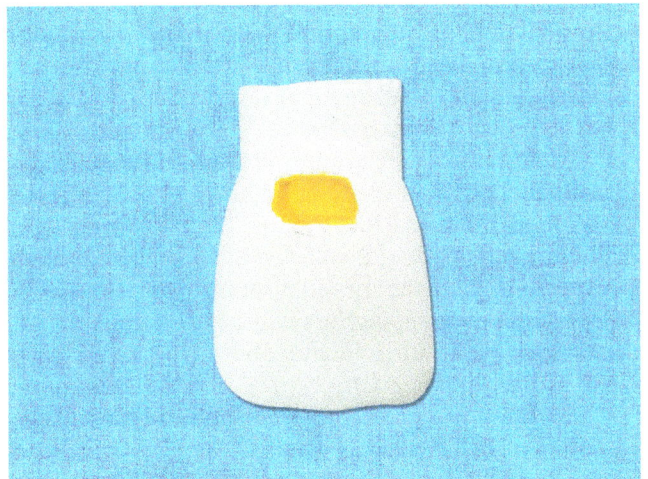
Class V cavity preparation in maxillary incisor.

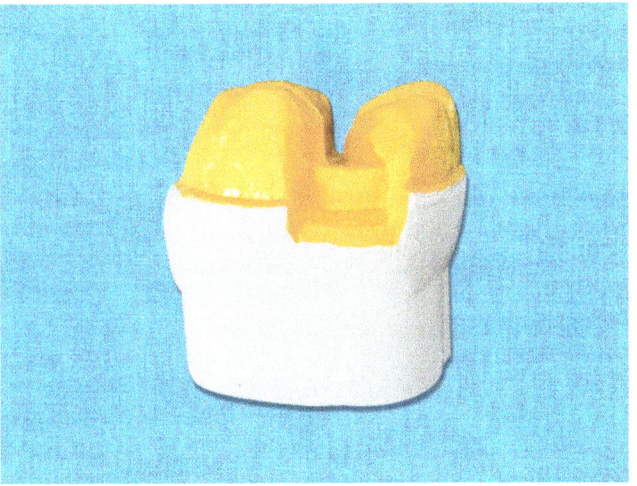
Tooth preparation for cusp capping-proximal view.

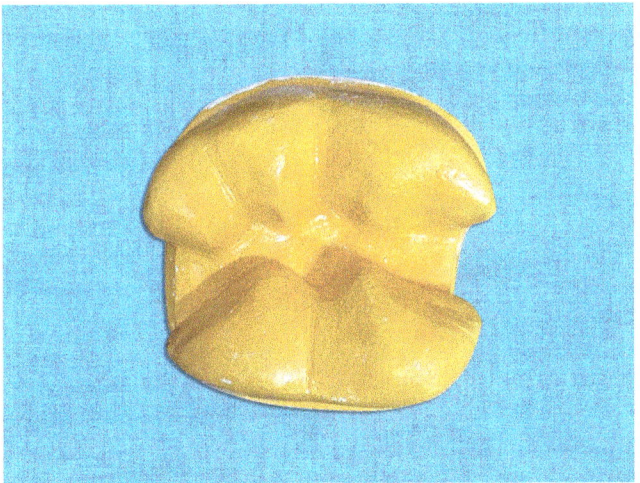
Tooth preparation for cusp capping-occlusal view.

Chapter 8: Tooth Preparation for Amalgam Restorations

Chapter Outline
- Class I cavity preparation for silver amalgam
- Class II cavity preparation for amalgam restoration
- Reverse curve
- Class III cavity preparation for amalgam restoration
- Class V cavity preparation

Dental amalgam as a material has been explained in detail in chapter 4 of this book. In this chapter, we'll be discussing the different tooth preparations for amalgam restorations. Amalgam has been used as a restorative material for more than 150 years due to its strength and user friendly properties.

The aim of tooth preparation for amalgam is not only to remove the fault present in the tooth but also to allow the amalgam material to function properly.

Tooth preparation form should allow the amalgam to:
- Have a uniform 1.5–2.0 mm of thickness for strength
- Produce a 90° amalgam angle (butt-joint form) at the margins
- Be mechanically retained in the tooth.

CLASS I CAVITY PREPARATION FOR SILVER AMALGAM

Definition
Tooth preparation involving:
- Pit and fissures of occlusal surfaces of premolars and molars
- Occlusal two-thirds of buccal and lingual surfaces of molars
- Lingual pits of maxillary anterior teeth.

Initial Cavity Preparation

Outline Form
Outline form means extending the preparation margins to the place they will occupy in the final preparation, avoid ending preparation margins in high-stress areas like cusp tip and crest of the ridges, and placing the margins on sound tooth structure.

Steps:
- Take number 245 bur for cavity preparation
- Its dimensions help in guiding ideal cavity preparation, i.e. depth of cavity preparation, 1.5 mm (half the length of bur, i.e., 3 mm), to preserve marginal ridge of width 1.6–2 mm (double the width of bur, i.e., 0.8 mm), rounded internal line angles, and convergent external walls (due to pear shape with rounded corners of the bur) **(Fig. 8.1)**
- Using number 245 bur oriented parallel to the long axis of tooth, make a punch cut in carious lesion **(Fig. 8.2A)**
- Maintain the initial depth of 1.5 mm from central fissure at least 0.2–0.5 mm in dentin.

If it is shallow preparation, it will not be able provide adequate bulk of the restoration, thus compromise the primary resistance form.

If depth is more, pulpal floor will be closer to the pulp resulting in sensitivity and postoperative pain
  - While maintaining the same depth and bur orientation, move the bur to include defective pits and fissures **(Figs. 8.2B and C)**
  - Extend the margin mesially and distally but do not involve marginal ridges. These walls should have dovetail shape to provide retention to the restoration.
- While working towards mesial and distal surface, orient the bur toward respective marginal ridge. This results in

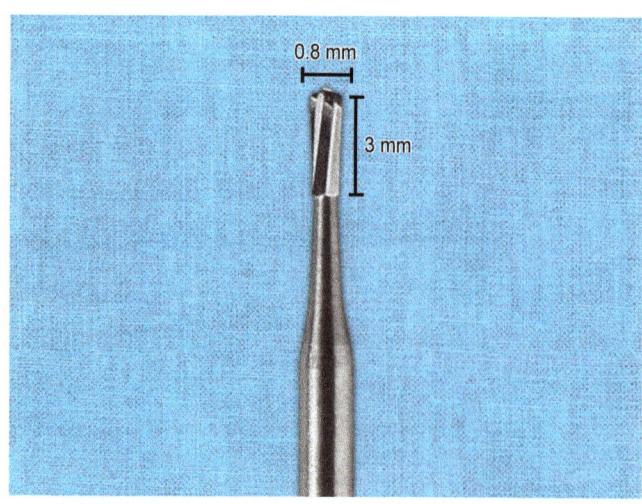

FIGURE 8.1: Dimensions of bur number 245 for cavity preparation.

slight divergence of mesial and distal walls, which helps to provide dentinal support for marginal ridges **(Fig. 8.4D)**
- Isthmus width should not be more than one-fourth of intercuspal distance
  If width is less, there will not be optimum convenience form
  If width is more, it will undermine the cuspal strength, thus reducing the resistance form
- Deep pit and fissure defects less than 0.5 mm apart should be included in outline form
- External outline form should have smooth curves, straight lines, and rounded angles. All unsupported and demineralized enamel should be removed
- Enameloplasty is done whenever required to remove sharp and irregular enamel margins by "rounding" or "saucering", thereby converting these into self- cleansable areas. Enameloplasty should not extend the outline form.

Primary Resistance Form

Primary resistance is achieved by having following features in the preparation:

- Box-shaped preparation with flat floors—This helps the tooth to resist occlusal masticatory forces without fracture. Though floor should be flat, but it should also follow the contour of occlusal surface
- Minimum occlusal depth of 1.5 mm, to provide adequate thickness of amalgam
- Cavosurface angle of 90° **(Fig. 8.2E)**
- Restricting the extension of external walls so as to have strong marginal ridge areas with sufficient dentin support
- Maintaining minimal width of cavity which is not more than 1/4th of intercuspal distance
- Keeping the pulpal floor 0.2 mm in dentin
- Inclusion of all the weakened tooth structure
- Rounding off all the internal line and point angles
- **Circumventing of cusps should be done** for preserving cuspal strength and achieving a smooth, free flowing outline form.

Primary Retention Form

Primary retention for amalgam is provided by following features:

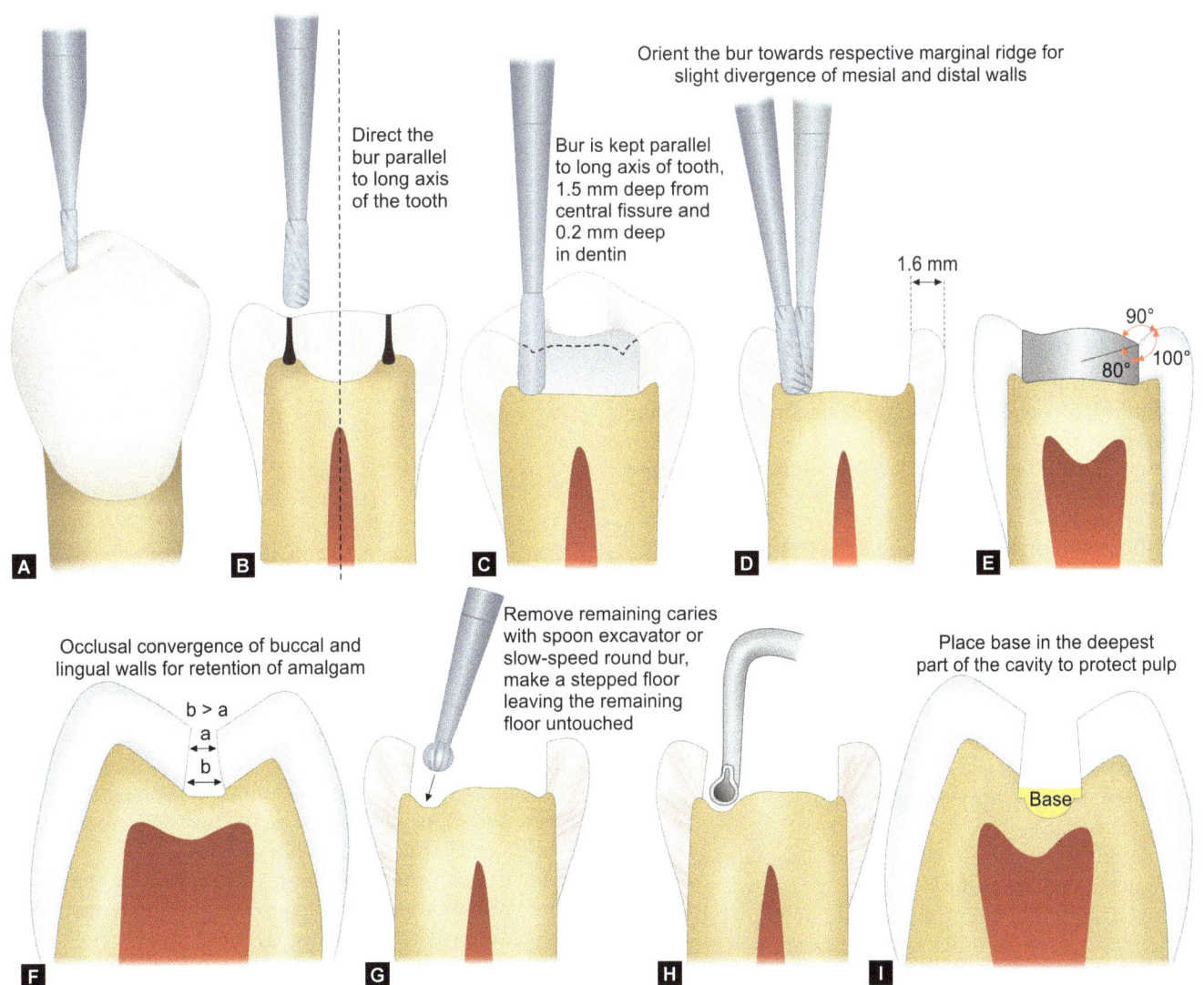

FIGURES 8.2A TO I: Steps of class I cavity preparation.

- Occlusal convergence (about 2–5%) of buccal and lingual walls **(Fig. 8.2F)**
- Occlusal dovetail.

Convenience Form

Convenience form is provided by having sufficient width of the preparation so as to have ease of accessibility and instrumentation.

Final Cavity Preparation

Removal of Remaining Carious Dentin

In this, remaining caries, old restorative material, and adjacent deep pits and fissures are removed and involved in the preparation.

In the large preparations with soft caries, the removal of carious dentin is done with spoon excavator or slow-speed round bur. In this, stepped or two-level pulpal floor is made, i.e., only portion of tooth which is affected by caries is removed, leaving the remaining floor untouched **(Figs. 8.2G and H)**.

Protection of Pulp, if Needed

Use of pulp protective materials depends upon following factors:
- Base is not required in shallow preparations (1.5–2.0 mm deep). In these cases, only varnish is used
- In a deep preparation, a base is placed in the deepest part in the thickness of 0.5–0.75 mm, so as to protect pulp **(Fig. 8.2I)**.

Be sure that no trace of the base material remains on enamel walls of preparation, as this would eventually dissolve in the oral fluids leaving a gap between the restoration and the tooth resulting in microleakage and recurrent caries.

Finishing of the Enamel Walls and Margins

Finishing of walls and margins is guided by the knowledge of dental histology. At this stage, all unsupported enamel is removed. Cavosurface angle should be made 90° butt joint type. This provides bulk to restoration, which in turn, provides maximum strength.

Final Cleaning and Inspection of the Preparation

Final stage of cavity preparation is to clean the preparation thoroughly with water and air spray. Then dry it with moist air and inspect it for final approval.

Cavity preparation on occlusal surface with buccal or palatal extension (Figs. 8.3A and B)
- For buccal or palatal extension, slight modification is required
- To prepare the lingual surface, hold the bur parallel to lingual surface
- Inclined the bur facially so as to establish the axial wall of lingual portion **(Fig. 8.4)**
- Axial wall should follow the contour of lingual surface of tooth and it should be 0.2 mm in the dentin
- Make a box shaped preparation with parallel mesial or distal walls

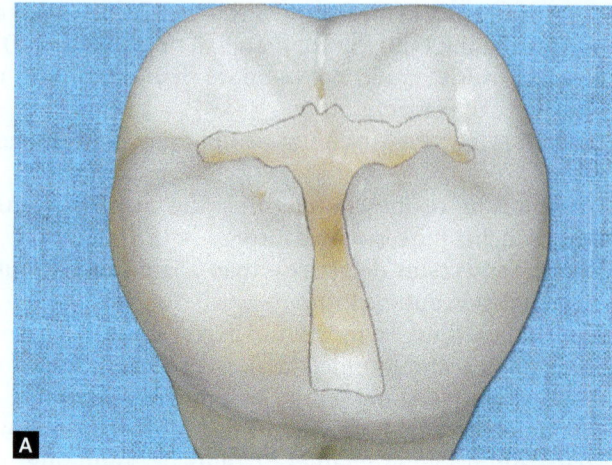
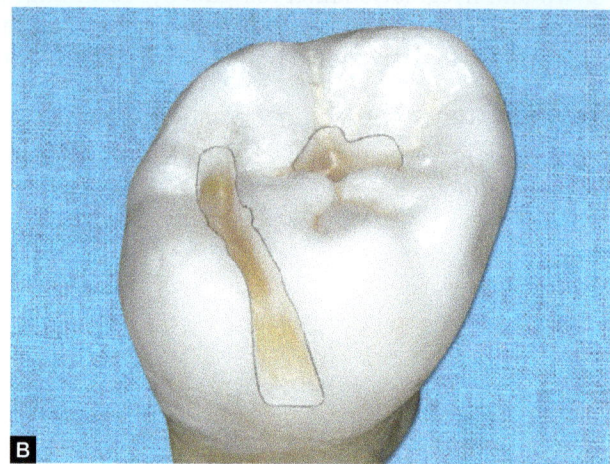

FIGURES 8.3A AND B: Photograph showing class I amalgam preparation; (A) Buccal extension; (B) Palatal extension.

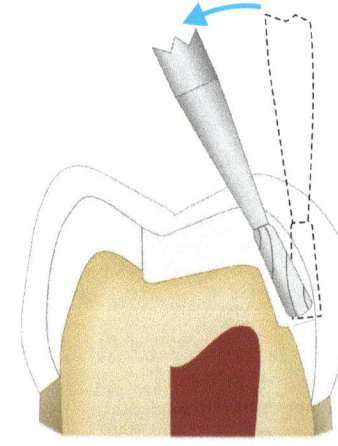

FIGURE 8.4: During lingual extension, inclined the bur facially so as to establish the axial wall of lingual portion.

- Round off the axiopulpal line angle. If additional retention is required, using No. 1/4 or 169 bur, place grooves into mesioaxial and distoaxial line angles
- Accomplish the final tooth preparation by removal of remaining caries and pulp protection. Finally, inspect the prepared cavity for amalgam restoration.

Cavity preparations on occlusal surfaces of different teeth (Figs. 8.5A to F)

Tooth Preparation for Amalgam Restorations

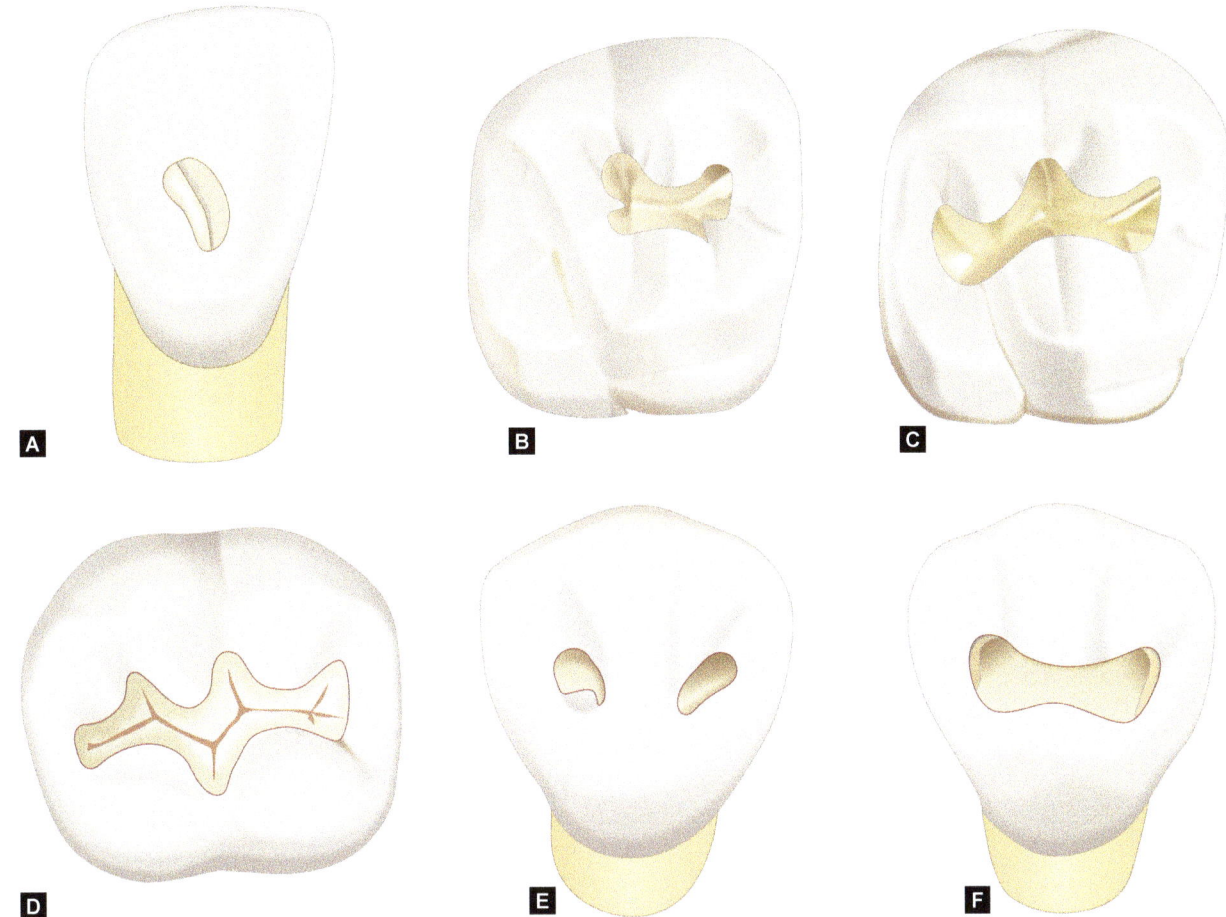

FIGURES 8.5 A TO F: Cavity preparations on occlusal surfaces of different teeth: (A) Cavity preparation on maxillary incisor; (B) Conservative preparation on occlusal surface of maxillary first molar; (C) Conventional preparation on occlusal surface of maxillary first molar; (D) Conventional preparation on occlusal surface of mandibular first molar; (E) Conservative preparation on occlusal surface of mandibular first premolar; (F) Conventional preparation on occlusal surface of mandibular premolar.

- Cavity preparation on maxillary incisors **(Fig. 8.5A)**
- Conservative preparation on occlusal surface of maxillary first molar **(Fig. 8.5B)**
- Conventional preparation on occlusal surface of maxillary first molar **(Fig. 8.5C)**
- Conventional preparation on occlusal surface of mandibular first molar **(Fig. 8.5D)**
- Conservative preparation on occlusal surface of mandibular first premolar **(Fig. 8.5E)**
- Conventional preparation on occlusal surface of mandibular premolar **(Fig. 8.5F)**.

CLASS II CAVITY PREPARATION FOR AMALGAM RESTORATION

Initial Cavity Preparation

Outline Form

Outline form for occlusal portion follows the same principles as given for pit and fissure lesions except that external outline is extended proximally towards defective proximal surface. For description, a mesio-occlusal preparation on mandibular second premolar is considered.

- ***Establishing the occlusal step:***
  - Using high-speed bur, make a punch cut in the pit closest to the involved proximal surface. Keep long axis of the bur parallel to the long axis of the tooth and maintain the initial depth of 1.5–2.0 mm **(Fig. 8.6A)**
  - Extend the outline to include the central fissure while maintaining uniformity in depth of pulpal floor **(Fig. 8.6B)**
  - Make isthmus width as narrow as possible, not more than one-fourth of the intercuspal distance
  - Give slight occlusal convergence to facial, lingual, and proximal walls to provide retention for amalgam
  - A dovetail is provided in the distal pit area to prevent mesial displacement of the restoration. Consider enameloplasty wherever required to conserve tooth structure.
- ***Extending occlusal step proximally:***
  - While maintaining established pulpal depth, extend the preparation toward proximal surface of tooth, ending 0.8 mm short of cutting through mesial marginal ridge **(Fig. 8.6C)**
  - Proximal cutting should be sufficiently deep into the dentin (0.5–0.6 mm) so that retentive locks are prepared into axiolingual and axiofacial line angles
- ***Preparation of proximal box:***
  - Widen the preparation faciolingually to just clear the contact areas
  - Proximal cut is diverged gingivally. It results in greater faciolingual dimension at gingival surface than occlusal surface

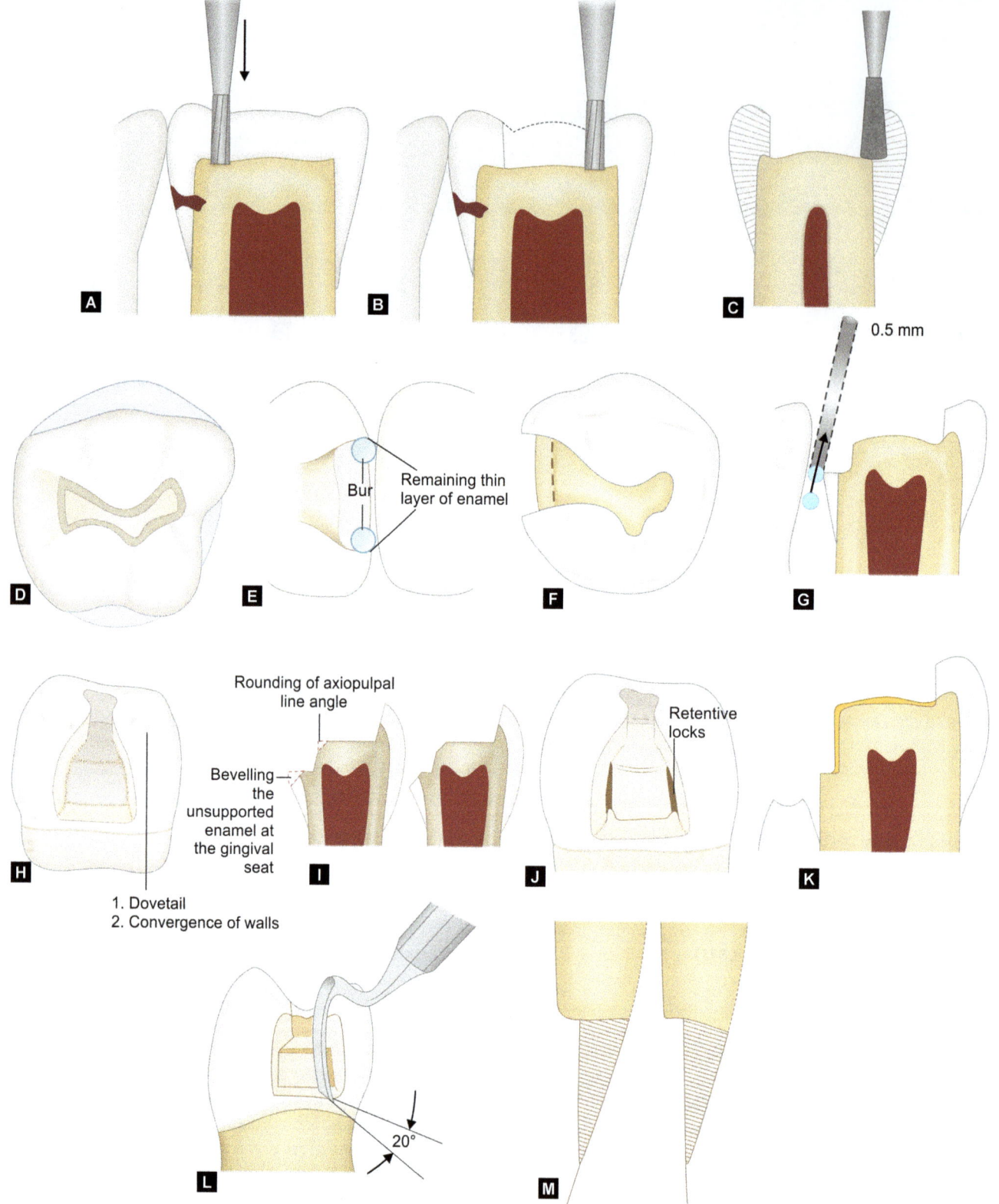

FIGURES 8.6A TO M: Steps of class II cavity preparation for amalgam restoration: (A) Keep long axis of bur parallel to the long axis of the tooth and maintain the initial depth of 1.5–2.0 mm; (B) Extend the outline to include the central fissure maintaining uniformity in depth of pulpal floor; (C) Extend the preparation toward proximal surface of tooth; (D) Diverge the proximal cut gingivally, resulting in greater faciolingual dimension at gingival surface than occlusal surface; (E) Keep a small slice of enamel at the contact area to prevent damage to adjacent tooth; (F) Make proximal cavosurface angle of 90° and proximal box converge occlusally; (G) Clearance of facial and lingual margins of the proximal box should be 0.2–0.5 mm from the adjacent tooth; (H) Occlusal convergence of buccal and lingual walls; (I) Rounding of axiopulpal line angle to reduce stress concentration and increase bulk of amalgam; (J) Retention locks at axiofacial and axiolingual line angles; (K) Providing pulp protection; (L and M) Beveling of gingival cavosurface angle for removing unsupported enamel rods.

- It provides good retention and conservation of marginal ridge (**Fig. 8.6D**)
- Keep a small slice of enamel at the contact area to prevent accidental damage to adjacent tooth (**Fig. 8.6E**)
- If there is any doubt that accidental damage to the adjacent tooth can occur, use a metal matrix band interdentally
- Fracture the slice of enamel in the region of the contact area with a small chisel or enamel hatchet
- Proximal margins should have a cavosurface angle of 90° and when completed, the walls of the proximal box should converge occlusally (**Fig. 8.6F**)
- Flatten the gingival floor so that masticatory forces are distributed equally
- Flattening of gingival floor is done using enamel hatchet
- Ideal width of gingival seat ranges from 0.6 to 0.8 mm for premolars and 0.8–1.0 mm for molars. It consists of 2/3rd of dentin and 1/3rd of enamel
- Ideal clearance of facial and lingual margins of the proximal box should be 0.2–0.5 mm from the adjacent tooth (**Fig. 8.6G**). If it is more than 0.5 mm, on facial aspect unesthetic display of amalgam occurs and on gingival aspect, damage to interdental papilla occurs. If clearance is less than 0.5 mm, it would be difficult to place matrix band and cavosurface margins do not end in self cleansable areas.

Primary Resistance Form

This can be obtained by incorporating the following features in the preparation:
- Providing enough depth of cavity to have sufficient bulk of amalgam
- Flat pulpal and gingival floor
- Cavosurface angle of 90°
- Maintaining minimal width of the preparation so as to preserve tooth structure
- Rounding the internal line and point angle
- Cusp capping for preserving cuspal strength.

Primary Retention Form

Retention is achieved by following features:
- Occlusal convergence (about 2–5%) of buccal and lingual walls (**Fig. 8.6H**)
- Occlusal dovetail.

Final Cavity Preparation

Removal of Remaining Caries or Old Restorative Materials

During final preparation, remove debris and examine for correction of all cavosurface angles and margins. Remove remaining caries, old restorative material, and adjacent deep pit and fissure involved in the preparation. In the large preparations with soft caries, the removal of carious dentin is done with spoon excavator or slow-speed round bur. In this, ***stepped or two-level pulpal floor*** is made, i.e., only portion of tooth which is affected by caries is removed, leaving the remaining preparation dentin untouched.

Secondary Retention and Resistance Form

Secondary resistance and retention is achieved by:
- Limit the extensions of external walls
- ***Rounding of axiopulpal line angle***: This reduces stress concentration and increases bulk of amalgam at that area (**Fig. 8.6I**)
- Providing retention locks at axiofacial and axiolingual line angles using 169 L bur, 0.2 mm into dentin (**Fig. 8.6J**)
- Placing retention grooves on axiofacial and axiolingual line angles with number 1/4 round bur or 1/8 bur. The grooves should extend in the proximal walls just inside the DEJ and not the corners of the box
- Circumferential slot 0.5–1.0 mm deep inside DEJ prepared by using number 33½ inverted cone bur
- Using pins like cemented, friction lock or threaded pins.
- Amalgapins.

Pulp Protection

Use pulp protective materials on pulpal floor and axial wall (**8.6K**).

Finishing of Enamel Walls and Margins

Finally finishing of walls and margins is done by removing all unsupported enamel. Beveling of enamel portion of gingival wall is done with the help of gingival margin trimmer. This helps to have full-length enamel rods at the gingival margin (**Figs. 8.6L and M**). Gingival cavosurface bevel is not indicated if gingival margin is placed gingival to cement oenamel junction (CEJ)
- Make cavosurface angle 90° butt joint to provide bulk to restoration, which in turn, provides maximum strength
- The final stage of cavity preparation is to clean the preparation thoroughly with water and air spray. Then dry it with moist air.

REVERSE CURVE

In class II preparations, extension of proximal area is important for elimination of caries and breaking proximal contacts. But in teeth with broader contacts, reversed S-shaped curve is given to both widen the box yet remove less tooth structure. Reverse curve is given to the proximal walls by curving them inward toward the contact area (**Fig. 8.7**). If excessive flare is given in these teeth, proximal walls will end past the axial

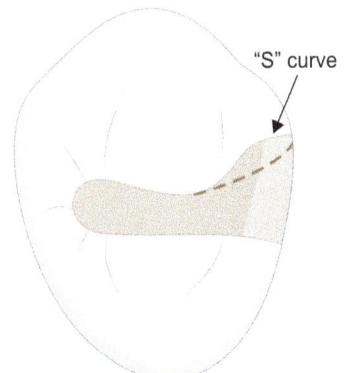

FIGURE 8.7: Reverse curve is given to the proximal walls by curving them inward towards the contact area to both widen the box yet remove the less tooth structure.

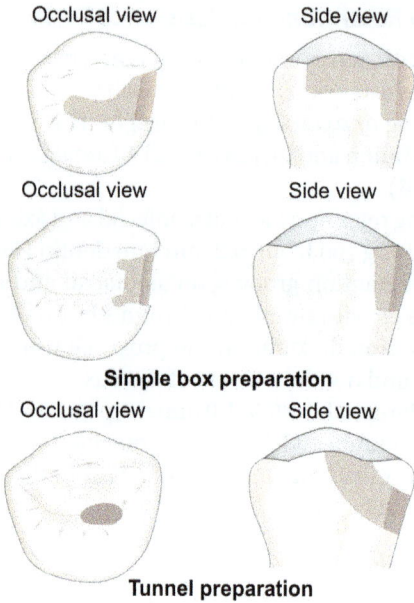

FIGURE 8.8: Modifications in class II design.

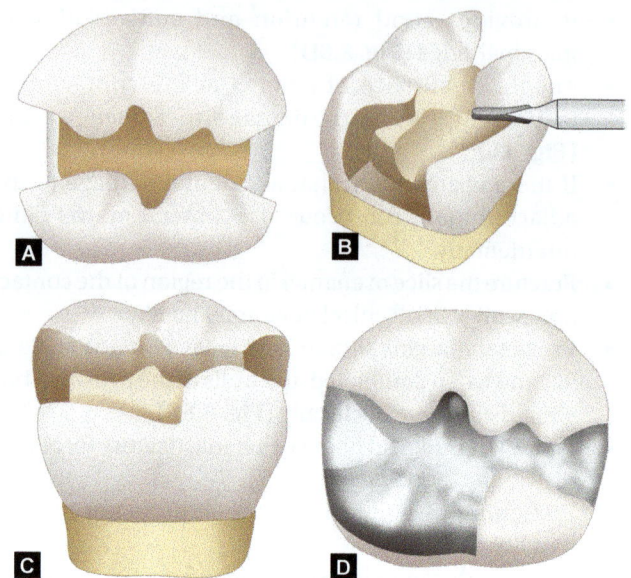

FIGURES 8.9A TO D: Schematic representation showing cusp capping for amalgam.

angle of tooth through the cusps resulting in weakening of tooth structure and fracture of restoration. Therefore, this S-shaped curve helps in increasing the resistance form of tooth and the amalgam restoration.

Advantages

- Conserves the sound tooth structure
- Preserves the triangular ridge of the affected cusp
- Flare of the proximal wall leaves the tangent to that outer tooth surface at 90° angle, this further increases the resistance form.

Modifications in Class II Design

Following modifications can be made in class II design (Fig. 8.8):
- *Slot preparation*
- *Simple box preparation*
- *Esthetic considerations*
- *Rotated teeth*
  Design features: They are similar as that of normally aligned teeth except that preparation depends on area of tooth which is in contact with adjacent tooth. Depending on angle of rotation, the proximal box is displaced facially or lingually.
- *Unusual outline form*
- *Conservative preparation for maxillary first molar and mandibular first premolar:*
  Conservative design in these teeth helps in the preservation of oblique ridge or the transverse ridge which protects the cuspal strength.
- Adjoining restoration
- Modification for abutment teeth
- *Cusp capping* (Figs. 8.9A to D):
  Cusp capping with amalgam is indicated if there is:
    - Faciolingual width of the cavity is more than 2/3rd of intercuspal distance.
    - Undermining of cusp by caries.

CLASS III CAVITY PREPARATION FOR AMALGAM RESTORATION (FIGS. 8.10A TO D)

Since amalgam is not esthetic restoration, it is not indicated for proximal surface of incisors and mesial surface of canines. *Amalgam for class III restoration is indicated in the distal surface of maxillary and mandibular canines especially, if:*
- The preparation is extensive with only minimal facial involvement
- The gingival margin primarily involves cementum
- Moisture control is difficult.

Contraindications

Class III amalgam restorations usually are contraindicated in esthetically important areas.

Advantages

- Amalgam restorations are stronger than other class III direct restorations.
- Easier to manipulate
- Less expensive to the patient.

Disadvantages

- Metallic color.
- Less conservative cavity preparation when compared to that of esthetic restorative materials

Initial Cavity Preparation

- Outline form includes only proximal surface. Shape of preparation is like a triangle with round corners. Labial side of triangle conforms more to the anatomy than with lingual side
- A punch cut is made using number 2 round bur on distolingual marginal ridge. Bur is positioned so that its long axis is perpendicular to the lingual surface of

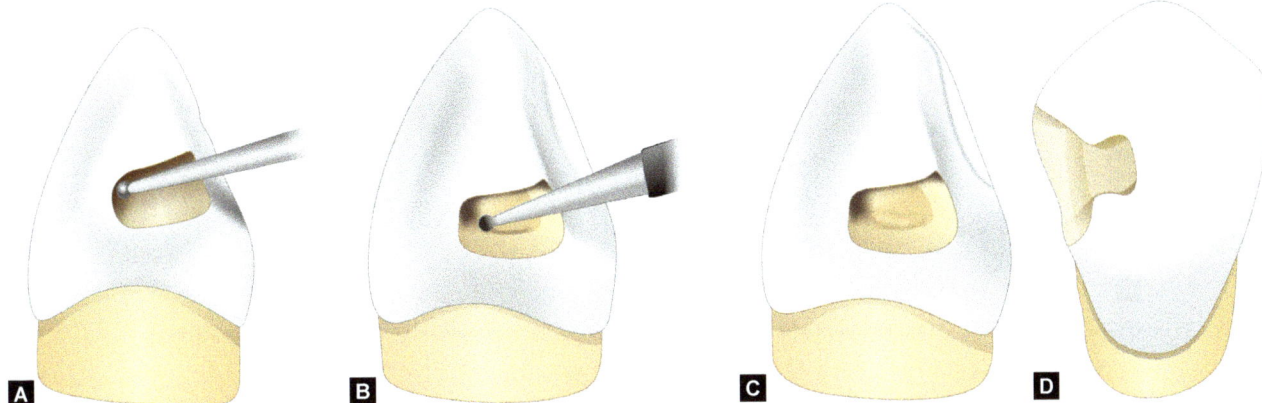

FIGURES 8.10A TO D: Schematic representation of Class III cavity preparation: (A) Class III cavity preparation; (B) Preparing the gingival retention form by placing round bur in axio-facio-gingival point angle and, moving the bur lingually to prepare the groove along the axiogingival line angle; (C) Completed gingival retention groove; (D) Completed class III preparation with lingual dovetail.

the tooth, but directed at a mesial angle as close to the adjacent tooth as possible **(Fig. 8.10A)**
- Preliminary shaping of preparation is completed with inverted cone bur with long axis of bur keeping perpendicular to the lingual surface of the tooth
- Penetration should be at a limited initial axial depth (i.e., 0.5–0.6 mm) inside the DEJ or at a 0.75–0.8 mm axial depth when the gingival margin is on the root surface (in cementum)
- This 0.75 mm axial depth on the root surface allows a 0.25-mm distance (the diameter of the No. 1/4 bur is 0.5 mm) between the retention groove and the gingival cavosurface margin
- Cavosurface angle should be about 90° at all margins. The facial, incisal, and gingival walls should meet the axial wall at approximately right angles
- Use a No. ½ round bur to accentuate the axial line angles, specially the axiogingival angle **(Figs. 8.10B and C)**.

Final Tooth Preparation

- Final tooth preparation involves removing any remaining infected dentin; protecting the pulp; developing secondary resistance and retention forms; finishing external walls; and cleaning, inspecting, and desensitizing or bonding.
- Remove any remaining infected carious dentin on the axial wall using a slow speed round bur and/or spoon excavators.
- **Resistance form is achieved by:**
  - Cavosurface margins of 90°
  - Enamel walls supported by sound dentin
  - Sufficient bulk of amalgam (minimal 1 mm thickness)
  - Rounded internal angles.
- **Retention form** is achieved by box-like preparation.
- **Secondary retention form** is provided by a gingival groove, an incisal cove, and lingual dovetail. The gingival retention groove is prepared by placing a No. ¼ round bur in the axio-facio-gingival point angle. Ideally, the direction of the gingival groove is slightly more gingival than axial and the direction of an incisal groove would be slightly more incisal than axial.

- Lingual dovetail is required for large preparations **(Fig. 8.10D)**. It is prepared only after completion of proximal portion because otherwise tooth structure needed for isthmus between proximal portion and dovetail might be removed when the proximal outline form is prepared.
- Pulp protection is provided by using base or liner on axial wall.
- Finishing of external walls is done to remove all unsupported enamel and to make cavosurface angle 90°. For rounding of junctions between different retentive grooves, angle former or GMT can be used.

CLASS V CAVITY PREPARATION

Class V lesion is present on the gingival third of facial and lingual surfaces of all teeth.

Indications
- Non-esthetic areas
- Areas where access and visibility are limited
- Areas where moisture control is difficult
- Subgingival lesions.

Contraindication
Esthetically important areas.

Initial Cavity Preparation
- Outline form is dictated by extension of caries. Outline resembles kidney or bean shape
- Preparation is started by keeping the bur perpendicular to long axis of tooth **(Fig. 8.11A)**
- Using an inverted cone bur of suitable size, enter the carious lesion (or existing restoration) to a limited initial axial depth of 0.5 mm inside the DEJ
- The depth is usually (1–1.25mm) total axial depth, depending on the incisogingival/occlusogingival location
- Extend the preparation incisally, gingivally, mesially and distally until the cavosurface margins are positioned in sound tooth structure to establish an initial axial depth of 0.5 mm inside the DEJ (if on the root surface, the axial

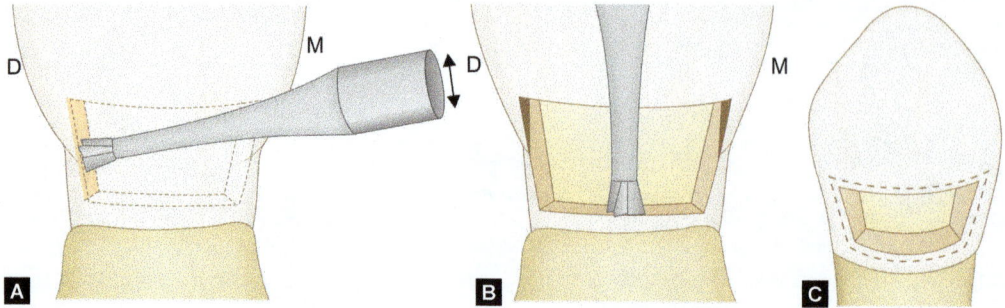

FIGURES 8.11A TO C: (A) Entry into lesion with the help of inverted cone bur; (B) Preparation of gingival wall; (C) Completed class V.

depth is 0.75 mm). A depth of 0.5 mm inside the DEJ will permit placement of necessary retention grooves without undermining the enamel **(Fig. 8.11B)**.

Final Cavity Preparation

- Final tooth preparation involves removal of any remaining infected dentin, pulp protection, retention form, finishing external walls, and final procedures of cleaning, inspecting, and desensitizing
- Remove any remaining infected axial wall dentin with a No. 2 or No. 4 bur
- For retention, give grooves incisally and gingivally along axioincisal and axiogingival line angles using a number 1/4th round bur, groove is prepared 0.2 mm into the dentin having depth of 0.25 mm
- Use hoe and chisel to finish the mesial, distal, and gingival walls.
- Finally, clean and inspect the cavity **(Fig. 8.11C)**.

VIVA QUESTIONS

Q.1 With which bur cavity preparation for amalgam is done?

Ans. Number 245 bur is used for cavity preparation because it's dimensions help in guiding ideal cavity preparation, i.e., depth of cavity preparation, 1.5 mm (half the length of bur, i.e., 3 mm), to preserve marginal ridge of width 1.6–2 mm (double the width of bur, i.e., 0.8 mm), rounded internal line angles, and convergent external walls (due to pear shape with rounded corners of the bur).

Q.2 What are features of primary resistance form for amalgam?

Ans.
- Box-shaped preparation with flat floors
- Minimum occlusal depth of 1.5 mm, to provide adequate thickness of amalgam
- Cavosurface angle of 900
- Restricting the extension of external walls so as to have strong marginal ridge areas with sufficient dentin support
- Maintaining minimal width of cavity which is not more than 1/4th of intercuspal distance
- Inclusion of all the weakened tooth structure
- Rounding off all the internal line and point angles
- Cusp capping in extensive caries for preserving cuspal strength.

Q.3 What are features of primary retention form for amalgam?

Ans.
- Occlusal convergence (about 2–5%) of buccal and lingual walls)
- Occlusal dovetail.

Q.4 How do you prepare the retention grooves?

Ans. By using No. 1/4 or 169 bur.

Q.5 What is reverse curve and what is it's significance?

Ans. Reverse curve is given to the proximal walls by curving them inward toward the contact area. If excessive flare is given in these teeth, proximal walls will end past the axial angle of tooth through the cusps resulting in weakening of tooth structure and fracture of restoration. Therefore, this S-shaped curve helps in increasing the resistance form of tooth and the amalgam restoration.

Significance:
- Conserves the sound tooth structure
- Preserves the triangular ridge of the affected cusp.

Q.6 What are different modifications in Class II design?

Ans.
- Slot preparation
- Simple box preparation
- Esthetic considerations
- For rotated teeth
- Adjoining restoration
- Modification for abutment teeth
- Cusp capping.

Q.7 When and where is class III preparation for amalgam is indicated?

Ans. Amalgam for class III restoration is indicated in the distal surface of maxillary and mandibular canines especially, if:
- Preparation is extensive with only minimal facial involvement
- Gingival margin primarily involves cementum
- Moisture control is difficult.

Q.8 What are indications of class V amalgam restorations?

Ans.
- Non-esthetic areas
- Areas where moisture control is difficult
- Subgingival caries.

Q.9 What should be the isthmus width of amalgam cavity?

Ans. 1/4th of intercuspal distance.

Q.10 What is ideal depth of amalgam cavity?

Ans. 1.5–2.0 mm total depth. 0.2–0.5 mm into the dentine.

Q.11 If class II tooth preparation involves only proximal surface, why do we make occlusal preparation also?

Ans. Occlusal preparation is done for convenience form. Since directly reaching the affected area with bur is difficult because of close proximity of the adjacent tooth therefore an occlusal preparation is made through which proximal surface is reached.

Q.12 What do you mean by breaking the contact?

Ans. In case of class II, III and IV caries, there is always a contact with the adjacent tooth. In these cases, whether caries are below or above the contact, the contact has to be broken so as to bring preparation margins into the embrasures for easy cleansability. If preparation margins end in non-cleansable areas, food stagnation in those areas may result in secondary caries.

Q.13 What should be ideal depth of the preparation?

Ans. Ideal depth should be 0.5 mm below DEJ, especially for non-adhesive materials. Since enamel is inelastic, it cannot be used for providing retentive and resistance form. So depth of preparation should be increased till elastic dentin is reached. Preparation should not end at dentino-enamel junction. This area is sensitive because of lateral branching of dentinal tubules and cytoplasmic extensions of odontoblasts.

Q.14 How is outline form affected by direction of enamel rods?

Ans. Enamel rods extend perpendicular from DEJ to enamel in a slightly wavy course. In vertical direction, they appear to converge towards a pit from DEJ, whereas they diverge as they move towards cusp tip from the DEJ.
In horizontal section, enamel rods flare out from DEJ towards outer surface.
Because of the direction of enamel rods, following walls are flared externally:
- Buccal and lingual walls of proximal box
- Mesial and distal walls of buccal and lingual boxes of class I extensions
- All walls of class V preparation
- If these walls are made to converge towards each other, this will result in unsupported enamel rods which may fracture later on.

Q.15 How does esthetics affect outline form?

Ans.
- For class III preparation, labial enamel is kept intact
- Preparation margins should be kept into embrasures for better esthetics
- Reverse curve is given in maxillary premolars.

Q.16 What is as isthmus and its significance?

Ans. Isthmus is the narrow connection between two portions of a preparation (occlusal and proximal). Most of the restoration failures occur at isthmus area. If it is very narrow, restoration will be very weak at that area. If isthmus is very wide, the remaining tooth structure will become very weak.

Q.17 When should two adjacent preparation be connected?

Ans. If healthy tooth structure between two preparations is less then 0.5 mm, the two adjacent preparations are joined to form one large preparation. For example, mesial and distal pits of maxillary first molar.

Q.18 How is retention achieved in amalgam restoration?

Ans.
- Occlusal convergence—inverted truncated shape
- Occlusal dovetail
- Undercuts.

Q.19 What is significance of dovetail?

Ans. It helps in retention in proximal direction. In other words, dovetail holds the proximal restoration from dislodging proximally.

Q.20 What precautions should be taken while removing deep carious lesion?

Ans. Use slow-speed handpiece with the round bur or spoon excavator that will fit in the carious lesion used with light force and a wiping motion.
Forces for removal of infective dentin should be directed laterally and not towards the center of the carious lesion.

Q.21 Which instrument is used for removal of unsupported enamel rods?

Ans. Chisel, hoe or hatchet is used for removal of unsupported rods.

Q.22 For smoothening the gingival seat which instrument is used?

Ans. GMT is used for making gingival seat.

Q.23 How do you check convenience form?

Ans. After tooth preparation, insert the small amalgam condenser into all parts of preparation. If even the small instrument does not enter some parts of tooth preparation, tooth preparation is widened.

Q.24 Where is gingival seat prepared for class II preparation?

Ans. Just beyond the caries or contact point whichever is more.

Q.25 What is ideal depth of tooth preparation for amalgam restoration? What happens with increase or decrease in depth?

Ans.
- 1.5-2 mm. If <1.5 mm: Inadequate space for amalgam: poor resistance and retention form
- If >1.5 mm: Results in decreased remaining dentin thickness: increased sensitivity and post operative pain.

Q.26 What is ideal width of tooth preparation for amalgam restoration? What happens with increase or decrease in width?

Ans.
- 1/3rd-1/4th of intercuspal distance. If <1/3rd-1/4th of intercuspal distance: reduces convenience form, i.e., accessibility for the instruments.
- If >1/3rd-1/4th of intercuspal distance: undermine cuspal strength: poor resistance and retention form.

Q.27 What is ideal width of marginal ridge?

Ans. 1.5 mm for premolars 2 mm for molars marginal ridge width lesser than 1.6 mm results in undermining of the marginal ridge and reduced resistance form.

Q.28 Where should be the gingival seat placed in class II tooth preparation?

Ans. It is placed cervical to the contact point so as to break contact with the adjacent tooth and to have restoration with self-cleansable margins.

Q.29 What will happen if gingival seat is placed very shallow at the same level with pulpal floor?

Ans. Inadequate removal of the proximal carious lesion and inadequate retention form.

Q.30 What should be the clearance from adjacent tooth in class II tooth preparation?

Ans. 0.5 mm. Clearance >0.5 mm: excessive loss of tooth structure, unesthetic display of amalgam facially and chances of damaging interdental gingival clearance <0.5 mm: inadequate caries removal and difficulty in placement of matrix band.

Chapter 9

Tooth Preparation for Direct Composite Resin and Glass Ionomer Cements

Chapter Outline

- General principles for tooth preparation for composite restorations
- Steps of composite restoration on teeth
- Repair of composite restorations
- Steps for placement of glass ionomer cement (GIC)

Resin composite is the most common alternative to dental amalgam. The use of composite to restore form and function for both anterior and posterior teeth has been widely suggested.

Direct composite resin has been discussed as a material in chapter 4. In this chapter we'll be discussing different tooth preparations for composite resin restorations.

GENERAL PRINCIPLES FOR TOOTH PREPARATION FOR COMPOSITE RESTORATIONS

- Conservation of tooth structure
- Variable depth of pulpal floor and axial wall
- Rough tooth preparation walls to facilitate bonding
- Enamel bevel to increase the surface area for etching and bonding
- Butt joint on root surface.

Pre-requisites to have a successful composite restoration:
- Tooth preparation according to size and location of the lesion
- Moisture control by rubber dam placement
- Thorough knowledge of etching and bonding
- Composite placement techniques and light curing
- Finishing and polishing of the restoration.

STEPS OF COMPOSITE RESTORATION ON TEETH

- Oral prophylaxis
- Shade selection
- Isolation
- Tooth preparation
- Pulp protection
- Matrix application
- Etching and bonding
- Composite placement
- Polymerization of composite resins
- Final contouring, finishing, and polishing of composite restoration.

Oral Prophylaxis

Operating site is cleaned using slurry of pumice in order to remove plaque, calculus, and superficial stains prior to the procedure and improves bonding to composite resins.

Shade Selection (Figs. 9.1A and B)

- Shade matching of wet teeth should be carried in natural daylight
- Dentin shade is selected from cervical third of tooth, and enamel shade is selected from its incisal third

TABLE 9.1: Indications and contraindications for composite restorations

Indications of composite restorations	Contraindications of composite restorations
I, II, III, IV, and V tooth preparations	Difficult moisture control
Esthetic improvement	Heavy occlusal stresses
Erosion, abrasion or hypoplastic defects	High caries susceptibility and poor oral hygiene
Core build up	Subgingival or root caries

TABLE 9.2: Advantages and disadvantages of composite restoration.

Advantages	Disadvantages
■ Good esthetics	■ Polymerization shrinkage can result in postoperative sensitivity and secondary caries
■ Conservation of tooth structure because of adhesive tooth preparation	
■ Low thermal conductivity	■ More technique sensitive than amalgam
■ Because of adhesion to tooth, there is increased retention and strengthening of remaining tooth structure	■ Less resistance to wear especially the microfilled composites
■ Since it does not contain metal, so no risk of galvanism	■ Takes more time for placement
	■ Expensive in comparison to amalgam restoration

- To confirm final shade, a small increment of selected composite is placed adjacent to the area to be restored and then light cured for matching.

Isolation

Isolation is best done by using rubber dam, though it can be done using cotton rolls, saliva ejector, and retraction cord.

Tooth Preparation

Designs of Tooth Preparation for Composites

Following three types of designs or their combination are most commonly prepared for composites:

Conventional

Conventional design is similar to the tooth preparation for amalgam restoration, except that there is less outline extension and preparation walls are made rough. It is *indicated for* preparations located on root surface.

Features:
- Prepared enamel margins should be 90 degree or greater.
- Butt joint cavosurface margin is made on root surfaces
- Prepared tooth surface is roughened to increase the bonding.

Beveled Conventional Tooth Preparation (Figs. 9.2A to F)

This design is almost similar to conventional design but enamel margins are beveled. It is indicated to restore large class III, IV, and V preparations **(Figs. 9.3 and 9.4)**.

Steps:
- Approach carious area palatally with round bur and move the bur in incisogingival direction
- Initial depth of axial wall should be 0.75 mm deep gingivally and 1.25 mm deep incisally. This results in the axial wall depth of 0.2 mm into the dentin
- Axial wall should follow contour of the tooth, i.e., shape of axial wall should be convex outwardly
- Keep external walls of tooth preparation perpendicular to the enamel surface with all enamel margins beveled.
- Prepare bevels using flat end tapering fissure diamond bur at cavosurface margins. Bevel should be 0.2–0.5 mm wide at an angle of 45° to external tooth surface.

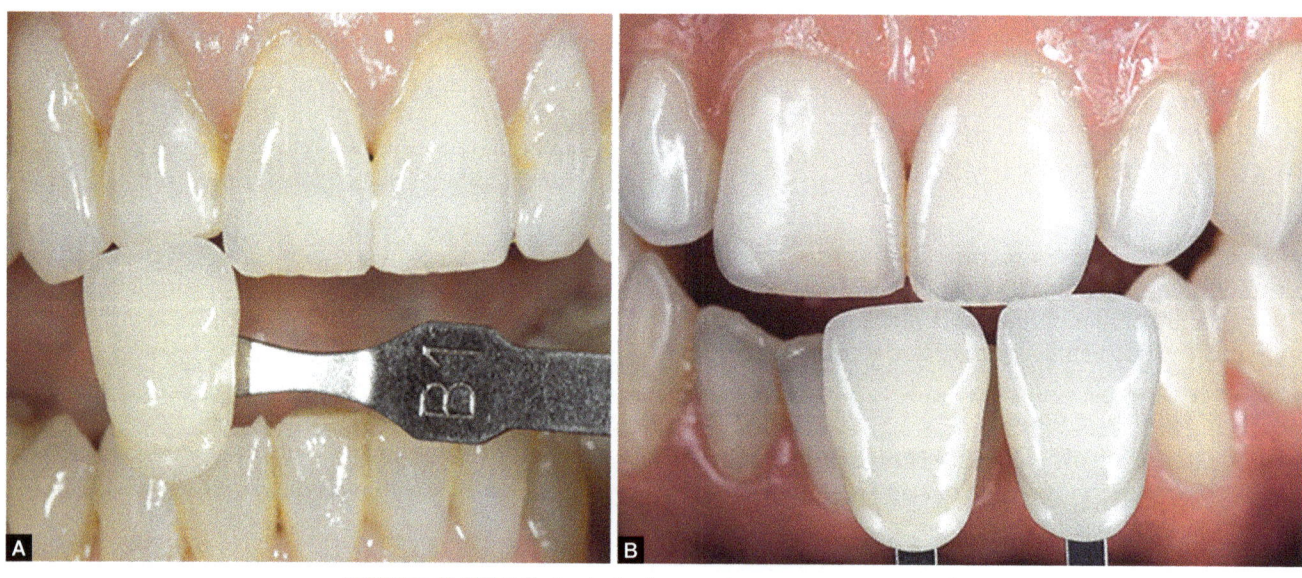

FIGURES 9.1A AND B: Shade selection for composite restoration in anterior teeth.

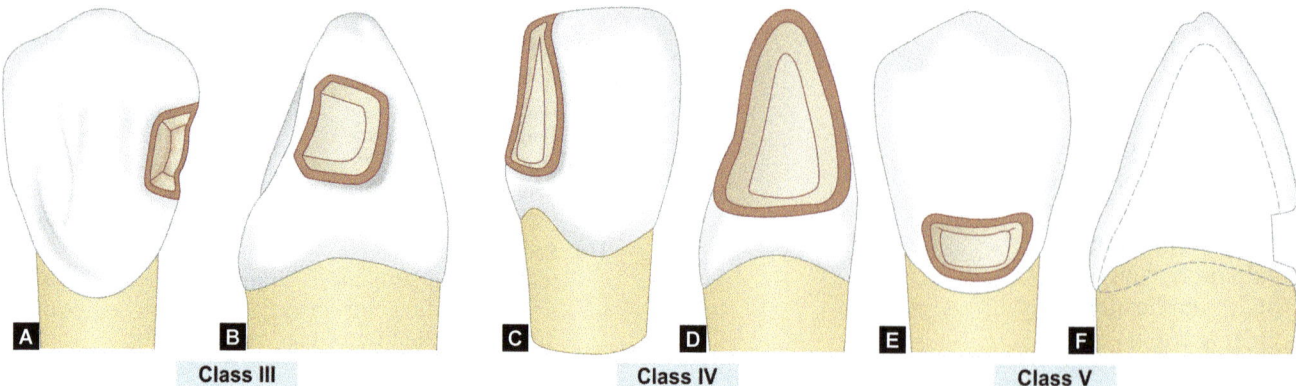

FIGURES 9.2A TO F: Beveled conventional tooth preparation (Dark brown outline of the tooth preparations represent beveled area).

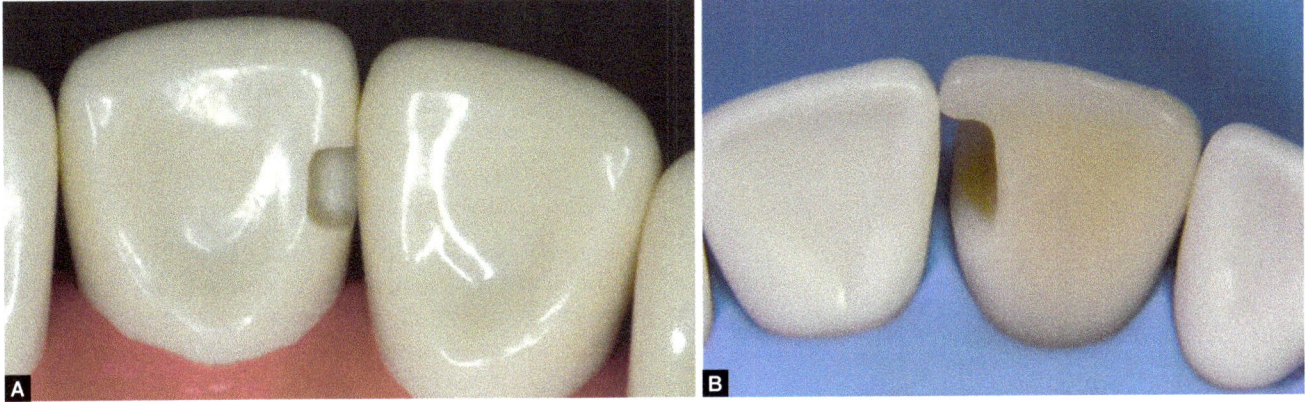

FIGURES 9.3A AND B: (A) Conventional box shape preparation; (B) Beveled conventional tooth preparation.

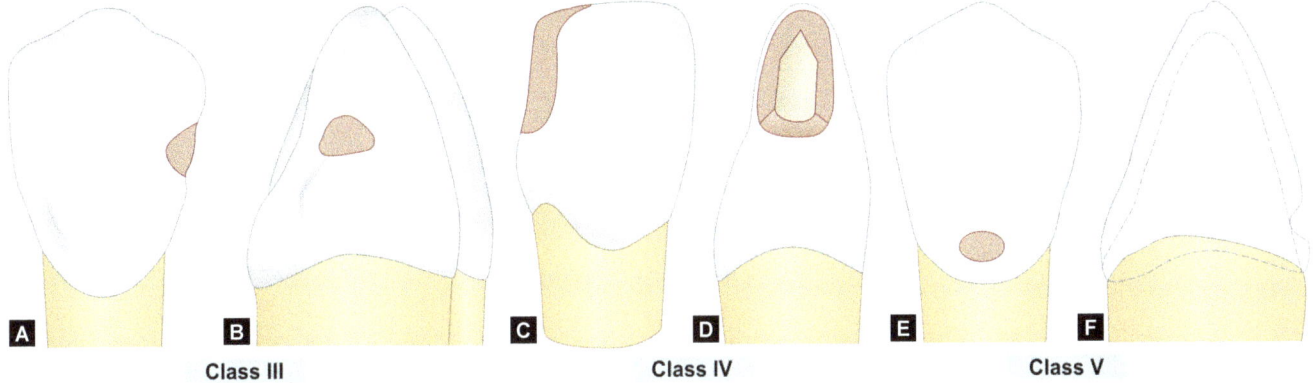

FIGURES 9.4A TO F: Modified conservative tooth preparation. It has scooped-out appearance without definite line angles. It is indicated for initial or small carious lesions.

Modified (Conservative Tooth Preparation) (Figs. 9.4A to F)

It has scooped-out appearance without definite line angles. It is indicated for initial or small carious lesions.

Features
- Preparation has scooped out appearance
- It does not have specified wall configuration or pulpal and axial wall depth
- Extent and depth of the preparation depends upon the extent and the depth of carious lesion.

While approaching a class III lesion, direction for **entry of bur is preferred from palatal side** because of the following reasons.
- Preservation facial enamel for esthetics
- Color matching not critical
- Unsupported facial enamel can be preserved for bonding with composite resin
- Future discoloration of composite is less visible.

Labial approach is indicated when:
- There is involvement of labial enamel
- Rotated teeth are present making palatal approach difficult
- Faulty old restoration placed facially needs replacement.

Pulp Protection
- In case of shallow cavities, application of bonding agent is sufficient for pulp protection
- In case of deep preparations, pulp protection is done using a light-cured calcium hydroxide base followed by GIC. Zinc oxide-eugenol should not be used as a sub-base because it inhibits the polymerization of resins.

Matrix Application
Following matrices can be used resin restorations:
- Tofflemire matrix retainer and band
- Clear polyester matrices
- Contact forming instruments
- Sectional matrices and contact rings like Palodent-BiTine Ring System, Composi-Tight matrix, precontoured sectional matrix bands, etc.

Etching and Bonding
- Apply 37% phosphoric acid etchant for 15–20 seconds with a syringe or brush on to the prepared surfaces. Properly etched surface shows frosted appearance
- After etching, apply a primer and bonding agent using disposable applicator tips and polymerize it with curing light.

Composite Placement Instruments and Method (Figs. 9.5A and B)

Hand instruments used for placing composites are usually made up of coating of Teflon, so as to avoid sticking of composite to the instrument. These instruments are simple and easy-to-use.

Irrespective of location of restoration, composites should be placed and polymerized in increments to ensure complete polymerization of the composite mass **(Figs. 9.6A to D)**.

Polymerization Using Curing Lamps (Fig. 9.7)

Most commonly used light source is quartz bulb with a tungsten filament in a halogen environment.

Tungsten-quartz halogen curing unit: Tungsten-quartz halogen (QHL) curing unit is conventional unit which consists of quartz bulb with tungsten filament. It uses visible light in the wavelength in the range of 410–500 nm.

It is inexpensive but intensity of its bulb decreases with time.

Plasma arc curing (PAC) unit: Plasma arc curing (PAC) produces high intensity light so it has short curing time due

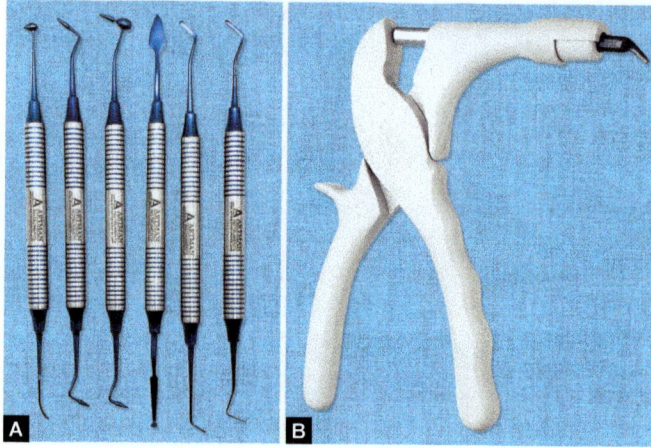

FIGURES 9.5A AND B: (A) Hand instruments; (B) Composite gun.

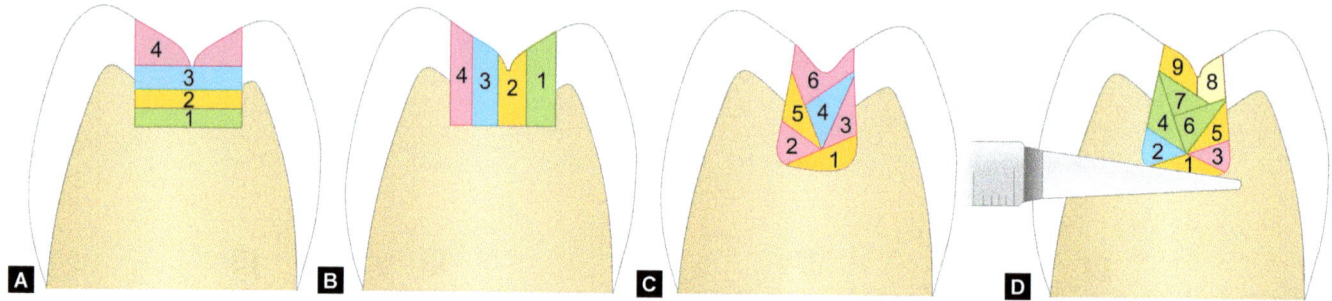

FIGURES 9.6A TO D: Incremental layering technique: (A) Horizontal layering technique; (B) Vertical layering technique; (C) Oblique layering technique; (D) Three-site technique.

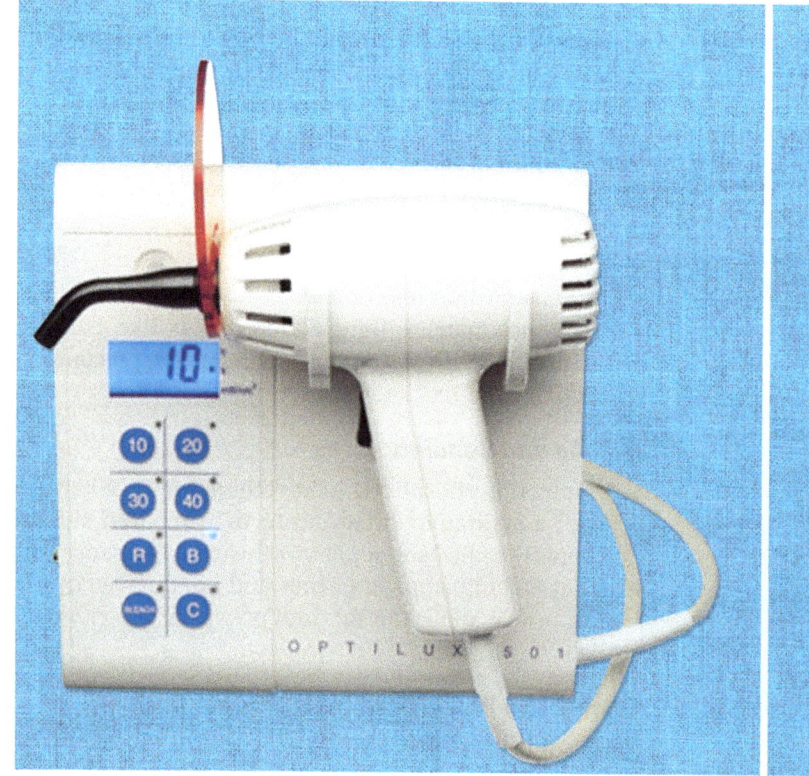
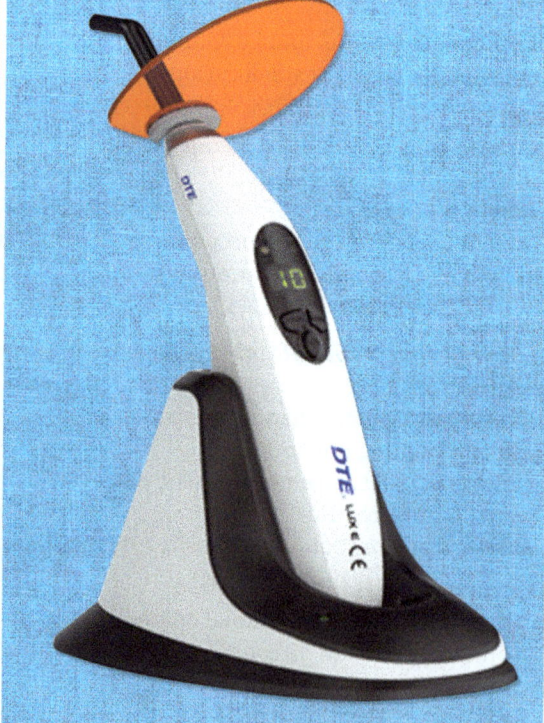

FIGURE 9.7: Curing lamps.

to high energy output but it is expensive and heat production need to be controlled.

Light-emitting diode unit: Light-emitting diode (LED) unit emits powerful blue light.

This light falls in narrow wavelength range of 440–480 nm. This corresponds to range of camphorquinone photoinitiator found in most of composite resins. Its low power consumption, does not require filter, causes minimal changes in light output over time but it is expensive

Argon laser curing unit: Argon laser light has wavelength of 490 nm, it causes uniform polymerization which is not affected by distance. It can cure to the greater depth but chances of damage to pulp can occur due to rise in temperature.

Final Contouring and Finishing

Final finishing and contouring can be done immediately after placement of restoration. Amount of contouring required after final curing can be minimized by careful placement technique. 12, 16, or 30 fluted carbide burs are used for gross finishing. Then, fine finishing diamond burs are used for final finishing. Scalpel blade and carving instruments are used to refine gingival margins and interproximal area. Flexible disks with soft flexible backing and rubber finishing and polishing points are used for finishing.

Features of Class II Composite Tooth Preparation (Figs. 9.8A to C)

- Tooth preparation for class II has decreased pulpal depth of axial wall
- Proximal box preparation has cavosurface angle at right angles to the enamel surface facially and lingually
- Bevels on occlusal surface are optional due to direction of enamel rods
- Gingival floors should clear the contact apically and they should be butt joined.

Figures 9.9 to 9.12 showing placement of composite restorations in different types of tooth preparations.

REPAIR OF COMPOSITE RESTORATIONS

- For repair, the roughen the old restoration with a diamond stone
- Etch the enamel margins
- Apply primer and adhesive
- Place composite and then finish and polish it.

TOOTH PREPARATION FOR GLASS IONOMER RESTORATION

Glass ionomer cement (GIC) has been discussed as a material in chapter 4, in this chapter we'll be discussing different tooth preparations for GIC restorations.

Table showing generalized indications and contraindications of using GIC as restoration.

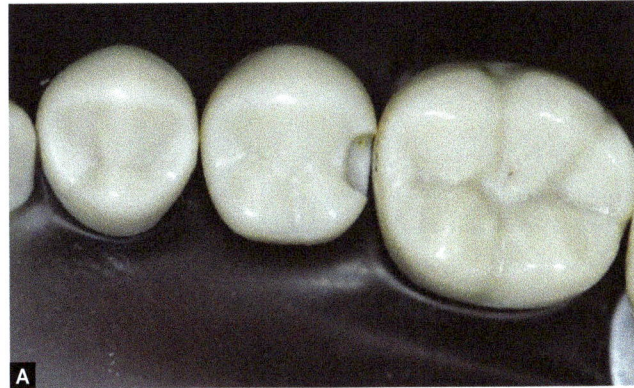
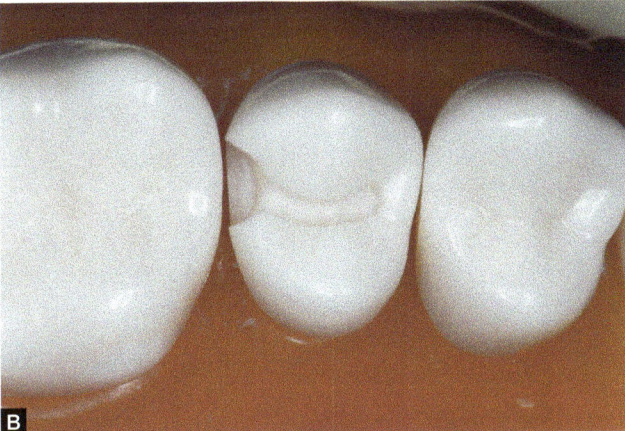
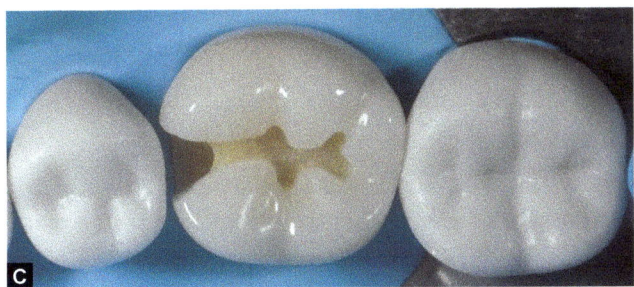

FIGURES 9.8A TO C: Tooth preparation for composite restoration: (A) Without involving occlusal surface; (B and C) Involving the occlusal surface.

Indications	Contraindications
For restorations of small class I (buccal and palatal pits), III and V lesions	In stress-bearing areas like class I, class II, and class IV preparations because glass ionomers lack fracture toughness
As luting agents	In mouth breathers because restoration may become opaque, brittle, and may fracture over time
As liners and bases	In patients with xerostomia because restorations can become opaque, brittle, and disintegrate over a short period of time
As pit and fissure sealants in high caries risk patients	In areas requiring esthetics like veneering of anterior teeth

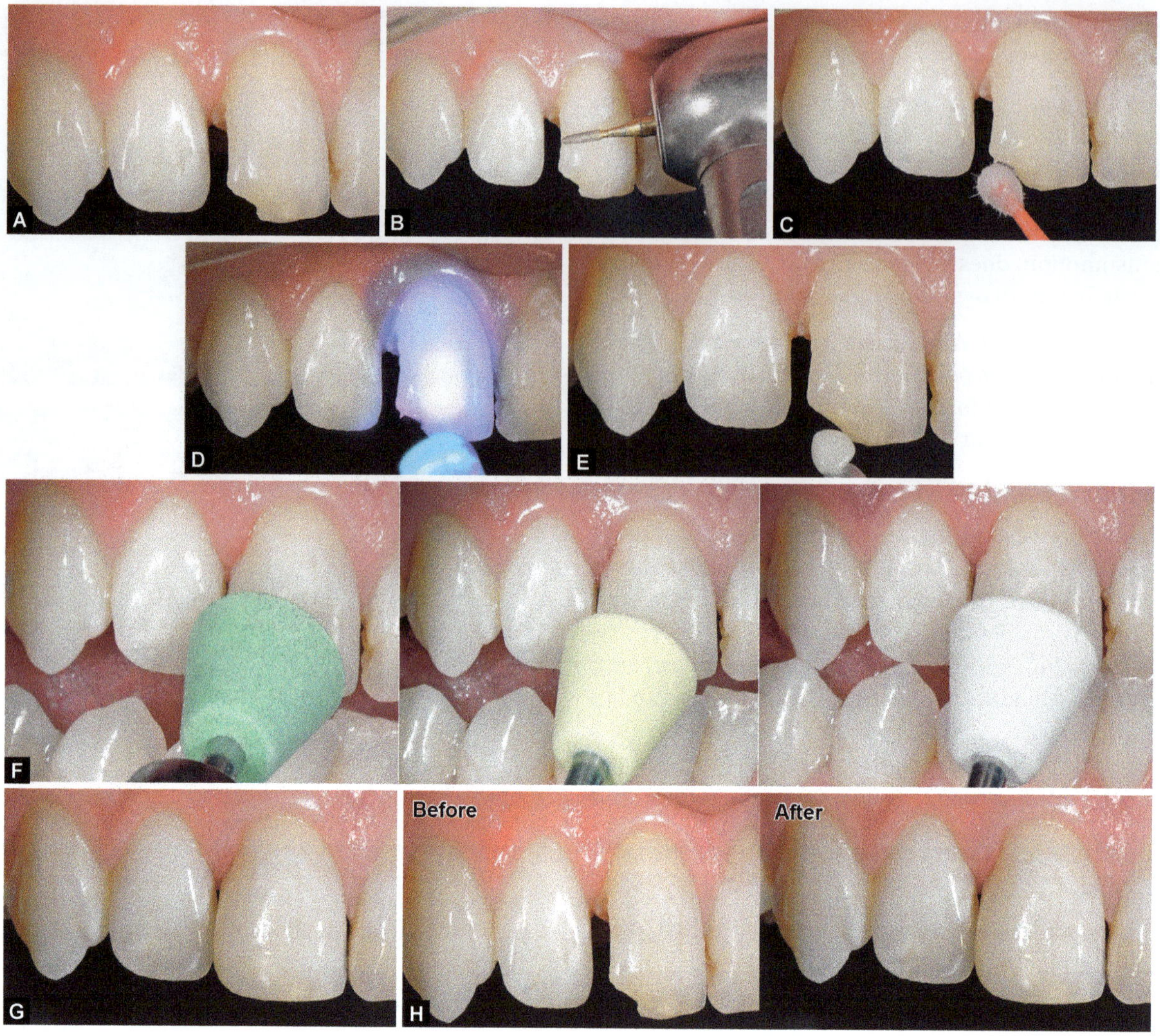

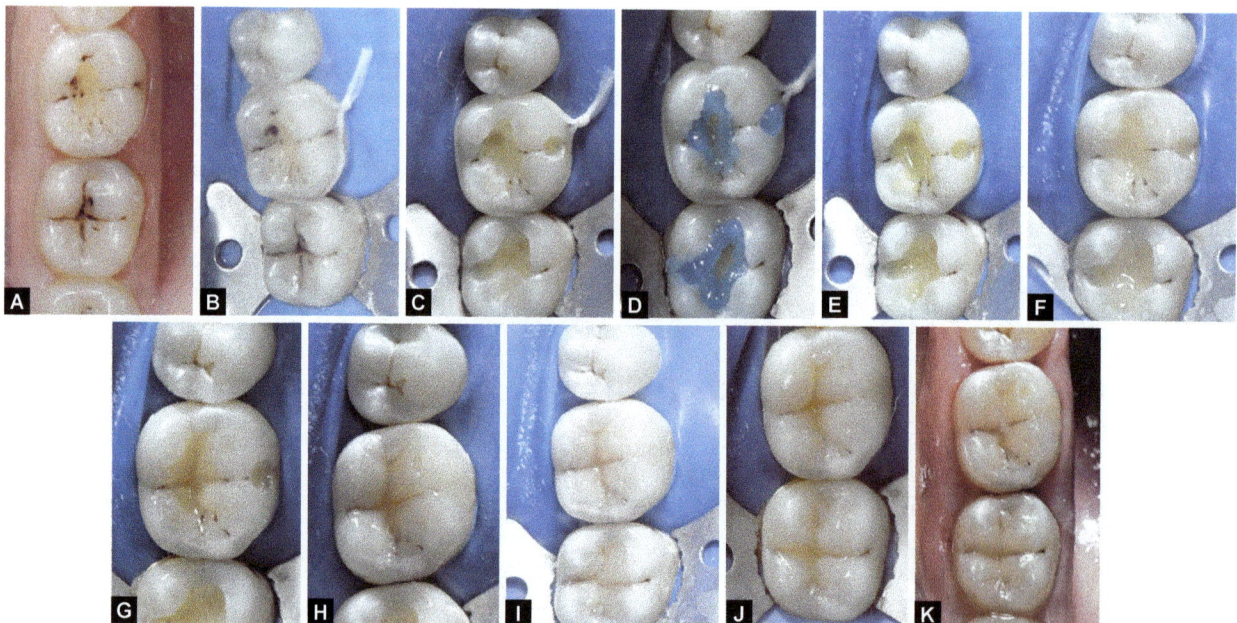

FIGURES 9.9A TO H: Restoration of maxillary central incisor with class IV lesion: (A) Preoperative photograph; (B) Tooth preparation; (C) Application of bonding agent after etching and rinsing; (D) Light curing; (E) Composite build-up; (F) Finishing and polishing of restoration; (G) Final restoration; (H) Photograph of before and after restoration of tooth.

FIGURES 9.10A TO K: Steps of class I cavity preparation and restoration using composite: (A) Preoperative photograph; (B) Isolation of teeth; (C) Tooth preparation; (D) Application of etchant; (E) Application of bonding agent; (F to J) Composite build-up; (K) Final restoration.

Tooth Preparation for Direct Composite Resin and Glass Ionomer Cements

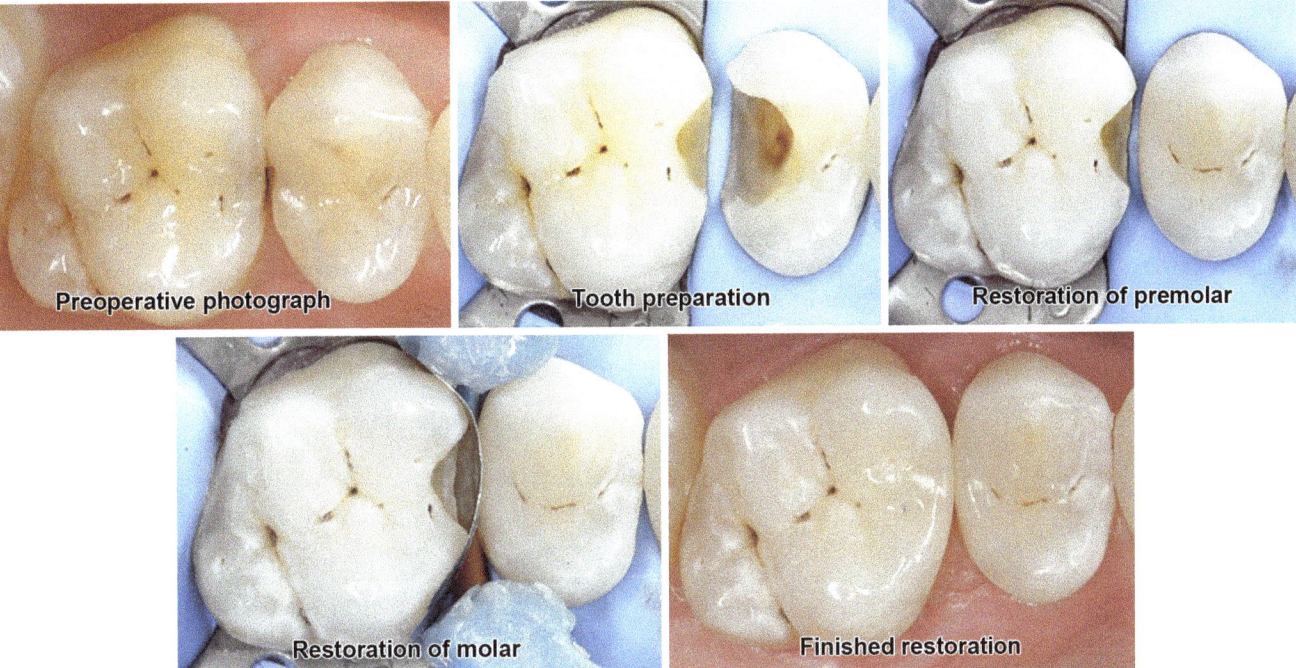

FIGURE 9.11: Class II composite preparation not involving the occlusal surface.

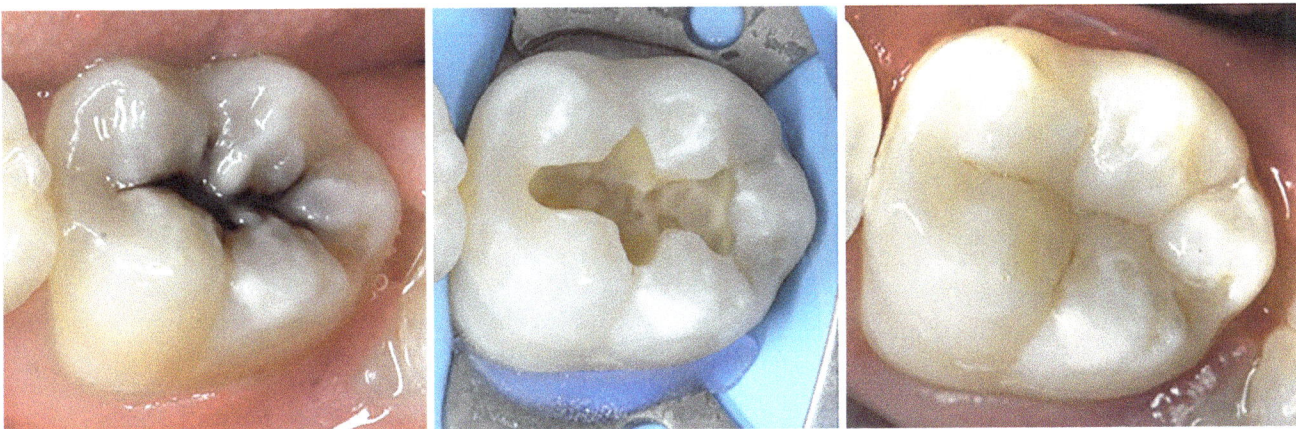

FIGURE 9.12: Moderate class I direct composite restorations.

STEPS FOR PLACEMENT OF GLASS IONOMER CEMENT (GIC)

1. Isolation
2. Tooth preparation
3. Surface conditioning
4. Manipulation of cement
5. Finishing and polishing
6. Surface protection.

Isolation

Saliva control is important for successful glass ionomer restorations. If moisture contaminates the cement during manipulation and setting, the gel will weaken and wash out prematurely. Commonly used methods for isolation are rubber dam, retraction cords, cotton rolls, and saliva ejectors.

Tooth Preparation

Tooth preparation for glass ionomer cement is done in two ways:

Cavity Preparation

Glass ionomer can be used for class III, class V, and small class I and II tooth preparations.

Class III Tooth Preparation

Glass ionomer is the material of choice to restore the class III lesion when caries extends onto the root surface.

Indications:
- In patients with high caries index
- When caries extend onto the root surface
- In areas with low occlusal stress.

Steps:
- ***Outline form:*** Using a small inverted cone bur, make an access through lingual marginal ridge. Extend the bur toward incisal or gingival area depending on caries.
- ***Retention and resistance form:*** Since retention in glass ionomer is chemical in nature, so placing undercuts and dovetail is not mandatory.
- ***Convenience form:*** Lingual wall is sometimes broken for access in maxillary teeth.
- ***Pulpal protection:*** If less than 0.5 mm of remaining dentin is present, calcium hydroxide liner is placed for pulp protection.

Class V Tooth Preparation
Indications:
- Patients with high caries incidence
- When esthetics is not of primary concern
- In root surface lesions.

Steps:
- ***Outline form:*** External outline form is limited to the extension of the lesion.
- ***Retention and resistance form:*** Retention is primarily achieved by chemical bonding, so nothing special is required for added retention.
- ***Pulp protection:*** Same as for class III.

Class I Tooth Preparation
Indications:
- Deep pits and fissures
- Recently erupted teeth in patients with high caries index.

Steps:
- ***Outline form:*** Use a small round bur to enter in the fissure and remove carious dentin. After this, use fine tapered fissure bur to widen the fissures.
- ***Retention form***: Since glass ionomer cement bonds chemically to tooth structure, so no special retention aid is required.
- ***Convenience form***: Widen the fissures properly for better flow of the glass ionomer.

Surface Conditioning
For better adhesion of GIC, many conditioning agents have been used. Polyacrylic acid is the most commonly used conditioner. It:
- Removes smear layer
- Promotes ion exchange
- Chemically cleans the dentin
- Increases surface energy.

Manipulation of the Cement
Manipulation of GIC has been explained in Chapter 4, page 42.

Finishing and Polishing
- During initial phase of cement setting, it is always preferred to delay finishing and polishing of glass ionomer cements.
- After placing the restoration, gross finishing is done following the matrix removal. Before starting the finishing procedure, the surface of restoration is coated with protective agent. Final finishing of restoration is done with the help of superfine diamond points, soflex disk, and abrasive strips in moist condition. After final finishing and polishing is done, surface of restoration is protected using petroleum jelly, varnish or bonding agent.

Surface Protection
Since glass ionomers show sensitivity to both moisture contamination and surface desiccation, the newly placed restoration should always be protected with the help of resin-bonding agent, cocoa butter, petroleum jelly or varnish.

VIVA QUESTIONS
Composite Restoration Technique

Q.1 Which chemical is used to etch enamel?
Ans. 37% phosphoric acid etchant for 15–20 seconds.

Q.2 How will you improve marginal adaptation in a composite restoration?
Ans. By beveling and acid etching.

Q.3 What is the approximate stress caused by polymerization shrinkage of composite?
Ans. 5MPa.

Q.4 Types of tooth preparation designs for composite restoration.
Ans.
- Conventional
- Beveled conventional
- Modified conservative
  - BOX
  - SLOT.

Q.5 Which cement is contraindicated under composite restoration and why?
Ans. Zinc oxide eugenol cement because it interferes with polymerization of composite restorations.

Q.6 Which laser light can be used for composite curing?
Ans. Argon.

Q.7 Name the technique for placement of composite restoration.
Ans. Composites should be placed and polymerized in increments to ensure complete polymerization of the composite mass.

Q.8 What are the different types of curing lamps used for composite restoration?
Ans.
- Tungsten-quartz halogen curing unit
- Plasma arc curing (PAC) unit
- Light-emitting diode unit
- Argon laser curing unit.

Q.9 What are the different methods to reduce polymerization shrinkage?
Ans.
- Incremental placement of composites
- Modifications in curing techniques.

Q.10 What region of tooth is more challenging to restore with composites?
Ans. Cervical third.

Q.11 What is the purpose of acid etching?
Ans. Etching is the process of increasing the surface reactivity by demineralizing the superficial calcium layer and thus creating the enamel tags.

Q.12 What are features of class II composite tooth preparation?
Ans.
- Tooth preparation for class II has decreased pulpal depth of axial wall
- Proximal box preparation has cavosurface angle at right angles to the enamel surface facially and lingually
- Bevels on occlusal surface are optional due to direction of enamel rods
- Gingival floors should clear the contact apically and they should be butt joined.

Q.13 What are the advantages of GIC restoration?
Ans.
- Chemical adhesion to the tooth surface, so conservative tooth preparation
- Anticariogenic effect due to fluoride release.

Q.14 What are general principles for tooth preparation for composite restorations?
Ans.
- Conservation of tooth structure
- Variable depth of pulpal floor and axial wall
- Rough tooth preparation walls to facilitate bonding
- Enamel bevel to increase the surface area for etching and bonding
- Butt joint on root surface.

Q.15 What are pre-requisites to have a successful composite restoration?
Ans.
- Moisture control by rubber dam placement
- Thorough knowledge of etching and bonding
- Composite placement techniques and light curing
- Finishing and polishing of the restoration.

Q.16 What are indications of composite restorations?
Ans.
- I, II, III, IV, and V tooth preparations
- Esthetic improvement
- Erosion, abrasion or hypoplastic defects
- Core build up.

Q.17 What are contraindications of composite restorations.
Ans.
- Difficult moisture control
- Heavy occlusal stresses
- High caries susceptibility and poor oral hygiene
- Subgingival or root caries.

Q.18 While approaching a class III lesion, why direction for entry of bur is preferred from palatal side?
Ans. Because of the following reasons:
- Preservation facial enamel for esthetics
- Color matching not critical
- Unsupported facial enamel can be preserved for bonding with composite resin
- Future discoloration of composite is less visible.

Q.19 When is labial approach is indicated?
Ans.
- Involvement of labial enamel
- Presence of rotated teeth making palatal approach difficult
- Faulty old restoration placed facially needs replacement.

Q.20 What are indications of GIC as restoration material in class III lesion?
Ans.
- In patients with high caries index
- When caries extend onto the root surface.

Q.21 What are indications of GIC as restoration material in class V lesion?
Ans.
- Patients with high caries incidence
- When esthetics is not of primary concern
- In root surface lesions.

Q.22 What is purpose of using conditioner before placing GIC restoration?
Ans.
- Removal of smear layer
- Chemically cleans the dentin
- Increase in surface energy.

Q.23 Why surface protection is needed in GIC restoration?
Ans. Since glass ionomers show sensitivity to both moisture contamination and surface desiccation, the newly placed restoration should always be protected with the help of resin-bonding agent, cocoa butter, petroleum jelly or varnish.

Chapter 10: Cast Metal Restorations

Chapter Outline

- Steps of inlay preparation
- Cavity preparation for class II gold inlays
- Wax pattern fabrication
- Spruing the wax pattern
- Washing of wax pattern
- Investing the wax pattern
- Burnout of wax pattern/wax elimination and heating
- Casting machines
- Melting the alloy
- Trying in the casting
- Cementation of the casting

DEFINITIONS (FIG. 10.1)

Inlay

It is an indirect intracoronal restoration fabricated extraorally and then cemented on prepared tooth.

Class II Inlay

This is an indirect restoration that caps one or more cusps of a posterior tooth but not all the cusps.

Onlay

It is an indirect restoration which is partly intracoronal and partly extracoronal that covers all cusps of a posterior tooth.

TABLE 10.1: Indications and contraindications for cast metal restorations.

Indications	Contraindications
■ Extensive tooth involvement	■ Not indicated in esthetic areas because of metallic color
■ Correction of occlusion	■ In patients with poor oral hygiene and high caries index
■ Already present cast metal restoration to prevent galvanic current	■ In young permanent teeth because of chances of iatrogenic pulp exposure due to high pulp horns
■ Proximal margins extending subgingivally	■ In patients having restorations with different metals since dissimilar metals cause galvanic currents when they come in contact with each other

TABLE 10.2: Advantages and disadvantages of cast metal restoration.

Advantages	Disadvantages
■ Optimal contacts and contours	■ Microleakage
	■ Technique sensitive
■ Good wear resistance	■ Unesthetic
■ Biocompatible	■ More number of appointments
■ Good strength	■ Expensive

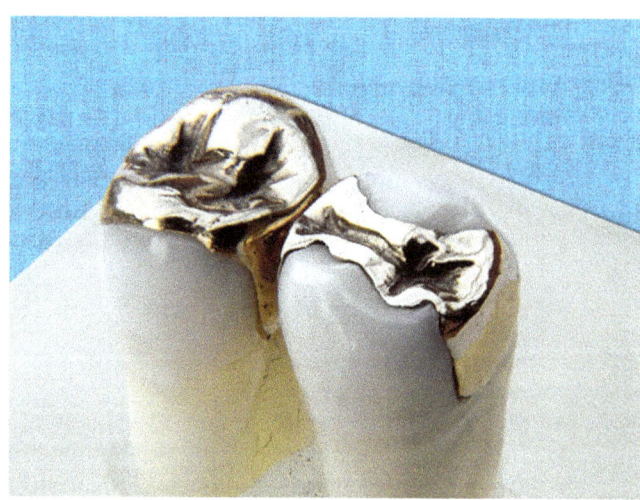

FIGURE 10.1: Inlay and onlay on posterior teeth.

STEPS OF INLAY PREPARATION

- Tooth preparation
- Impression taking
- Die making
- Wax pattern
- Investing of the pattern and creating the mold
- Gold casting.

CAVITY PREPARATION FOR CLASS II GOLD INLAYS (FIGS. 10.2A TO L)

Instruments Used for Cavity Preparation for Cast Metal Restorations

- No. 271. Tungsten carbide tapering fissure bur with 0.8 mm width
- 169L Tapered fissure bur with 0.5 mm width
- No. 8865 slender fine grit flam shaped diamond for preparing cavosurface bevels

Cast Metal Restorations

- Chisel, hatchet and wedelstaedt for removal of undermining enamel and producing primary and secondary bevels
- Spoon excavator for removal of remaining soft caries
- Gingival margin trimmer for creating gingival bevels.

Initial Tooth Preparation
Occlusal Outline Form

- Penetrate the tooth with No. 271 bur held parallel to long axis of the tooth to initial depth of 1.5 mm
- Keeping the bur parallel, extend the tooth preparation while maintaining the initial pulpal depth of 1.5 mm
- Give dovetail on mesial side of occlusal preparation to resist distal displacement of final restoration
- Conserve the mesial marginal ridge and if any faulty shallow fissure is present, manage it by enameloplasty or including it in cavosurface bevel
- Maintain the isthmus width of 1/3rd of intercuspal distance.

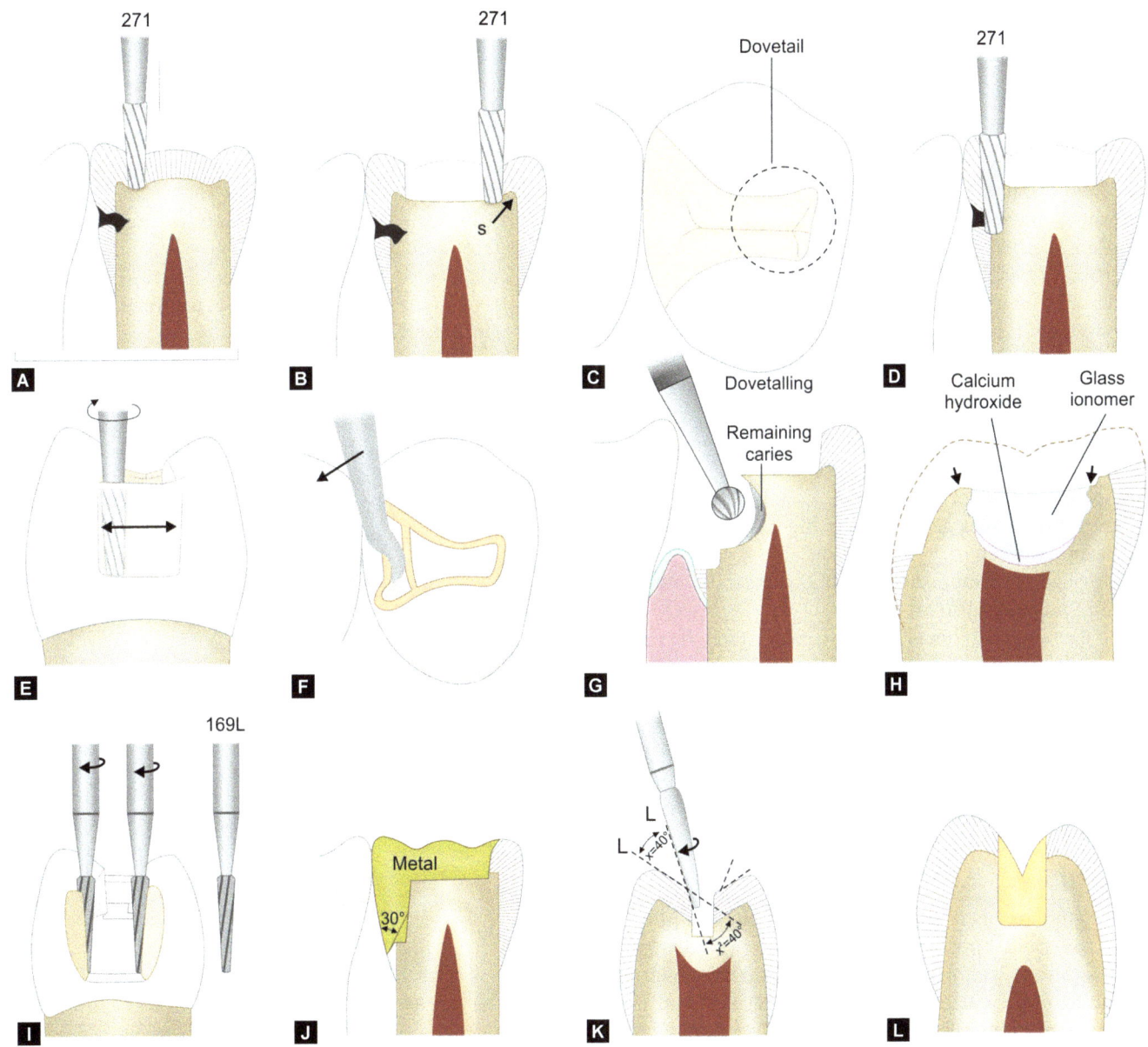

FIGURES 10.2A TO L: Tooth preparation for class II gold inlays: (A) Penetrate the tooth with No. 271 bur held parallel to long axis of the tooth to initial depth of 1.5 mm; (B) Extend the tooth preparation while maintaining the initial pulpal depth of 1.5 mm, uniform taper and flat pulpal floor; (C) Give dovetail to resist displacement of final restoration; (D) Make proximal ditch cut, 0.8 mm wide with 0.5 mm in dentin and 0.3 mm in enamel. Extend this ditch facially and lingually and proceed gingivally; (E) To break contact from adjacent tooth, make two cuts with no. 271 bur; one on facial limit and other at lingual limit of the proximal box; (F) Remove the remaining thin slice of unsupported enamel using spoon excavator; (G) Remove remaining caries, and using spoon excavator or slow speed round bur; (H) Use pulp protective agents whenever indicated; (I) Place retention grooves in axiofacial and axiolingual line angles using number 169 L carbide; (J) Prepare gingival bevel of 30–45° to remove unsupported enamel and provide a stronger obtuse angle of tooth structure for lap sliding fit and sealing of margins of the restoration; (K) Give occlusal bevel of 30–40° using flame-shaped bur; (L) When cusps are steep, little or no bevel is placed

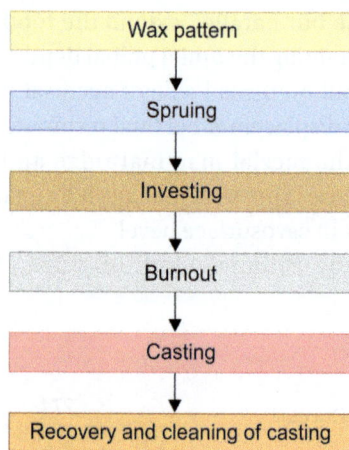

Proximal Box Preparation

- While maintaining the same pulpal depth and holding the bur parallel to long axis of tooth, extend the preparation towards contact area of the tooth
- Isolate the distal enamel by proximal ditch cut. Width of this cut should be 0.8 mm with 0.5 mm in dentin and 0.3 mm in enamel. Extend this ditch facially and lingually to the sound tooth structure and proceed gingivally
- Gingival extension should remove any caries present on the gingival floor and it should provide at least 0.5 mm clearance from the adjacent tooth
- To break contact from adjacent tooth, make two cuts with no. 271 bur; one on facial limit and other at lingual limit of the proximal box
- Extend these cuts gingivally till the bur is through the proximal surface
- Thin slice of unsupported enamel wall can be removed using spoon excavator
- Using enamel hatchet or binangle chisel, plan the ragged enamel margins of proximal surface.

Removal of Remaining Carious Dentin and Pulp Protection

Remove remaining caries using spoon excavator or slow speed round bur. Use pulp protective agents whenever indicated.

Gingival Bevels

Prepare gingival bevel of 30–45° with the help of gingival margin trimmers. It removes weak or unsupported enamel, provides a stronger obtuse angle of tooth structure which aids in finishing of the casting and lap sliding fit and sealing of margins of the restoration.

Occlusal Bevels

Give occlusal bevel of 30–40° using flame shaped bur to remove any irregularities in the preparation or unsupported enamel rods at the cavosurface margin.

Final Cleaning, Drying and Inspection of the Cavity

Final stage of inlay preparation is to clean the preparation thoroughly with water and air spray. Then dry it with moist air.

WAX PATTERN FABRICATION

There are two methods for wax pattern fabrication:
- **Direct wax pattern method (Fig. 10.3):**
  - In this, wax pattern is prepared directly on to the prepared tooth using type I wax
  - Apply separating media like Vaseline uniformly on prepared tooth surface
  - Soften the inlay wax by heating and moving it over alcohol flame. Wax is rotated to heat till it becomes shiny, soft and can be compressed between the fingers
  - Compress the softened inlay wax into the prepared tooth for few minutes with finger pressure
  - Remove excess of wax using warm carving instrument.
  - Once the satisfactory wax pattern is formed, attach sprue former at 45° to the thickest point of the wax pattern.
- **Indirect wax pattern method (Figs. 10.4A to D):**
  - In this wax pattern is fabricated on a die of the prepared tooth by using type II inlay wax
  - Lubricate the die using separating media like petroleum jelly
  - Adapt the inlay wax to the die and do the carving using a warm instrument, and attach a sprue former to the wax pattern.

SPRUING THE WAX PATTERN (FIG. 10.5)

- **Purpose of sprue former:** Sprue former provides a channel so that molten metal flows into mold space after the wax pattern has been eliminated
- **Types of sprue former:** A sprue former can be made up of wax, resin or metal
- **Sprue diameter:** Sprue diameter should be either equal or greater than the thickest part of wax pattern
- **Attachment of sprue former:** Sprue former should be attached to the thickest portions of wax pattern
- **Sprue length:** Length of sprue former should be long enough so that the end of wax pattern is 1/8th to 1/4th of an inch (3 to 6.5 mm) away from the open end of casting ring.

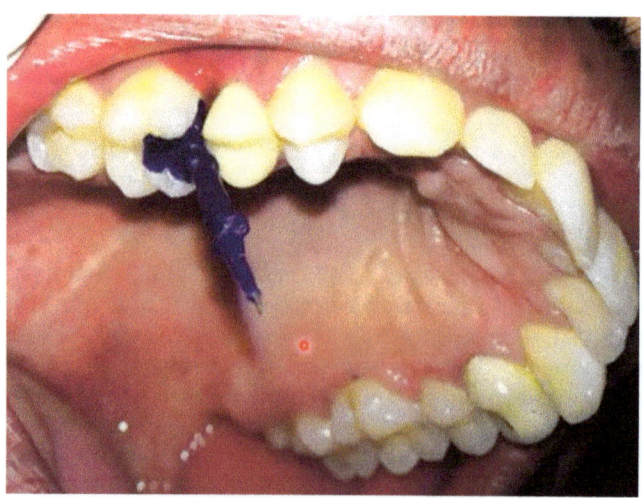

FIGURE 10.3: Direct wax pattern.

Cast Metal Restorations

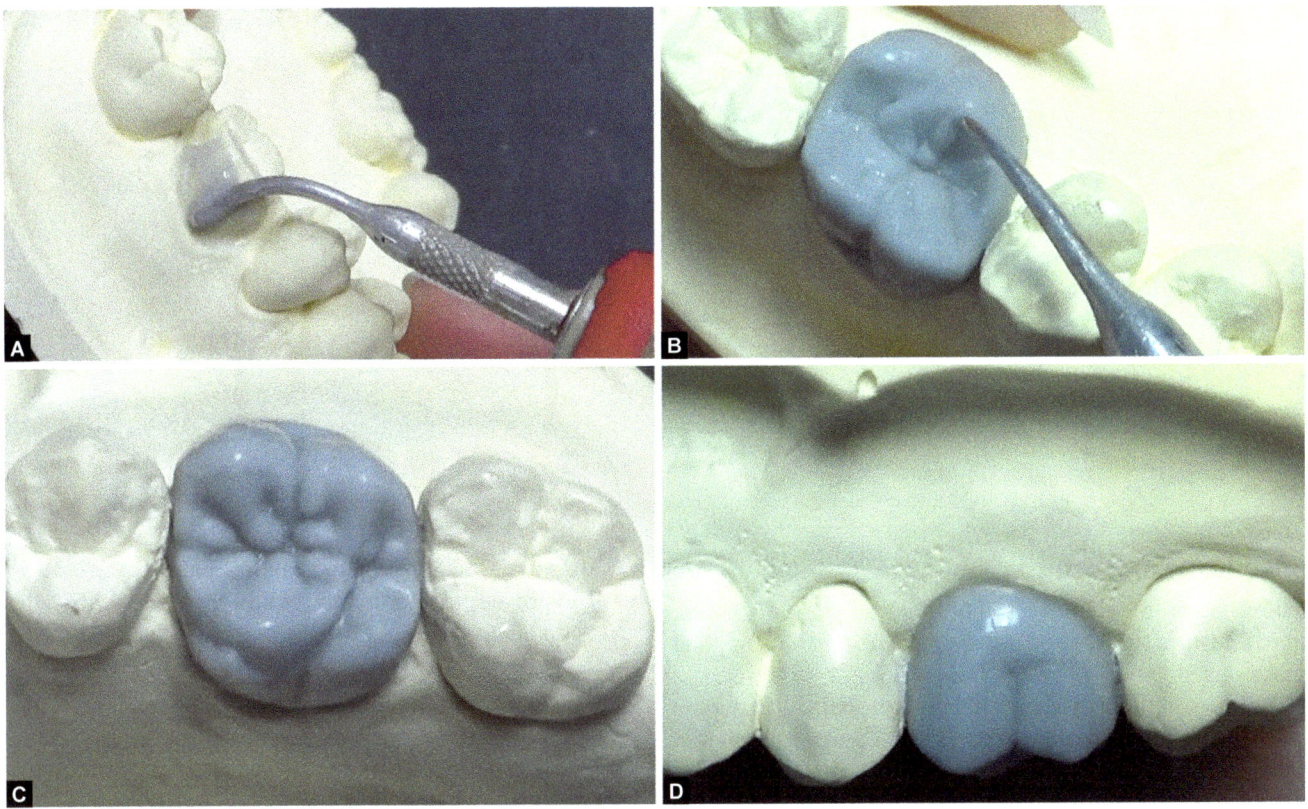

FIGURES 10.4A TO D: Photographs showing making of an indirect wax pattern.

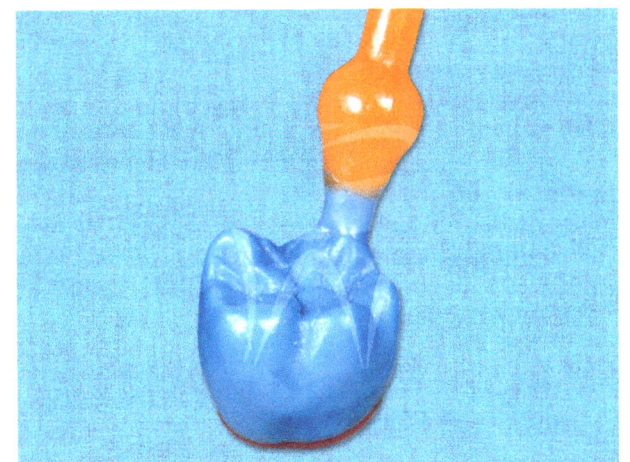

FIGURE 10.5: Photograph showing sprue former attached to the wax pattern, note the angle, thickness and reservoir on sprue former.

- **Angulation of the sprue former:** Sprue should always be attached at an angle of 45° to the bulkiest portion of the wax pattern
- **Reservoir:** Reservoir is added around sprue former and close to wax pattern, i.e., 1–2 mm away from wax pattern to provide constant supply of molten metal to fill the mold space

WASHING OF WAX PATTERN

Before investment, the wax pattern should be washed and covered with detergent. Soap and 3% hydrogen peroxide is applied with a brush to remove cavity debris and blood which could result in rough casting. It is then rinsed with water. After washing, a layer of detergent is applied to reduce surface tension and aid in flow of the investment material over the wax pattern eliminating small bubbles that may remain. These agents are also called wetting agents. Soap is not a good wetting agent as it reacts with calcium sulphate of the binder forming a precipitate. Synthetic detergents are common like lissapol, teepol, cetavlon cetrimide, etc. Pattern must be left to dry for 10 minutes before investing takes place.

INVESTING THE WAX PATTERN (FIGS. 10.6A AND B)

Once the wax pattern is cleaned, it is surrounded by an investment that hardens and forms the mold in which casting is made.

Investment materials basically consist of:
- **Refractory material:** Silica is main refractory material in form of quartz and cristobalite
- **Binder:** It binds the refractory materials together. Types of investment materials based on nature of binder are:
  - **Gypsum bonded investment:** Used for casting gold, can withstand temperature of 700°C
  - **Phosphate bonded investment:** Used for metal ceramic and cobalt-chromium alloys, can withstand higher temperature (850–1100°C)
  - **Ethyl silica bonded investment:** Used for base metal alloy partial dentures, can withstand higher temperature (1100°C).
- **Additives:** Sodium chloride, boric acid, graphite, copper powder are added to improve physical properties of the investment.

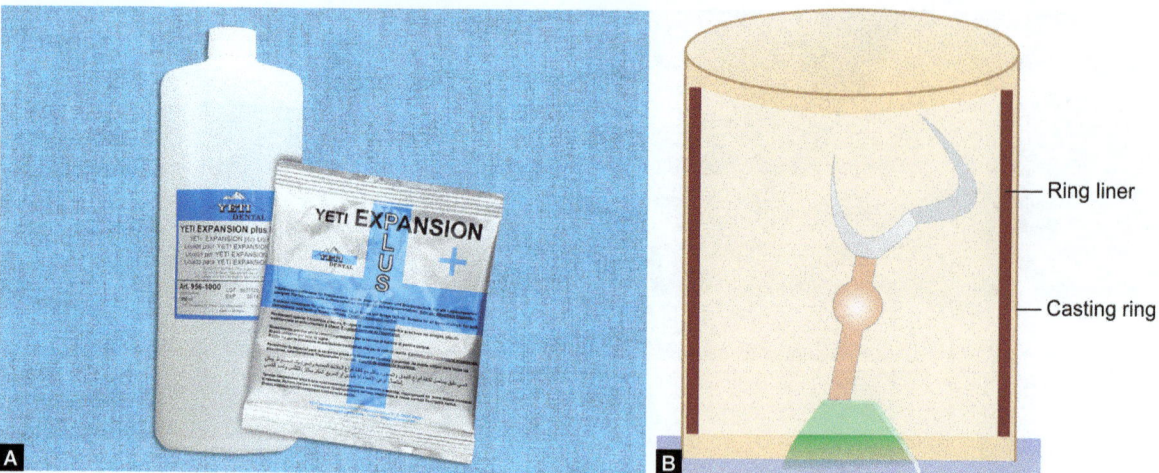

FIGURES 10.6A AND B: (A) Gypsum investment material; (B) Schematic representation of investment pattern.

Principles of Investing

In order to confine the investment material around the wax pattern, casting ring is used. Most commonly, stainless steel tings are used.

To allow mold expansion, uniform setting and hygroscopic expansion of investment, a liner is placed inside the ring. Commonly, ring liners are made up of asbestos, non-asbestos (Cellulose or ceramic) and combination of above.

Casting ring liner is kept 3 mm short at each end of the ring. Minimum liner thickness is 1 mm. liner can be used either dry or wet. But wet is preferred because it affords greater setting expansion along with hygroscopic expansion of the investment.

Two main methods of investing the wax pattern are:
1. Hand investing
2. Vacuum investing.

Hand Investing

- Investment powder is incorporated to the liquid in the mixing bowl in the proper powder-liquid ratio. Here, the mixing for the investment material is done by hand followed by mechanically mixing under vacuum (as in case of phosphate bonded investments)
- Mixing is done in accordance with the manufacturer's instructions
- Pattern is painted with a layer of investment and the remainder is vibrated slowly into the ring
- Ring is tilted once the investment reaches the level of pattern, minimizing entrapment of air

> **Box 10.1: Investing**
>
> There are three types of investing materials for dental castings:
> 1. **Gypsum bonded:** Type 2, 3 and 4 gold alloys, with stand temperature up to 7000°C
> 2. **Phosphate bonded:** Metal ceramic framework, withstand higher temperature
> 3. **Silica bonded:** High melting base metal alloy in CPD, withstand higher temperature

- After that, the investment is allowed to set
- If hygroscopic expansion technique is used, the ring is placed in 37°C water bath for one hour.

Disadvantages
- Increased porosity in investment
- Less reproduction of detail than vacuum investing
- Less tensile strength
- Less smooth cast than that obtained by vacuum investing.

Vacuum Investing

For prevention of air entrapment during investing, vacuum investing is done.

Vacuum investing is further of two types:
1. **Mechanical vacuum investing:** In this type, mixing of investment and its filing into ring is done mechanically under vacuum.
2. **Manual vacuum investing:** Here investment is spatulated by hand under vacuum and then ring is filled. Manual investing is more appropriate as greater control during addition of investment.

BURNOUT OF WAX PATTERN/WAX ELIMINATION AND HEATING (FIG. 10.7)

Once the investment has set for an about one hour, it is ready for burn out. If delayed, it is kept in 100% humidor. It is recommended to begin the burnout procedure while the mold is still wet because water trapped in pores of investment reduces the absorption of wax, as water vaporizes, it flushes wax from the mold.

For proper elimination, the mold is placed in the furnace with sprue hole placed downwards. This allows wax elimination as liquid, more circulation of oxygen into the cavity to react with wax and form gases rather than fine carbon.

Heating should be gradual as 400°C in 20 min and maintained for 30 min. For next 30 min, temperature is increased to 700°C and maintained for 30 min (1 hr 20 min). The casting procedure should be completed without permitting the mold to cool.

Cast Metal Restorations

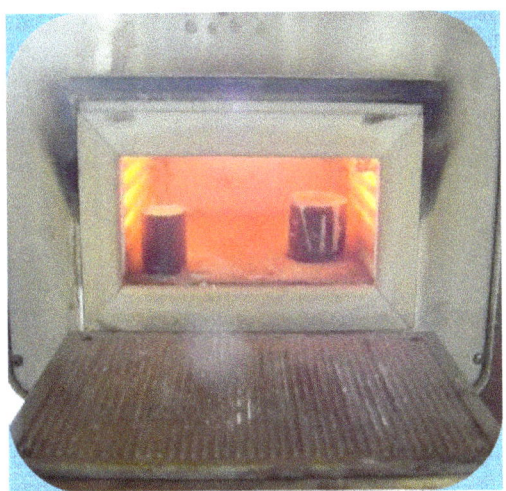

FIGURE 10.7: Burnout of wax pattern.

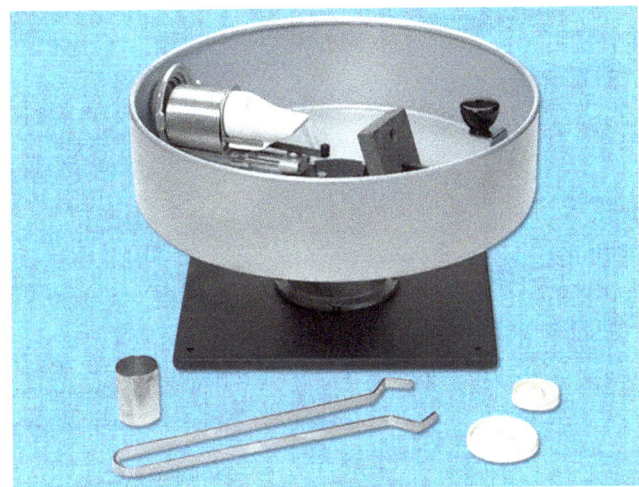

FIGURE 10.8: Centrifugal casting machine.

Temperature Requirements for Various Investments

For gypsum bonded investment:
- In hygroscopic low heat technique – temperature required – 468°C for 60 to 90 mins. Casting done immediately after investment
- In high heat thermal expansion technique-slow heating to 650°C in 60 mins, held for 15 to 20 mins.

  Gypsum investments disintegrate at 700°C to release sulphur gas which causes black and brittle castings.

For phosphate bonded investments:
- Heated to 315°C for 30 mins and usually burn out takes place between 750 to 900°C.

CASTING MACHINES

Different types of casting machines are used for casting of dental alloys.

Basically two types of casting machines are used:
1. Centrifugal casting machine
2. Air pressure casting machine.

Centrifugal Casting Machine (Fig. 10.8)

It is very popular and cheap in cost, giving good results for small castings. Here, the centrifugal force is used to accelerate the flow of molten metal into the mold space. Sequence of steps to be followed in gold alloy casting is as follows:
- Heat the ring in which wax pattern has been invested to 1200°F and keep it at this temperature for 15 minutes in the furnace
- Move the arm of the casting machine by 2 to 3 turns in clockwise direction and lock it so that the arm does not rotate back
- Heat the gold alloy in the crucible of the casting machine until it becomes bright orange in color and has a shiny appearance
- Place the casting ring in the cradle of the casting machine. The end of the ring with the sprue should be towards the crucible. Move up the crucible as close as possible to the casting ring
- When the gold alloy is fully melt, release the lock of the casting arm so as to force the molten gold into the mold by centrifugal force
- Remove the ring from the casting machine and keep it in the water keeping sprue end upward and above the water level, and dry, till the ring is cooled
- Recover the casting and clean it with a bristle toothbrush and water to remove investment from the casting.

Advantages
- Simplicity of design and operation
- Opportunity to cast both small and large castings on same machine.

Air Pressure Casting Machine

In this, compressed air or gases such as carbon dioxide or nitrogen is used to force the molten alloy into the mold. This type of machine is preferred for small castings.

Other Casting Machines
- Electrical resistance heated casting machine
- Induction casting machine
- Direct current arc melting machine
- Titanium casting.

MELTING THE ALLOY (FIGS. 10.9A TO E)

Various devices are used for melting of alloys. These can either be by torch or by electrical means.

Torch melting: It uses—
- ***Gas/air***: The gas used is mainly propane and has the lowest temperature of all sources. Used for small inlays and type I and II alloys
- ***Natural gas/oxygen***: Has high temperature and can be used for PFM alloys
- ***Acetylene/oxygen***: It has the highest temperature and is used for base metal alloys
    - ***Zones of flame***: There are four zones in a flame:
      i. ***Mixing zone:***
         - Dark in color
         - Air and gas are mixed here before combustion
         - No heat is present.

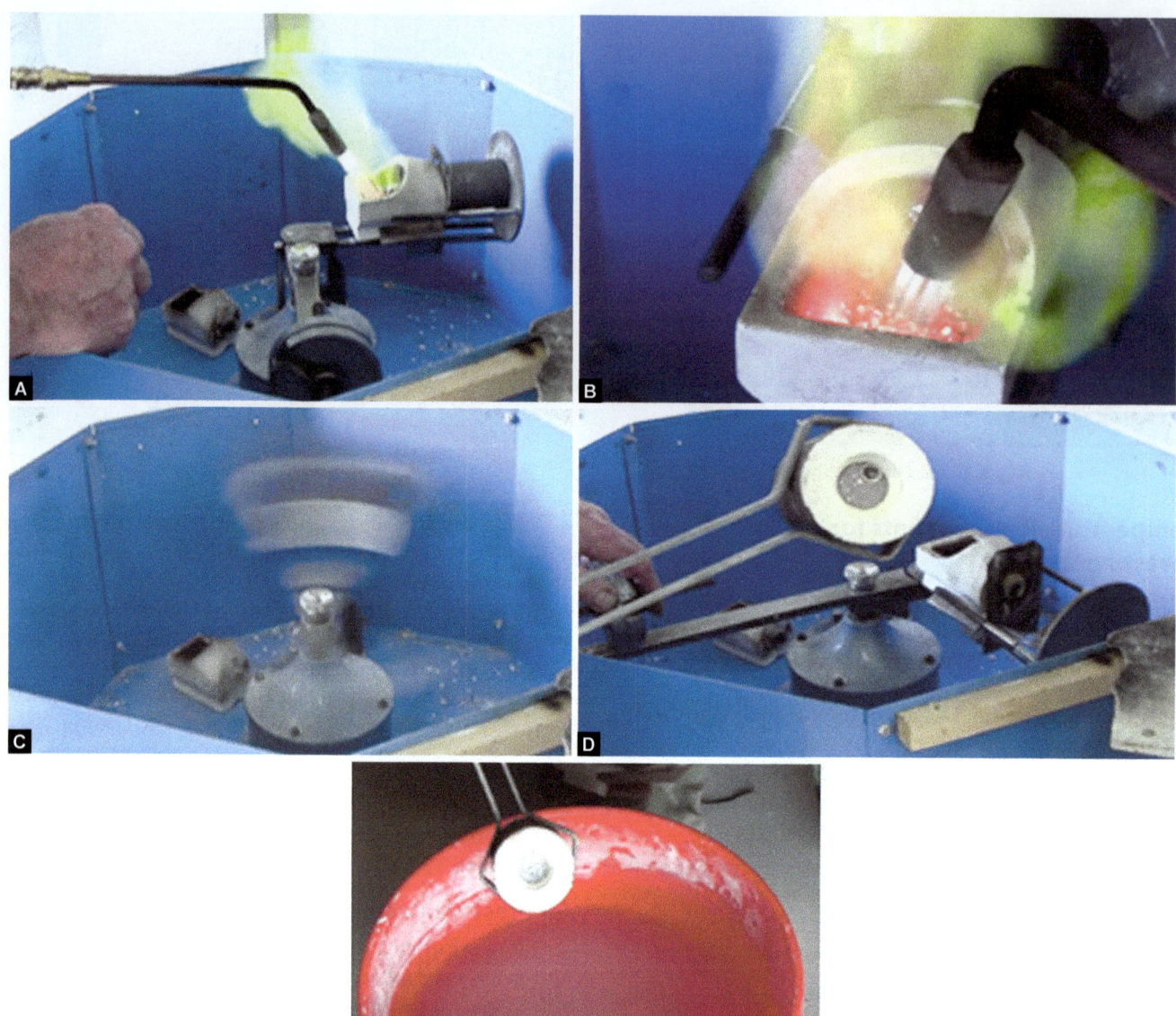

FIGURES 10.9A TO E: (A and B) Melting of alloy using torch method; (C) Casting of restoration using centrifugal machine; (D) Removal of casting ring; (E) Quenching of casting in cold water.

ii. **Combustion zone:**
   - Surrounds the inner zone
   - Green in color
   - Here, the gas and air is partially burned. This zone is definitely oxidizing in nature
   - Should always be kept away from the molten alloy during fusion.

iii. **Reducing zone:**
   - Dimly blue and located just beyond the tip of the green combustion zone is the reducing zone
   - Hottest part of the flame and it should be kept constantly on the alloy during melting.

iv. **Oxidizing zone:**
   - Zone in which final combustion between gas and surrounding air occurs
   - Not used for fusion of alloys
   - This portion of the flame should not be used to melt the alloy.

- **Electric melting units:** These machines use resistance or induction heating system for alloy melting.

Cleaning of Casting

After completion of casting, casting ring is removed from casting machine and quenched.

Quenching

Quenching involves rapid cooling at room temperature water bath or ice water bath. It does not allow sufficient time for atomic movements to form an ordered structure. This disordered structure is retained at room temperature, making it soft and ductile. This helps in final adjustments easier.

Advantages

- When water comes in contact with hot investment, a violent reaction ensues. The investment becomes soft, granular and facilitates easy removal of casting from casting ring
- Keeps the gold alloy in annealed state for easy burnishing and polishing.

Pickling

Surface of casting usually appears dark due to presence of oxides and other contaminants. This type of film can be removed by method known as 'pickling'. Pickling is a process in which discolored casting is heated with an acid in test tube or beaker.

Solution preferred for pickling are—

- 50% HCl solution (best suited for gypsum bonded investment)
- 50% sulphuric acid.

Precautions to be taken during pickling

- Best method for pickling is to place casting in a test tube and pour acid over it. Acid solution should not be boiled rather it should be heated
- Use fresh pickling solution every time, because copper from previous casting can contaminate the new casting
- Casting should not be heated and then dropped into the pickling solution as margins of casting may be distorted during heating
- Casting should not be held with steel instruments as this may contaminate pickling solution and casting. Instead of steel tweezer, rubber coated or Teflon tweezer should be used.

Finishing and Polishing

Examine the fitting of restoration for any nodules or defects. If present, these can be removed using carbide bur. Try in the casting with sprue button. It should fit the prepared tooth passively. If found satisfactory, remove the sprue close to inlay/onlay using carborundum disc. Burnish the inlay margins of die with ball burnisher. Refine occlusal anatomy using dull round bur at slow speed. Check occlusion and remove any prematurities. Polish the casting using rubber abrasive points. Finally, using Tripoli or rough with felt wheel polish the casting for final luster.

TRYING IN THE CASTING

- Before 'trying in' procedure, remove temporary restoration and cement completely and carefully. Place a four-layered gauze piece as a throat screen during trying in and removal of small indirect restoration till the cementation of casting
- Place casting on tooth using light pressure. If it does not seat properly, do not force it in the preparation. Overcontoured proximal surfaces may also prevent seating of casting
- Check occlusion by asking patient to bite on bite paper. High points in restoration result in perforation of articulating paper. Improper occluding contacts make the tooth unstable and tend to deflect it
- Evaluate the embrasures and judge the points where proximal recontouring is required. Contacts can be present too occlusally, broad faciolingually or occlusocervically
- Pass dental floss through contact to find out the tightness of the contact and its locations
- Adjust contact area so that casting seats passively. Fine carborundum particles, impregnated rubber disks or wheels can be used for adjusting the proximal contact and contours.

CEMENTATION OF THE CASTING

- Clean the casting thoroughly before cementation
- Isolate the prepared tooth, clean it and apply a thin layer of varnish in the preparation
- Apply warm air to the gingival sulcus of the prepared tooth to dry it
- Apply a thin layer of luting cement on the surfaces of the casting which will be in contact with the tooth surface and on the tooth preparation surface
- Seat the casting with the help of hand pressure using a suitable instrument
- Ask the patient to bite on a small cotton pellet which is placed on the occlusal surface of the casting
- Clean the area with dry cotton for removing the remnants of set cement
- Recheck the occlusion for harmony of centric occlusion.
- Finally, check the gingival sulcus for any remnants of cement to avoid irritation to the supporting tissues.

To Prevent Post-cementation Pain

- Do not desiccate the tooth
- Use the proper powder-to-liquid ratio of luting cement.
- Do not remove the smear layer
- Use a base material on deep areas of the preparation
- Apply a resin dentin-desensitizer
- Avoid overfilling the casting with cement
- Seat the casting gently
- Protect the cement from moisture contamination
- Clean up excess cement only after it has fully set; this prevents the cement from being pulled out from underneath margins.

Figure 10.10 showing cavity preparation and cast metal restoration on maxillary second premolar.

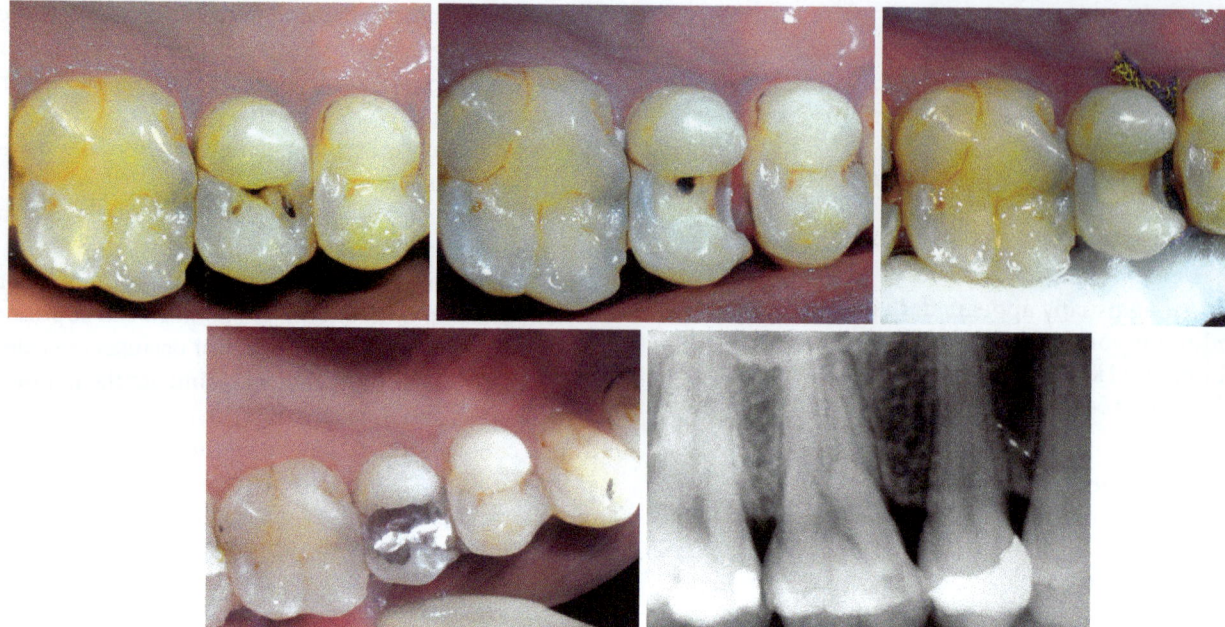

FIGURE 10.10: Cavity preparation and cast metal restoration on maxillary second premolar.

■ VIVA VOCE

Q.1 Define inlay.
Ans. It is an indirect intracoronal restoration fabricated extraorally and then cemented on prepared tooth.

Q.2 Define class II Inlay.
Ans. This is an indirect restoration that caps one or more cusps of a posterior tooth but not all the cusps.

Q.3 Define onlay.
Ans. It is an indirect restoration which is partly intracoronal and partly extracoronal that covers all cusps of a posterior tooth.

Q.4 What are indications of cast metal restorations?
Ans.
- Extensive tooth involvement
- Correction of occlusion
- Already present cast metal restoration to prevent galvanic current
- Proximal margins extending subgingivally.

Q.5 What are contraindications of cast metal restorations?
Ans.
- In a esthetic cases because of metallic color
- In patients with poor oral hygiene and high caries index
- In young permanent teeth because of chances of iatrogenic pulp exposure due to high pulp horns
- In patients having restorations with different metals since dissimilar metals cause galvanic currents when they come in contact with each other.

Q.6 What are advantages of cast metal restorations?
Ans.
- Optimal contacts and contours
- Good wear resistance
- Biocompatible
- Good strength.

Q.7 Which instruments used for cavity preparation for cast metal restorations?
Ans.
- No. 271. Tungsten carbide tapering fissure bur with 0.8 mm width
- 169L Tapered fissure bur with 0.5 mm width
- No. 8865 slender fine grit flam shaped diamond for preparing cavosurface bevel
- Chisel, hatchet and wedelstaedt for removal of undermining enamel and producing primary and secondary bevels
- Spoon excavator for removal of remaining soft caries
- Gingival margin trimmer for creating gingival bevels.

Q.8 What are steps of inlay preparation?
Ans.
- Tooth preparation
- Impression taking
- Die making
- Wax pattern
- Investing of the pattern and creating the mold
- Gold casting.

Q.9 What are advantages of giving bevels in cast metal restorations?
Ans.
- Remove weak or unsupported enamel
- Provide a stronger obtuse angle of tooth structure which aids in finishing of the casting
- Provide lap sliding fit and sealing of margins of the restoration.

Q.10 What is purpose of using a sprue former?
Ans. Sprue former provides a channel so that molten metal flows into mold space after the wax pattern has been eliminated.

Q.11 Where should be the attachment of sprue former?
Ans. Sprue former should be attached to the thickest portions of wax pattern.

Cast Metal Restorations

Q.12 What should be the length of sprue former?

Ans. Length of sprue former should be long enough so that the end of wax pattern is 1/8th to 1/4th of an inch (3 to 6.5 mm) away from the open end of casting ring.

Q.13 At what angle should be the sprue former attached?

Ans. Sprue should always be attached at an angle of 45° to the bulkiest portion of the wax pattern.

Q.14 What is the purpose of reservoir and where is it attached?

Ans. Reservoir is added around sprue former and close to wax pattern, i.e., 1–2 mm away from wax pattern to provide constant supply of molten metal to fill the mold space.

Q.15 What are different types of investment materials?

Ans. Types of investment materials based on nature of binder are:
- Gypsum bonded investment
- Phosphate bonded investment
- Ethyl silica bonded investment.

Q.16 How is melting of alloy done?

Ans.
- Torch melting
- Electric melting units.

Q.17 What is quenching?

Ans. Quenching involves rapid cooling at room temperature water bath or ice water bath. It does not allow sufficient time for atomic movements to form an ordered structure. This disordered structure is retained at room temperature, making it soft and ductile. This helps in final adjustments easier.

Q.18 What is pickling?

Ans. Pickling is a process in which discolored casting is heated with an acid in test tube or beaker.

Solution preferred for pickling are:
- 50% HCl solution (best suited for gypsum bonded investment)
- 50% sulphuric acid.

Q.19 What should be done if casting is short of proximal contact with adjacent tooth?

Ans. To treat this problem, a solder of 650 or higher is added to the casting. The difference between solidus temperature of inlay and liquidus temperature of solder should be 100°F.

Steps of soldering
1. Treat the proximal surface of casting with abrasive wheel to remove traces of any polishing agents, as they may act as antiflux.
2. Cut a strip of solder, it should extend 1 mm beyond contact area.
3. Apply borax type flux on the contact area of the casting and on both the surfaces of the piece of solder.
4. Place the solder at proper place on the contact area requiring build-up and direct the pinpoint flame of bunsen burner to the solder with the help of blow pipe so that the solder melts and flows.
5. Apply melt solder on to the casting.
6. Trim and polish the contact.

Chapter 11: Basics of Endodontics

Chapter Outline

- Etiology of pulpal diseases
- Progression of pulpal pathologies
- Endodontic instruments
- Access cavity preparation
- Access cavity of anterior teeth
- Access cavity preparation for premolars
- Working length determination
- Significance of working length
- Irrigation of root canal system
- Cleaning and shaping
- Basic principles of canal instrumentation
- Techniques of root canal preparation

INTRODUCTION

Endo is a Greek word for "inside" and odont is Greek word for "tooth". Endodontic treatment deals inside of the tooth.

Endodontics is the branch of clinical dentistry associated with the prevention, diagnosis and treatment of pathosis of the dental pulp and their sequelae.

Thus, the main aim of the endodontic therapy involves to:
- Maintain vitality of the pulp
- Preserve and restore the tooth with damaged and necrotic pulp
- Preserve and restore the teeth which have failed to the previous endodontic therapy.

Features of pulp which distinguish it from tissue found elsewhere in the body:
- Pulp is surrounded by rigid walls and so is unable to expand in response to injury as a part of the inflammatory process. Therefore, pulpal tissue is susceptible to change in pressure affecting the pain threshold
- There is minimal collateral blood supply to pulp tissue which reduces its capacity for repair following injury
- Pulp is composed almost entirely of simple connective tissue. At its periphery there is a layer of highly specialized cells, the odontoblasts. Secondary dentin is gradually deposited as a physiological process which reduces the blood supply and therefore, the resistance to infection or trauma
- Innervation of pulp tissue is both simple and complex. Simple in that there are only free nerve endings and consequently the pulp lacks proprioception. Complex because of innervation of the odontoblast processes which produces a high level of sensitivity to thermal and chemical change.

Pulp Cavity (Fig. 11.1)

Pulp cavity is the cavity present in center of tooth and enclosed by dentin except at apical foramen. In coronal portion, part of cavity is called pulp chamber and in root portion, it is called root canal.

Pulp Chamber

It occupies the coronal portion of pulp cavity and acquires the shape according to external form of crown. Floor of pulp chamber merges into root canal at orifices. Roof of chamber consists of dentin covering pulp chamber incisally or occlusally.

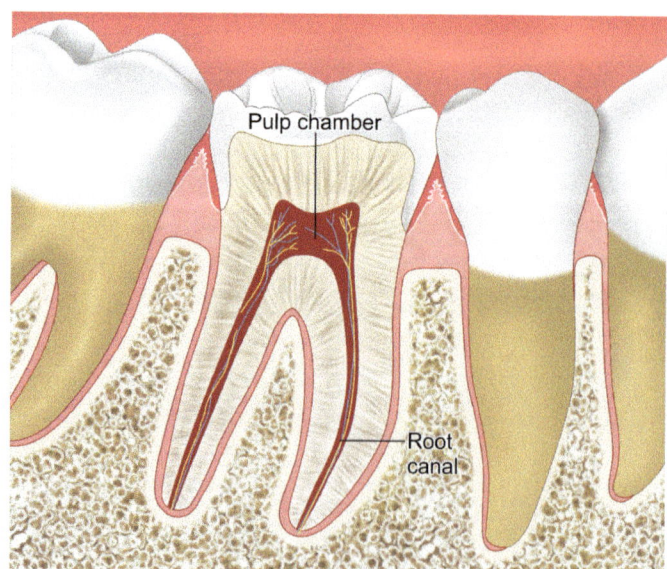

FIGURE 11.1: Schematic representation of pulp cavity showing pulp chamber and root canal.

Root Canal

Root canal extends from canal orifice to apical foramen. Usually canal has curvature or constriction before terminating at the apex.

ETIOLOGY OF PULPAL DISEASES

- Dental caries
- Trauma like fracture, or avulsion of tooth
- Pathologic wear, e.g. attrition, abrasion, etc.
- Thermal injury like heat generated by cutting and restorative procedures
- Microleakage around a restoration
- Periodontal pocket and abscess
- Anachoresis.

PROGRESSION OF PULPAL PATHOLOGIES

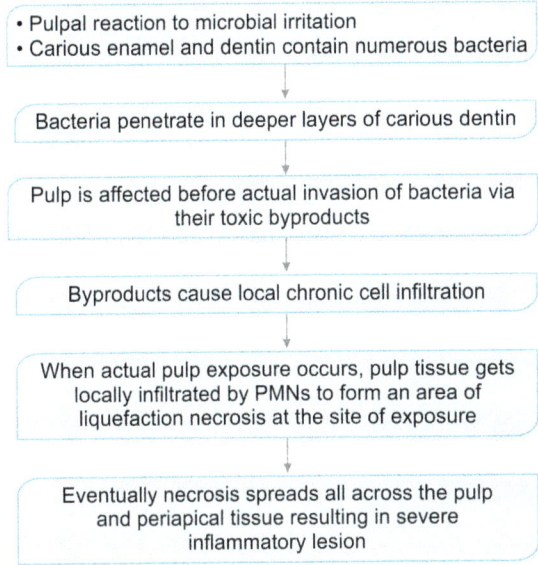

ENDODONTIC INSTRUMENTS

Although variety of instruments are used in general dentistry, are applicable in endodontics, yet some special instruments are unique to endodontic purpose **(Table 11.1)**.

Standardization of Instruments Given by Ingle and Levine

Ingle and Levine suggested following guidelines for instruments for having uniformity in instrument diameter and taper **(Figs. 11.2A to E)**

- Instruments are numbered from 10 to 100. There is increase in 5 units up to size 60 and in 10 units till they are size 100. This has been revised to include numbers from 6 to 140
- Each number should represent diameter of instrument in 100th of millimeter at the tip. For example, a No. 25 reamer shall have 0.25 mm at D_1 and 0.57 mm (0.25 + 0.32) at D_2. These sizes ensure a constant increase in taper, i.e., 0.02 mm/mm of the instrument regardless of the size
- Working blade shall begin at tip (D_1) and extend 16 mm up the shaft (D_2). D_2 should be 0.32 mm greater than D_1, ensuring that there is constant increase in taper, i.e, 0.02 mm/mm of instrument

TABLE 11.1: Grossman's classification of endodontic instruments.

Function	Instruments
Exploring	Smooth broaches and endodontic explorers (to locate canal orifices and determine patency of root canal)
Debriding or extirpating	Barbed broaches (to extirpate the pulp and other foreign materials from the root canal)
Cleaning and shaping	Reamers and files (Used to shape the canal space)
Obturating	Pluggers, spreaders and lentulos pirals (To pack gutta-percha points into the root canal space)

- Instrument handles should be color coded for their easier recognition **(Fig. 11.3)** (pink, gray, purple, white, yellow, red, blue, green, black, white.............)
- Instruments are available in 21 mm, 25 mm, 28 mm, 30 mm and 40 mm of length. 21 mm length is commonly used for molars, 25 mm for anterior teeth, 28 and 30 mm for canines and 40 mm for endodontic implants.

Barbed Broach

- Broach is short handled instrument meant for single use only
- Here smooth surface of wire is notched to form barbs bent at an angle from the long axis **(Fig. 11.4)**
- Broach does not cut the dentin but can effectively be used to remove cotton or paper points which might have lodged in the canal.

Reamer

- Reamer is used to ream the canals. It cuts by inserting into the canal, twisting clockwise one quarter to half turn and then withdrawing, i.e., penetration, rotation and retraction
- Reamer has triangular blank and lesser number of flutes than file **(Fig. 11.5A)**.

Files

- Kerr manufacturing company was first to produce files, so these were also called K-files
- Files are predominantly used with filing or rasping action in which there is little or no rotation in the root canals
- File is placed in root canal and pressure is exerted against the canal wall and instrument is withdrawn while maintaining the pressure.

K-file

- It is triangular, square or rhomboidal in cross-section, manufactured from stainless steel wire, which is grounded into desired shape.
- K-file has 1½–2½ cutting blades per mm of their working end (more than reamer) **(Fig. 11.5B)**.

Hedstrom File (H-file)

- Hedstrom file has flutes which resemble successively triangles set one on another **(Fig. 11.5C)**

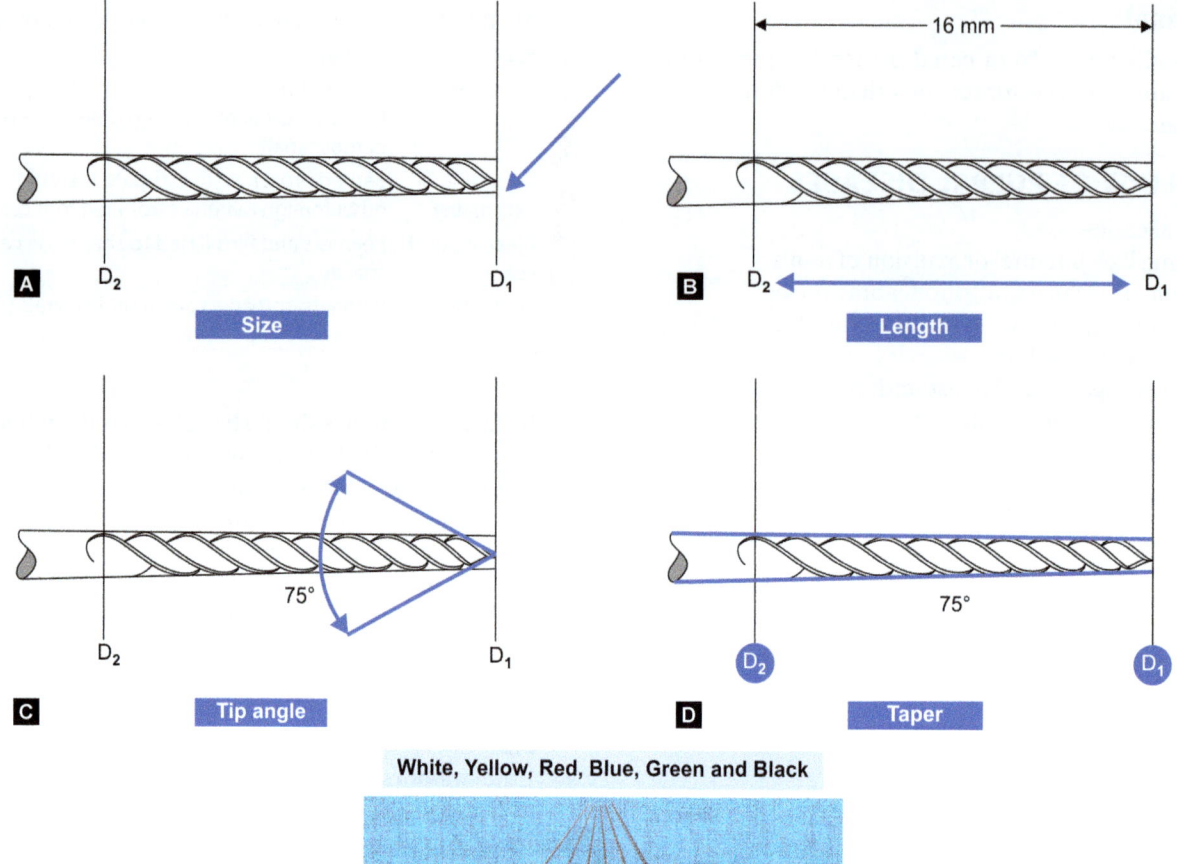

FIGURES 11.2A TO E: Ingle Levine specifications of size, length, tip angle, taper and color for endodontic instruments.

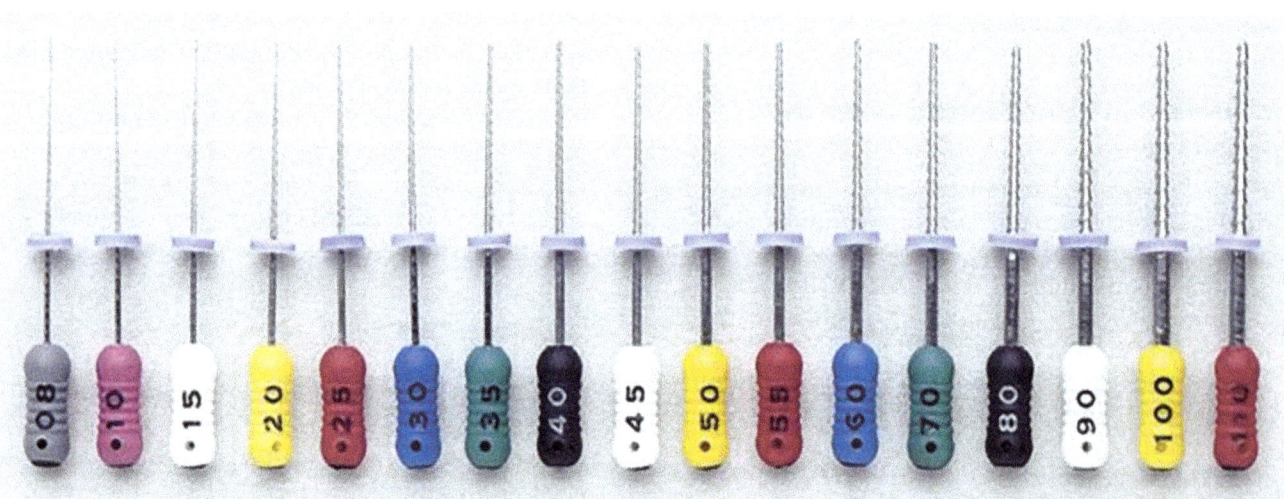

FIGURE 11.3: Color coding and numbers of different instruments.

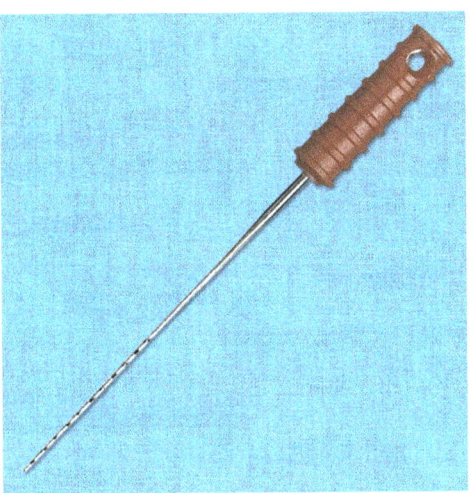

FIGURE 11.4: Barbed broach.

- Hedstrom file cuts only when instrument is withdrawn because its edges face the handle of the instrument
- When used in torquing motion, its edges can engage in the dentin of root canal wall, causing H-files to fracture
- Hedstrom file should be used to machine the straight canal because it is strong and aggressive cutter
- Since, it lacks the flexibility and is fragile in nature, the H-file tends to fracture when used in torquing action.

NiTi Rotary Instruments

NiTi alloys contain 55% weight Ni and 45% Ti.

Advantages of NiTi instruments	Disadvantages of NiTi instruments
■ Shape memory ■ Superelasticity ■ Good resiliency ■ Corrosion resistance ■ Softer than stainless steel	■ Poor cutting efficiency ■ NiTi files do not show signs of fatigue before they fracture

ACCESS CAVITY PREPARATION

Access cavity preparation is defined as an endodontic coronal preparation which enables unobstructed access to the canal orifices, a straight-line access to apical foramen, complete control over instrumentation and accommodate obturation technique.
- An ideal access preparation should have following qualities
- An unobstructed view into the canal
- A file should pass into the canal without touching any part of the access cavity
- No remaining caries should be present in access cavity
- Obturating instruments should pass into the canal without touching any portion of the access cavity.

ACCESS CAVITY OF ANTERIOR TEETH (FIGS. 11.6A TO G)

- Remove all the caries and any defective restorations so as to prevent contamination of pulp space and have a straight-line access into the canals

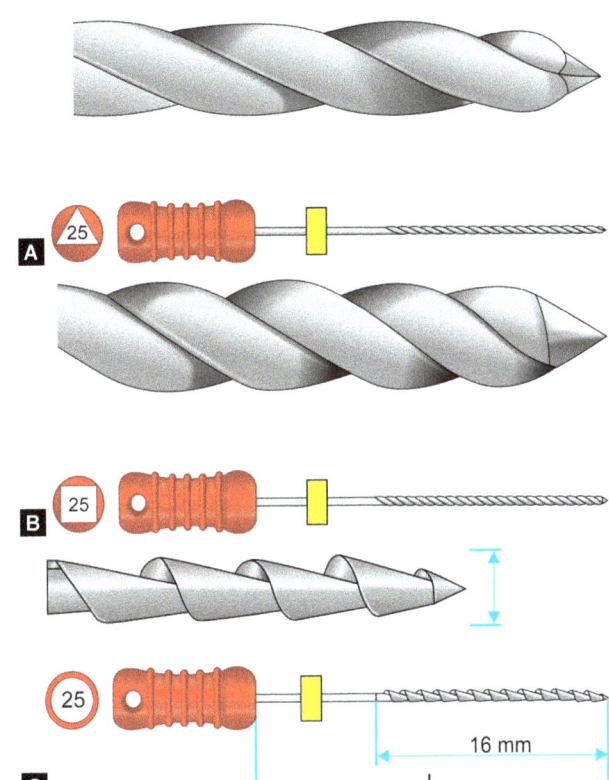

FIGURES 11.5A TO C: (A) Triangular cross section and lesser number of flutes in reamer; (B) Line diagram showing square cross section and more number of flutes in file; (C) H-file resembles successive triangles set on one another.

- Access opening is initiated at the center of the lingual surface by directing a round bur perpendicular to the lingual surface. Once enamel is penetrated, bur is directed parallel to the long axis of the tooth, until 'a drop' in effect is felt
- When pulp chamber has been penetrated, the remainder of chamber roof is removed by working a round bur from inside to outside. This is done to remove all the obstructions of enamel and dentin overhangs that would entrap debris, tissues and other materials
- Now locate the canal orifices using endodontic explorer. Sharp explorer tip is used to locate the canal orifices, to penetrate the calcific deposits if present, and to evaluate the straight-line access
- Once the canal orifices are located, remove the lingual shoulder using Gates–Glidden drills or safe-tipped diamond or carbide burs
- Finally smoothening of the cavosurface margins of access cavity is done to allow better and précised placement of final composite restoration with minimal coronal leakage.

ACCESS CAVITY PREPARATION FOR PREMOLARS (FIGS. 11.7 A TO F)

- Site of access opening in premolars is in center of the occlusal surface between buccal and the lingual cusp tips
- Penetrate the enamel with No. 4 round bur in high-speed contra-angle handpiece. The bur should be directed parallel to the long axis of tooth and perpendicular to the

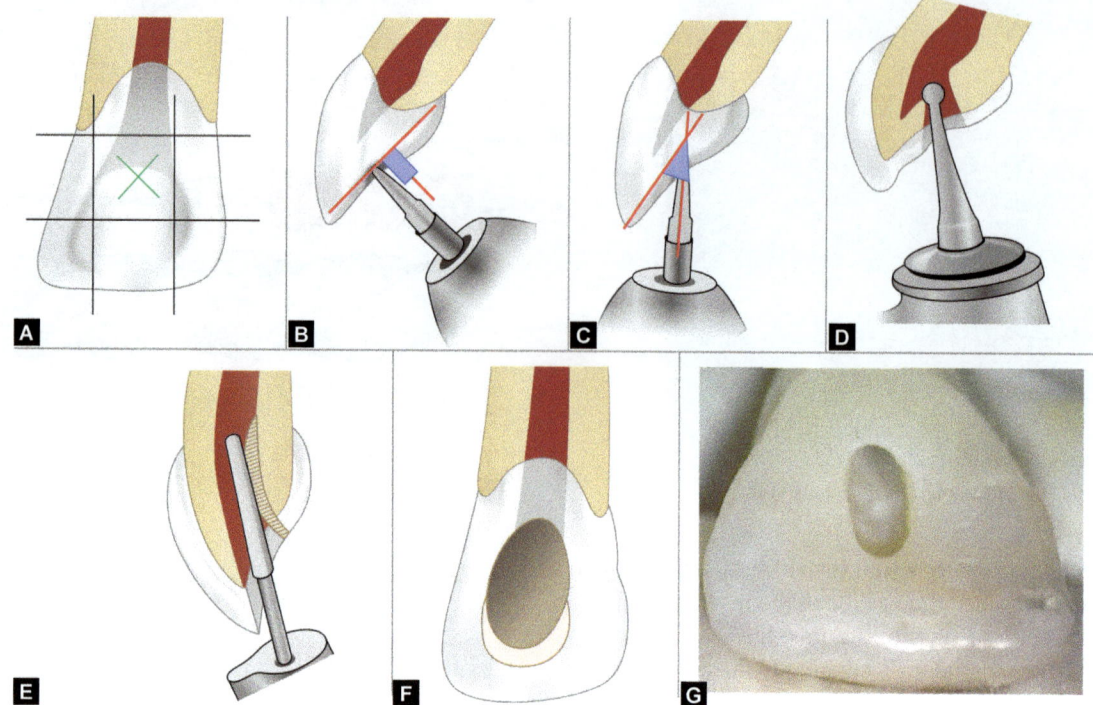

FIGURES 11.6A TO G: Schematic representation of access cavity preparation for maxillary anterior teeth: (A) Initial point for entry of bur is middle of middle third of palatal surface; (B) Keep round bur perpendicular to the long axis of the tooth; (C) Bur is directed 45° to the long axis of the tooth to penetrate the pulp chamber; (D) Removal of chamber roof; (E) Removal of lingual shoulder; (F and G) Final access cavity shape of maxillary incisor.

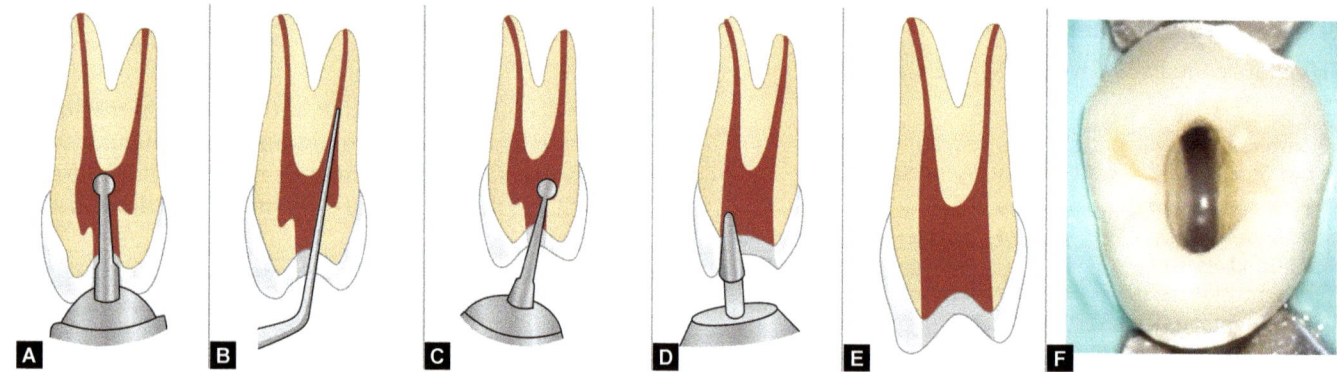

FIGURES 11.7A TO F: Schematic representation of access cavity preparation for premolars: (A) Penetrate the enamel using round bur and move it in buccolingual direction; (B) Locate the canal orifice using endodontic explorer; (C) Move the bur inside to outside for removing roof of the pulp chamber; (D) Removal of coronal bulges for straight line access; (E and F) Final preparation with coronal flare and larger dimensions buccolingually.

occlusal table. External outline form for premolars is oval in shape with greater dimensions on buccolingual side
- Once the clinician feels "drop" into the pulp chamber, penetrate deep enough to remove the roof of pulp chamber without cutting the floor of pulp chamber. To remove the roof of pulp chamber place a bur (round, tapered fissure or safety tip) alongside the walls of pulp chamber and work from inside to outside
- After removal of roof of pulp chamber, locate the canal orifices with the help of sharp endodontic explorer
- Walls of access cavity are smoothened and sloped slightly towards the occlusal surface.

Figures 11.8 and 11.9 showing access cavity preparation for maxillary molars, and mandibular molars.

WORKING LENGTH DETERMINATION

Working length is defined as "the distance from a coronal reference point to a point at which canal preparation and obturation should terminate". A reference point is chosen which is stable and easily visualized during preparation. Reference point is that site on occlusal or the incisal surface from which measurements are made. Usually, it is incisal edge of anterior teeth and buccal cusp of posterior teeth.

Definitions Related to Working Length (Fig. 11.10)
- **Anatomic apex** is "tip or end of root determined morphologically".
- **Radiographic apex** is "tip or end of root determined radiographically".

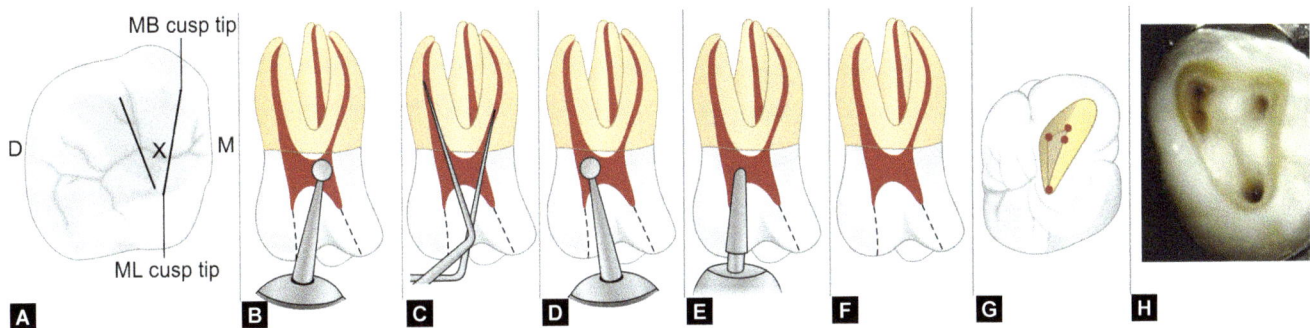

FIGURES 11.8A TO G: Schematic representation of access cavity preparation for maxillary molars: (A) Mesial boundary is a line joining the mesial cusps and distal boundary is the oblique ridge. Initial point of bur penetration is on the central groove midway between mesial and distal boundaries; (B) Penetrate the enamel with No. 4 round bur in the central groove directed palatally until "drop" into the pulp chamber is felt; (C) Explore the canal orifices with sharp endodontic explorer; (D) De-roof the pulp chamber moving bur from inside to outside; (E) Remove any cervical bulges or obstructions if present; (F) Final access cavity shows confluent walls of pulp chamber and occlusal surface; (G) Occlusal view showing rhomboid shaped pulp chamber with acute mesiobuccal angle, obtuse distobuccal angle and palatal right angle; (H) Access cavity preparation of maxillary first molar.

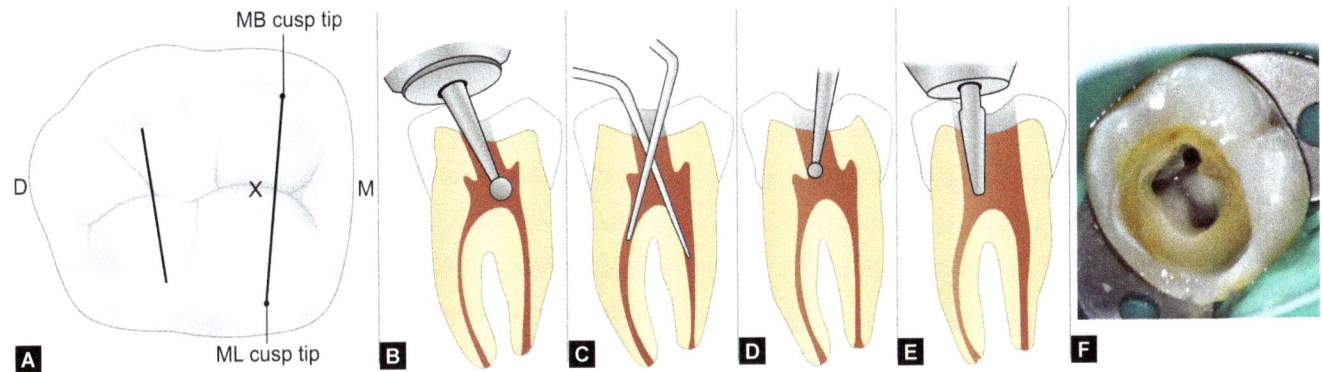

FIGURES 11.9A TO F: Access cavity preparation for molars: (A) Sectioned tooth showing pulp cavity; (B) Initial point of entry of bur; (C) Explore canal orifices with sharp endodontic explorer; (D) Deroofing of pulp chamber; (E) Removal of coronal ledges or obstructions; (F) Final shape of access cavity with chamber walls flared occlusally; (G) Access cavity preparation of mandibular molar.

- **Apical foramen** (major diameter) is main apical opening of the root canal which may be located away from anatomic or radiographic apex.
- **Apical constriction** (minor diameter) is apical portion of root canal having narrowest diameter. It is usually 0.5–1 mm short of apical foramen.
- **Cemento-dentinal junction** is the region where cementum and dentin are united, the point at which cemental surface terminates at or near the apex of tooth. Location of CDJ ranges from 0.5 to 3 mm short of anatomic apex.

SIGNIFICANCE OF WORKING LENGTH (FIGS. 11.10 AND 11.11)

- Working length determines how far into canal instruments can be placed and worked
- Failure to accurately determine and maintain working length may result in length being over than normal which will lead to postoperative pain, prolonged healing time and lower success rate because of incomplete regeneration of cementum, periodontal ligament and alveolar bone
- When working length is made short of apical constriction, it may cause persistent discomfort because of incomplete cleaning and underfilling. Apical leakage may occur into uncleaned and unfilled space short of apical constriction.

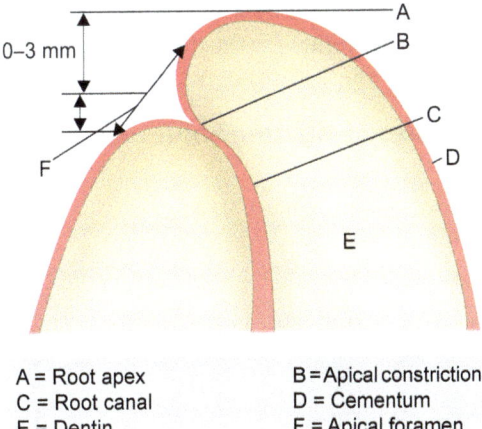

A = Root apex   B = Apical constriction
C = Root canal   D = Cementum
E = Dentin   F = Apical foramen

FIGURE 11.10: Schematic representation of apical root anatomy.

It may support continued existence of viable bacteria and contributes to the periradicular lesion and thus, poor success rate.

Radiographic Method of Length Determination (Figs. 11.12A to D)

- Measure the estimated working length from preoperative periapical radiograph
- Adjust stopper of instrument to this estimated working length and place it in the canal up to the adjusted stopper

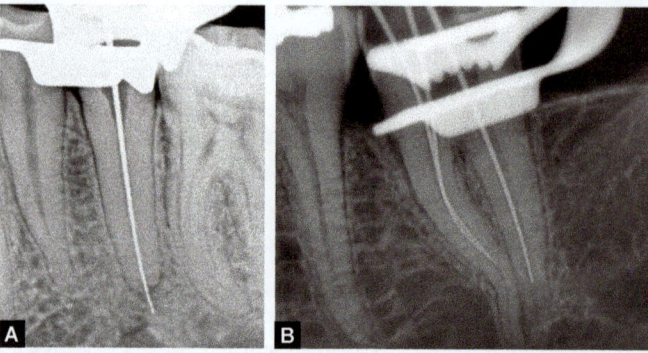

FIGURES 11.11A AND B: (A) Radiograph showing working length beyond the apex; (B) Radiograph showing working length short of apex.

- Take the radiograph
- On the radiograph, measure the difference between the tip of the instrument and root apex. Add or subtract this length to the estimated working length to get the new working length
- Correct working length is finally calculated by subtracting 1 mm from this new length.

IRRIGATION OF ROOT CANAL SYSTEM (FIG. 11.13)

Every root canal system has spaces that cannot be cleaned mechanically. The only way we can clean webs, fins and anastomoses is by effective use of an irrigation solution.

Functions of Irrigants

- Irrigants perform physical and biologic functions. Dentin shavings get removed from canals by irrigation
- Instruments are less likely to break when canal walls are lubricated with irrigation
- Irrigants help in removing the debris from accessory and lateral canals where instruments cannot reach.

Commonly used Irrigating Solutions

- Saline
- Sodium hypochlorite 0.5–5.25%

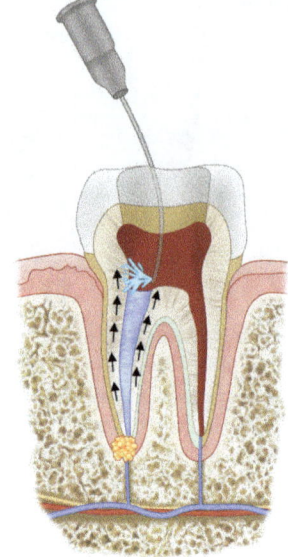

FIGURE 11.13: Irrigation of root canal.

- Ethylenediaminetetraaceticacid (EDTA)
- Hydrogen peroxide
- Chlorhexidine.

CLEANING AND SHAPING

Cleaning and shaping is one of the most important step in the root canal therapy for obtaining success in the root canal treatment. Cleaning comprises removal of all potentially pathogenic contents from the root canal system. Shaping is establishment of a specifically shaped cavity which performs dual role of three dimensional progressive access into the canal and creating an apical preparation which permits obturation.

BASIC PRINCIPLES OF CANAL INSTRUMENTATION (FIGS. 11.14A AND B)

- There should be a straight line access to the canal orifices. Create a straight line access by removing overhang dentin

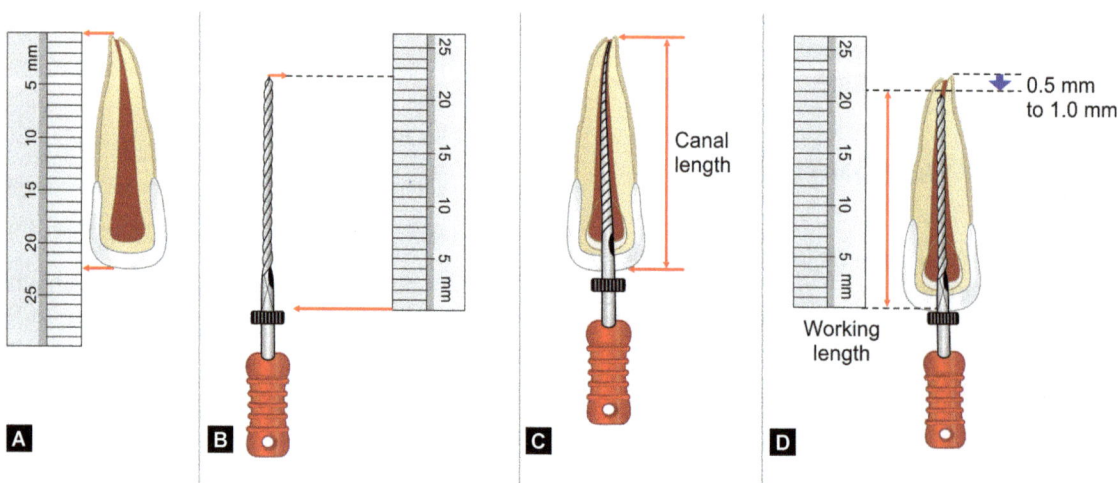

FIGURES 11.12A TO D: Working length measurement by Ingle's method: (A) Measure estimated working length from preoperative radiograph; (B) Adjust stopper of instrument to this length; (C) Place it in canal up to the adjusted stopper; (D) Take the radiograph and measure the difference between tip of the instrument and root apex. Add or subtract this length to estimated working length to get the new length.

Basics of Endodontics

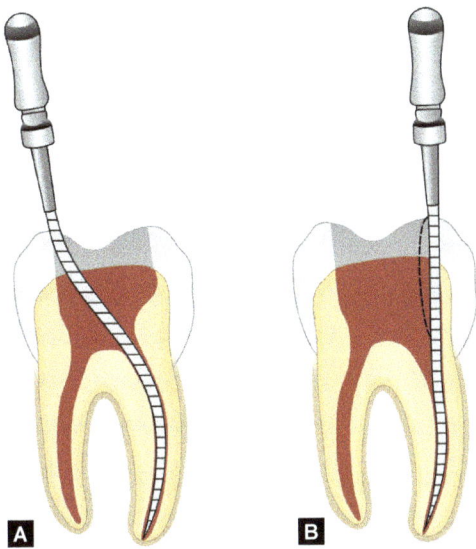

FIGURES 11.14A AND B: (A) Not removing dentin from mesial wall causes bending of instrument while inserting in canal leading to instrumental errors; (B) Removal of dentin interference from access opening gives straight line access to the canal without any undue bending.

influences the forces exerted by a file in apical third of the canal
- Files are always worked with in a canal filled with irrigant. Therefore, copious irrigation is done in between the instrumentation, i.e., canal must always be prepared in wet environment
- Canal enlargement should be done by using instruments in the sequential order without skipping sizes
- All the working instruments should be kept in confines of the root canal to avoid any procedural accidents
- Recapitulation is regularly done to loosen debris by returning to working length. The canal walls should not be enlarged during recapitulation
- Never force the instrument in the canal. Forcing or continuing to rotate an instrument may break the instrument.

Schilder's objectives for cleaning and shaping of root canal system:
- **Root canal preparation should develop a continuously tapering cone:** This mimics the natural funnel-shaped preparation of canal
- **Making the preparation in multiple planes which introduces the concept of "flow":** It preserves the natural curve of the canal
- **Making the canal narrower apically and widest coronally:** To create a continuous taper up to apical third which creates the resistance form to hold gutta-percha in the canal
- **Avoid transportation of the foramen:** There should be gentle and minute enlargement of the foramen while maintaining its position
- **Keep the apical opening as small as possible:** This is done to avoid number of iatrogenic problems.

TECHNIQUES OF ROOT CANAL PREPARATION (FIGS. 11.15A TO C)

There are **two approaches** used for **biomechanical preparation**, either starting at the apex with fine instruments and working up to the orifice with progressively larger instruments, this is **step back technique** or starting at the orifice with larger instrument and working up to apex with larger instruments, this is **crown down technique**.

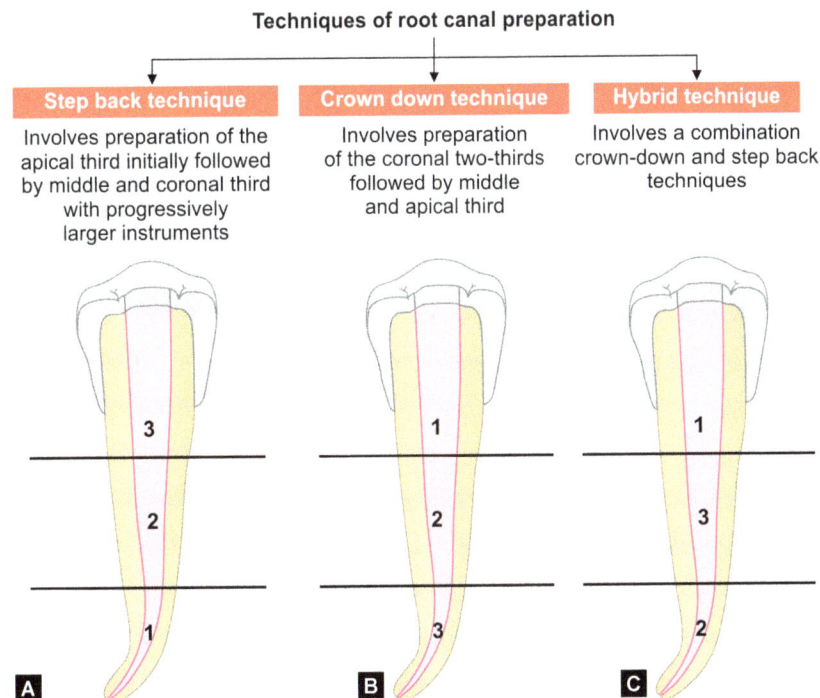

No.1, 2, 3 tell the sequence of canal preparation

FIGURES 11.15A TO C: Line diagram showing sequence of canal preparation in step back, crown down and hybrid technique.

VIVA QUESTION

Q.1 What is the main aim of the endodontic therapy?
Ans.
- To maintain vitality of the pulp
- To preserve and restore the tooth with damaged and necrotic pulp.

Q.2 How is pulp different from other dental tissues?
Ans.
- It has minimal collateral blood supply, it reduces its capacity for repair following injury
- Pulp is surrounded by rigid dentin so is unable to expand in response to injury as a part of the inflammatory process.

Q.3 What are the causes of pulpal diseases?
Ans.
- Dental caries.
- Trauma like fracture, or avulsion of tooth
- Pathologic wear, e.g., attrition, abrasion, etc.
- Periodontal pocket and abscess.

Q.4 What is barbed broach used for?
Ans. Barbed broach is used to remove pulp, cotton or paper points which might have lodged in the canal.

Q.5 What are the differences between a reamer and a file?
Ans.

	Files	Reamers
Flutes	More (1½–2/mm)	Less (½–1/mm)
Cutting motion	Rasping and penetration (push and pull)	Rotation and retraction
Transport of debris	Poor because of tighter flutes	Better because of space present in flutes

Q.6 What are the advantages of NiTi alloys?
Ans.
- Superelasticity
- Good resiliency
- Corrosion resistance
- Softer than stainless steel.

Q.7 What is the shape of access cavity of maxillary incisors?
Ans. It is triangular in shape with base towards incisal surface.

Q.8 What is the shape of access cavity of premolars?
Ans. It is oval in shape with greater dimensions on buccolingual side.

Q.9 What is the shape of access cavity of maxillary first molar?
Ans. It is rhomboid in shape.

Q.10 What is the shape of access cavity of mandibular molar?
Ans. It is trapezoidal or rhomboidal in shape.

Q.11 Why do we measure working length?
Ans. It determines how far into canal instruments should be placed and worked. If not properly calculated, it can get short of the apex or may go beyond apex.

Q.12 What are the functions of irrigants?
Ans. Irrigants help in removing the debris from accessory and lateral canals where instruments cannot reach. Instruments are less likely to break when canal walls are lubricated with irrigants.

Q.13 Name commonly used irrigating solutions?
Ans.
- Saline
- Sodium hypochlorite (0.5–5.25%)
- Hydrogen peroxide
- Chlorhexidine.

Q.14 How is step back technique performed?
Ans. It involves two phases. Phase I, involves the preparation of apical constriction and phase II involves preparation of the remaining canal.

Chapter 12: Examination Spotters

INSTRUMENTS

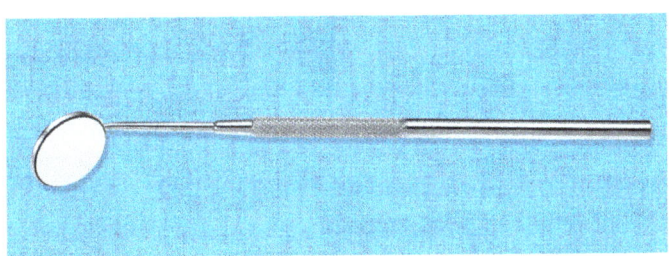
Spotters: 1

Spotter 1: Mouth Mirror
- It is used as diagnostic instrument and to improve access to instrumentation
- It has handle, shank and a mirror attached to a round metal disk at one end
- It is used for: Direct vision, indirect vision, retraction, transillumination.

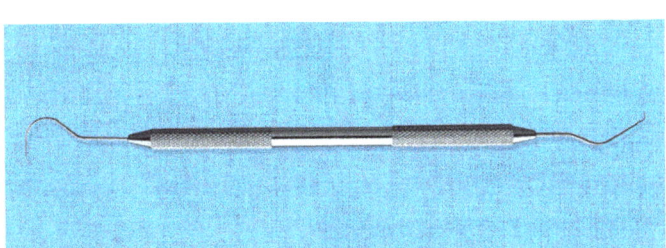
Spotters: 2

Spotter 2: Explorer
- Explorer is used as a diagnostic aid
- It has straight handle which can be plain or serrated
- Shank is curved with one or more angles
- Working tip is pointed
- Used for examining pit and fissure caries
- Interproximal explorer is used for examination of interproximal caries and assessing marginal fit of the restoration.

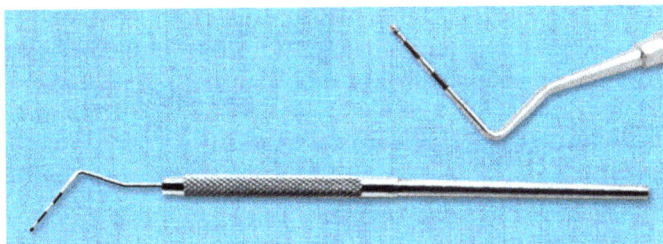
Spotters: 3

Spotter 3: CPITN Probe
- It is a also called as WHO probe
- It has 0.5 mm ball ended probe tip with color coding between 3.5 to 5.5 markings
- It is used to check the dimensions of tooth preparations.

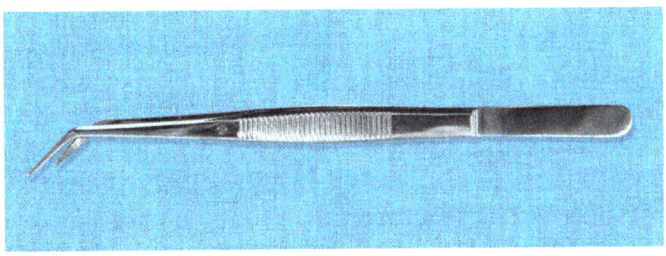
Spotters: 4

Spotter 4: Tweezer
- Tweezer has angled end with inner serrations
- It has inner guide pin which provides stability
- It is available in different sizes
- Used to place and remove cotton rolls and other small materials to and from the mouth.

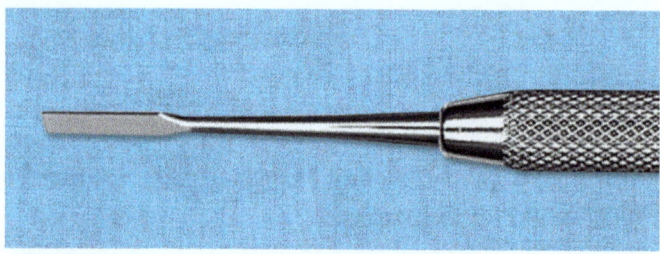

Spotters: 5

Spotter 5: Chisel

- Straight chisel has straight shank and blade with bevel only on one side
- Cutting edge is perpendicular to plane of instrument
- Used with straight thrust force and push motion
- It is mainly used for cutting enamel, smoothen and sharpen the tooth preparations.

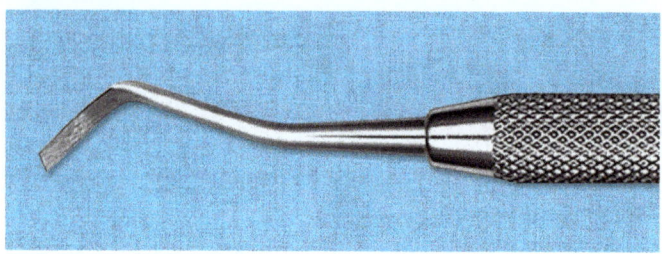

Spotters: 6

Spotter 6: Gingival Margin Trimmer

- Available in paired double planed instrument
- Available as mesial and distal gingival margin trimmer
- Used for:
  - Planing gingival cavosurface margin
  - Removal of unsupported enamel
  - To bevel axiopulpal line angle in the class II tooth preparation.

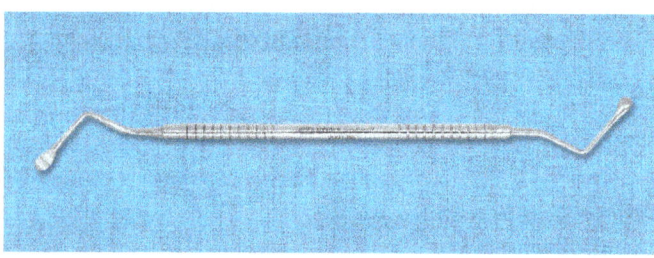

Spotters: 7

Spotter 7: Spoon Excavator

- A double-ended instrument with a spoon shaped blade
- Cutting edge of blade is directed in the same plane as that of long axis of the handle
- Used for:
  - To remove soft caries in scooping motion
  - For carving amalgam restorations and wax patterns.

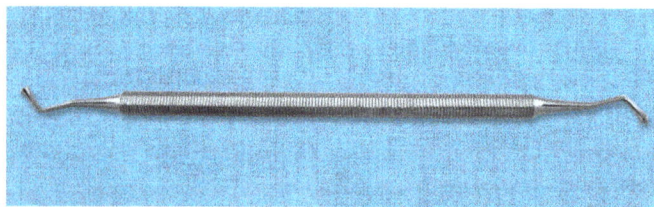

Spotters: 8

Spotter 8: Burnisher

- Burnisher is a double ended-instrument which has smooth rounded ends available in different types
- Used for:
  - To smoothen and polish the restoration
  - For giving initial occlusal anatomy
  - For final condensation of amalgam
  - For burnishing margins of cast gold restoration
  - Shaping matrix bands according to tooth anatomy.

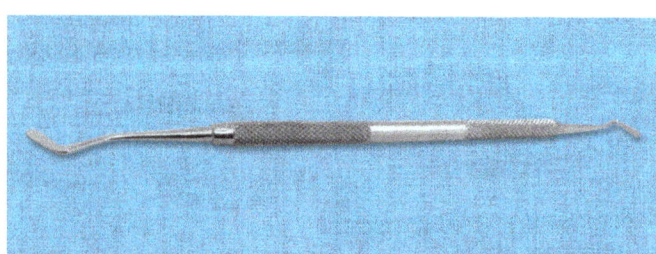

Spotters: 9

Spotter 9: Plastic Filling Instrument

- It is double ended instrument which is used to carry the mixed cement which is plastic stage
- It is used to convenience form of the prepared cavities.

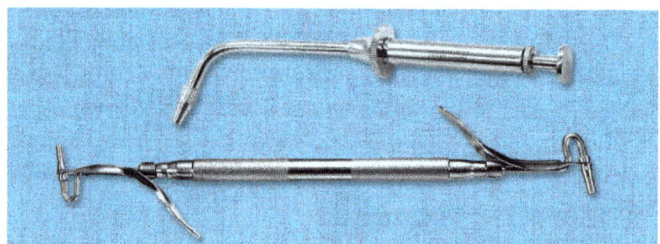

Spotters: 10

Spotter 10: Amalgam Carrier

- It is used to place mixed amalgam in the prepared cavity. It is available as both single and double ended carrier
- It has a hollow cylinder in to which the triturated amalgam can be loaded to dispense in the cavity.

Spotter 11: High-speed Diamond Point

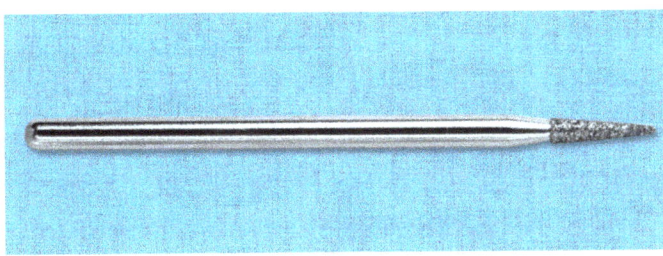

Spotters: 11

- Used with high-speed airotor handpiece
- Has head, neck and friction lock type shank
- Used for tooth preparations and removal of old restorative materials
- Named on the basis of shape of head like round, inverted, straight, tapered, etc.

Spotter 12: Slow-speed Dental Bur

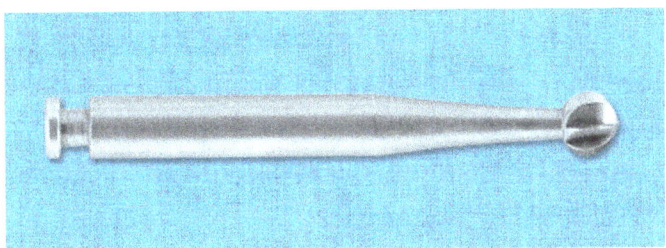

Spotters: 12

- Slow-speed dental bur used with micromotor handpiece
- Has head, neck and latch-type shank
- Used for finishing and polishing purposes
- Named on the basis of shape of head like round, inverted, straight, tapered, etc.

Spotter 13: Wooden Wedges

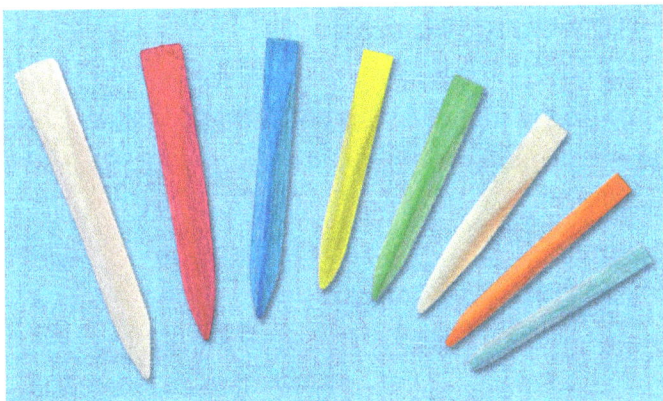

Spotters: 13

- Used for adaptation of matrix band closely to the tooth and thus prevent overhanging of the restoration
- Used for rapid separation during tooth preparation and restoration
- Available as triangular and round shapes, triangular is preferred over round shape.

Spotter 14: Plastic Wedges

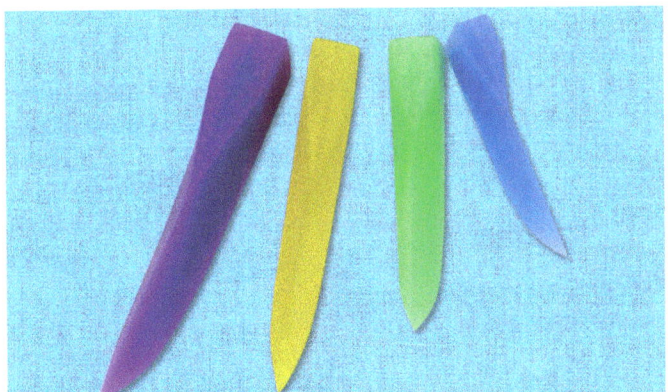

Spotters: 14

- These are ready made wedges which are available in different sizes and colors
- Used for adaptation of matrix band closely to the tooth and thus prevent overhanging of the restoration
- Used for rapid separation during tooth preparation and restoration

Spotter 15: Tofflemire Retainer

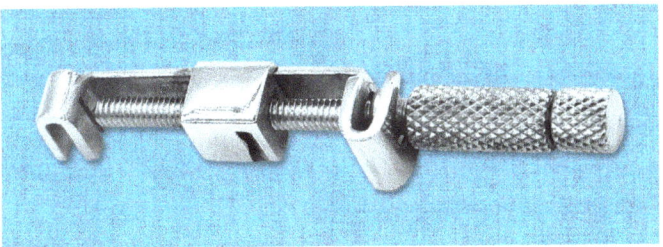

Spotters: 15

- Also known as 'universal' matrix because it can be used in all types of tooth preparations of posterior teeth
- Has head, slot, small and large knurled nuts as its components
- Used for class I tooth preparations with buccal or lingual extensions and class II (MOD) tooth preparations
- Easy to use, provides good contact and contours.

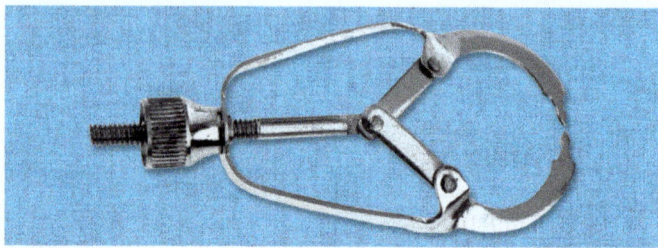

Spotters: 16

Spotter 16: Ivory No. 1 Matrix Retainer

- Most commonly used matrix band holder for unilateral class II tooth preparations
- It has a claw at one end with two flat semicircle arms having a pointed projection at the end
- On other end, there is a screw which is when rotated clockwise, brings ends of both claws closer to each other
- Keeping the matrix band around the tooth, screw is tightened so as to fit the band snugly around the tooth
- Used for restorations of unilateral class II tooth preparations, especially when the contact on the unprepared side is very tight.

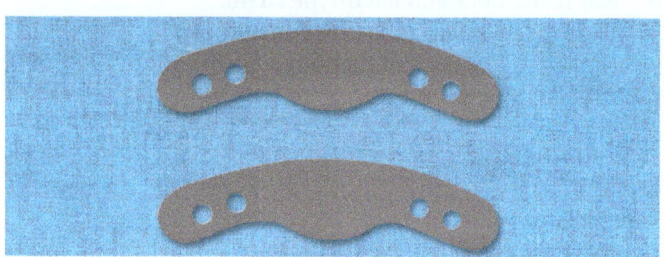

Spotters: 17

Spotter 17: Ivory No. 1 Matrix Band

- Used with matrix retainer no.1
- Band is slightly convex in its middle part
- This projected margin is kept towards the gingiva on the side of tooth preparation
- It has holes into which retainer is inserted and adjusted according to the tooth.

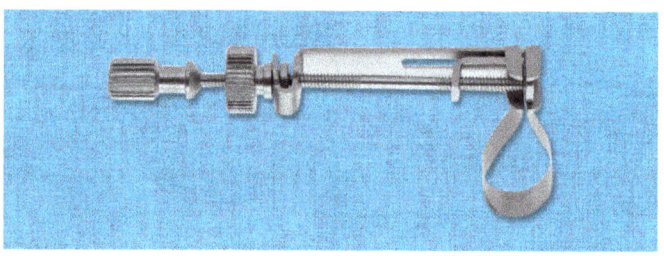

Spotters: 18

Spotter 18: Ivory No. 8 Matrix Retainer

- It holds the matrix band that encircles the tooth to provide missing walls on both proximal sides
- Circumference of the band can be adjusted using the screw present in the matrix band retainer
- Used for:
  - Unilateral or bilateral class II preparations (MOD)
  - Class II compound tooth preparations having more than two missing walls

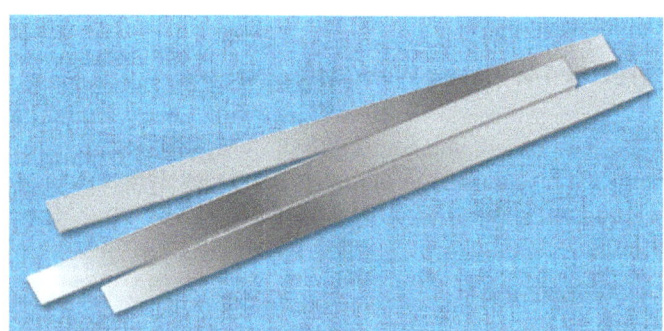

Spotters: 19

Spotter 19: Ivory No. 8 Matrix band

- Used with ivory matrix band retainer no. 8
- It is made up of thin sheet of metal so that it can pass through the contact area of the unprepared proximal side of the tooth
- Used for class II restorations.

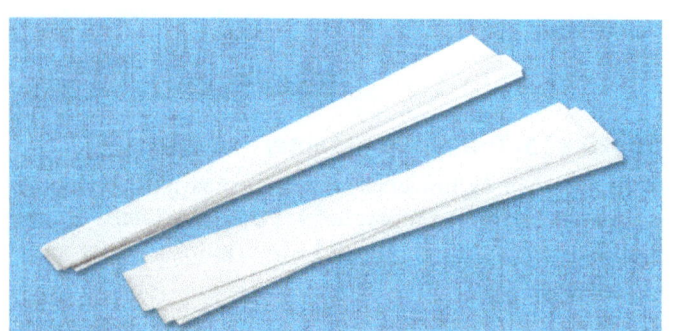

Spotters: 20

Spotter 20: Mylar Strips

- Cellophane (Cellulose acetate) strips are used during tooth-colored restorations
- Specially used during Class III and IV composite restorations because they allow light to be transmitted during polymerization.

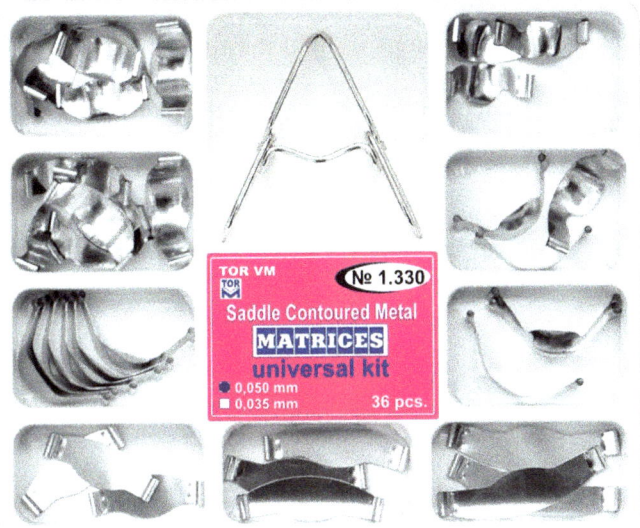

Spotters: 21

Spotter 21: Sectional Matrix

Sectional matrix system is used during placement of interproximal amalgam or composite restorations. Kit contains pre-contoured metal matrix forms and rings for matrix retention and tooth separation.
- This matrix system offers accurate contacts and seal. It is easy to place and remove
- It minimizes chances of overhangs.

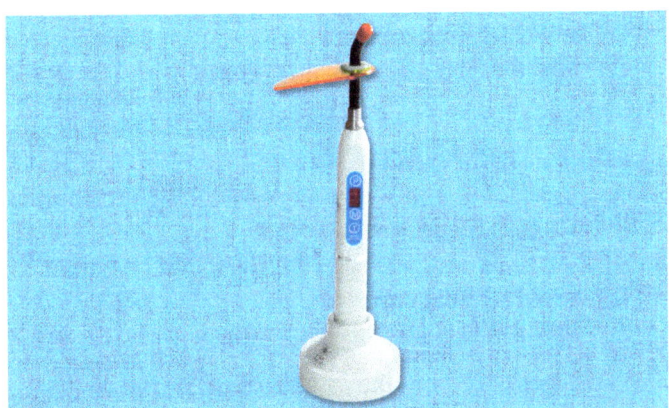

Spotters: 22

Spotter 22: Light Cure Unit

- Light curing unit is used to initiate the polymerization of composite resins
- It has a light source and optical fibers
- In this visible light with the wavelength ranging from 400–500 nm is used to polymerize the resin.

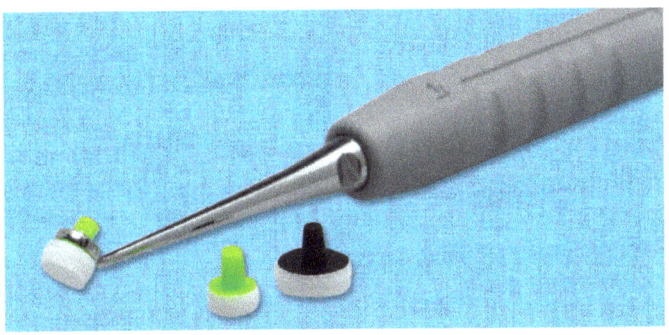

Spotters: 23

Spotter 23: Optrasculpt Pad

- OptraSculpt is a contouring instruments used for the non-stick shaping and contouring of surfaces.
- It does not stick to composites, and its working angles are adjusted to the anterior and posterior regions.

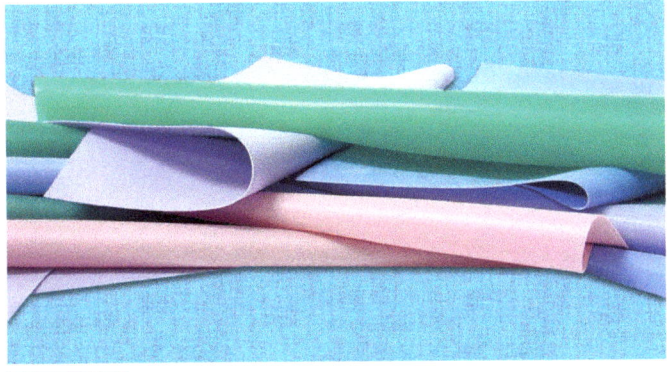

Spotters: 24

Spotter 24: Rubber Dam Sheet

- Rubber dam sheet is normally available in size 5 × 5 or 6 × 6 sq inches in light and dark colors
- Dark colors are preferred (green or black) for good contrast
- Sheet has dry and shiny sides. Dull side faces the occlusal surface of isolated teeth because it is less reflective than shiny surface
- It is available in three thicknesses: light, medium, and heavy. Thicker dam is effective in retracting the tissues and is more resistant to tearing. Thinner dam can easily pass through the contacts easier, so used in cases of tight contacts.

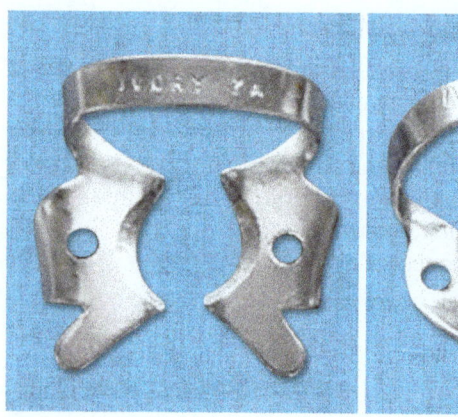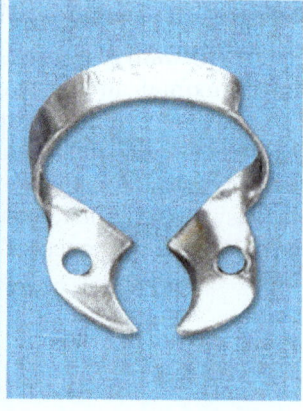

Spotter 25: Rubber Dam Clamp

- Rubber dam clamps to hold the rubber dam onto the tooth are available in different shapes and sizes.
  - They anchor the rubber dam to the tooth
  - Help in retracting the gingiva.

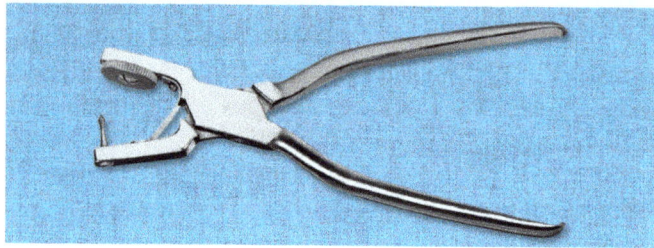

Spotter 26: Rubber Dam Punch

- Rubber dam punch is used to make the holes in the rubber sheet through which the teeth can be isolated
- Working end is designed with a plunger on one side and a wheel on the other side. This wheel has different sized holes on the flat surface facing the plunger.

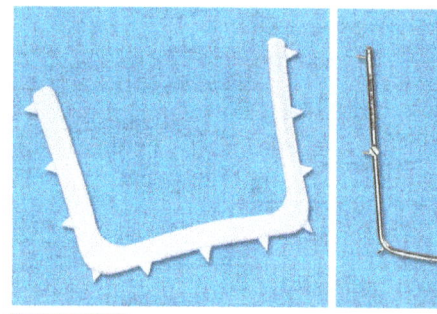

Spotter 27: Rubber Dam Frame

- Rubber dam frame supports the edges of rubber dam.
- It serve following purposes:
  - Support the edges of rubber dam
  - Retract the soft tissues
  - Improve accessibility to the isolated teeth.

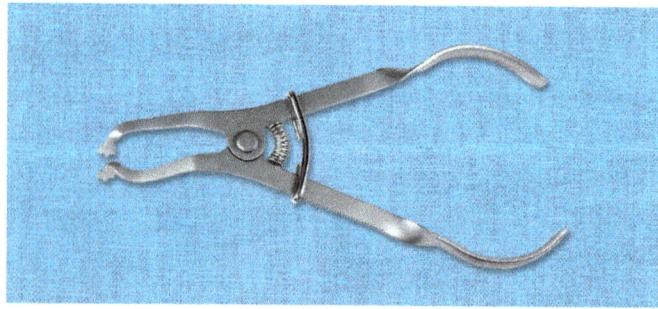

Spotter 28: Rubber Dam Forceps

Rubber dam forceps is used to carry the clamp to the tooth.

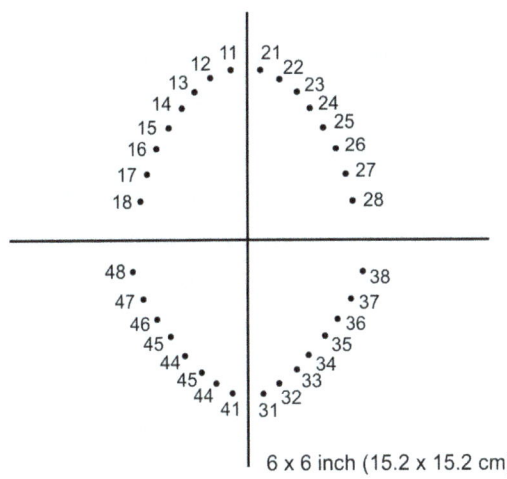

Spotter 29: Rubber Dam Template

- It is an inked rubber stamp which helps in marking the dots on the sheet according to position of the tooth
- Holes should be punched according to arch and missing teeth.

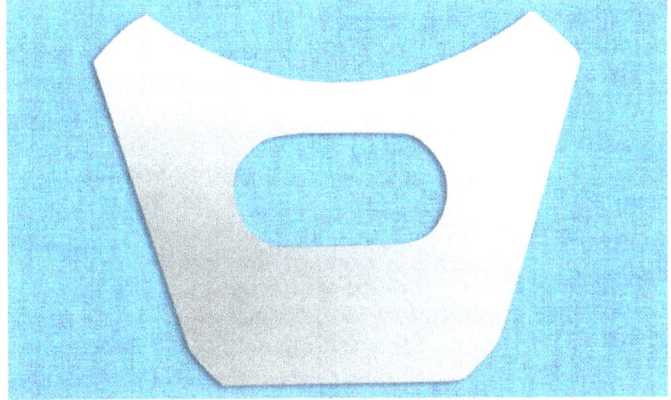

Spotter 30: Rubber Dam Napkin

This is a sheet of absorbent materials usually placed between the rubber sheet and soft tissues. It absorbs saliva from corner of patient's mouth.

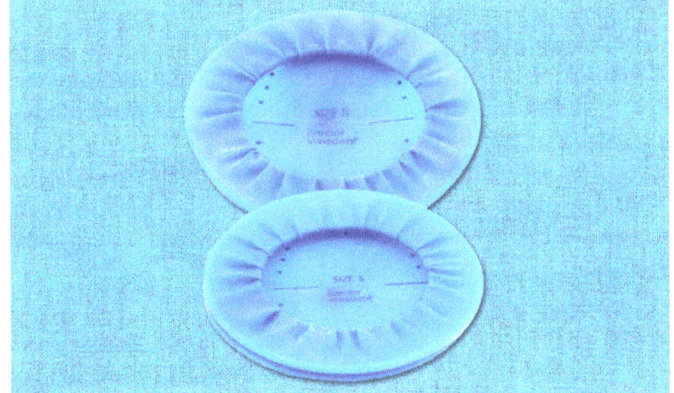

Spotter 31: Optra Dam

- It is an anatomically shaped rubber dam for isolation.
- It is made up of flexible latex.
- For use, intraoral ring is positioned in gingivobuccal fold and outer ring remains outside the mouth.

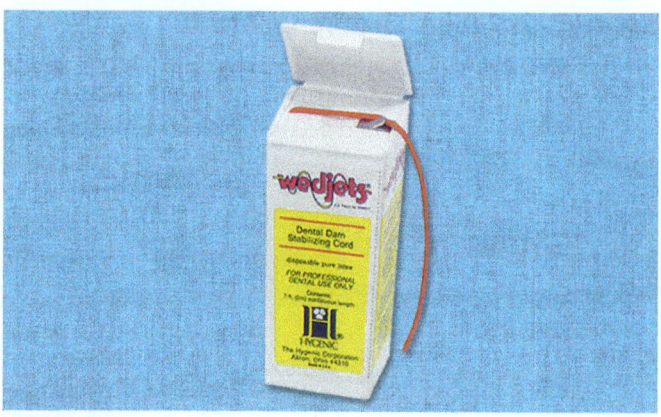

Spotters: 32

Spotter 32: Wedjets

Wedjet cord is made up of natural latex to stabilize the dam with little chances of tissue trauma.

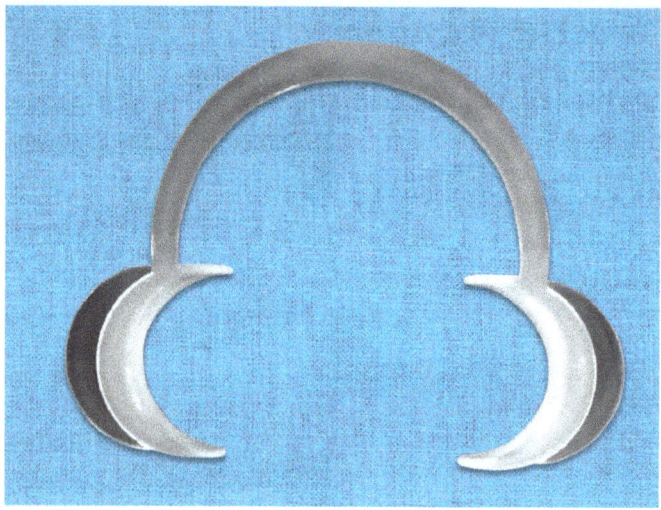

Spotters: 33

Spotter 33: Cheek Retractor

- It pulls tissue away to expose an area that needs dental work.
- It keeps the tissue in a retracted position during the procedure.

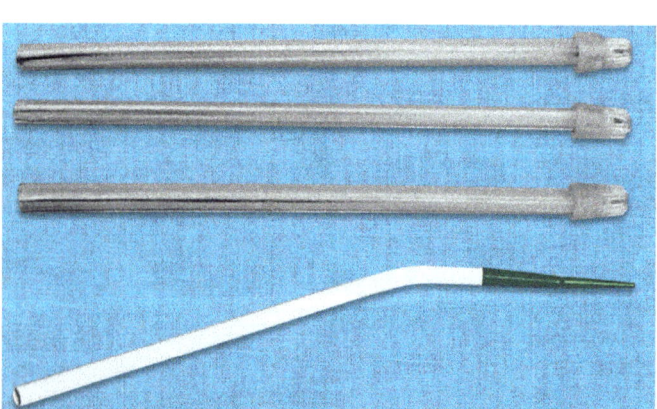

Spotters: 34

Spotter 34: Low-volume Evacuator

- Saliva ejector is best used to remove small amounts of moisture and saliva collected in the oral cavity during clinical procedure.
- Tip of saliva ejector should be smooth to prevent any tissue injury.
- To avoid any interference with working, it can be bent to place in the required area of mouth.

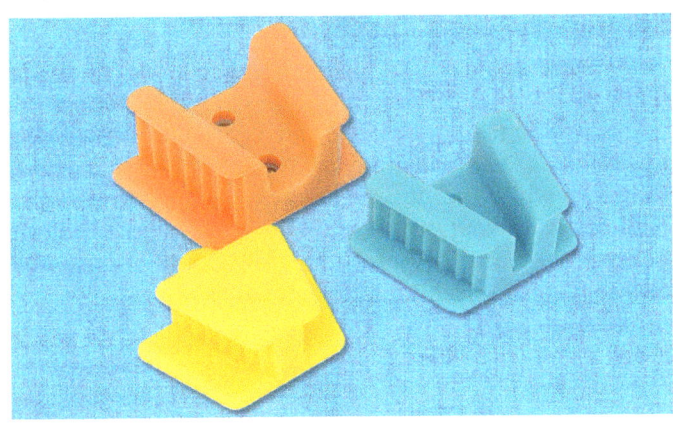

Spotters: 35

Spotter 35: Mouth Prop
- Mouth prop establishes and maintains suitable mouth opening
- It is placed on the side opposite to treatment. It offers muscle relaxation to patient, provides sufficient mouth opening for long durations.

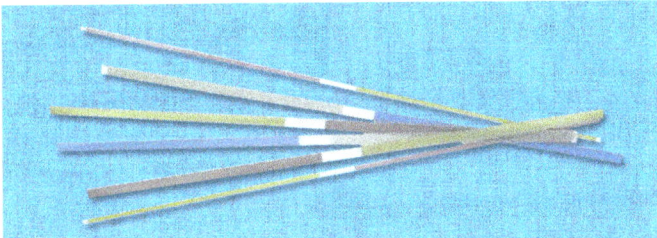

Spotters: 36

Spotter 36: Interproximal Finishing Strips
These are made from metal or plastic, have an abrasive side that can be used for interproximal reduction, contouring or finishing the restoration. These are available in different grits and colors coding to make them easy to identify.

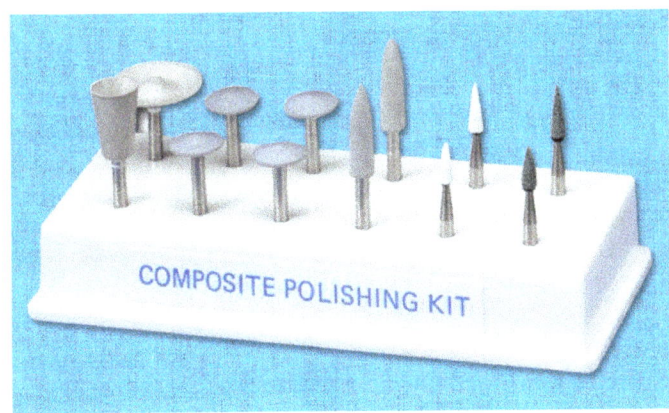

Spotters: 37

Spotter 37: Composite Polishing Kit
Composite kit contains all instruments for contouring, finishing and polishing of composite restorations: Green stones to reduce excess material, white stones for finishing, fine instruments for high gloss without damage to the enamel.

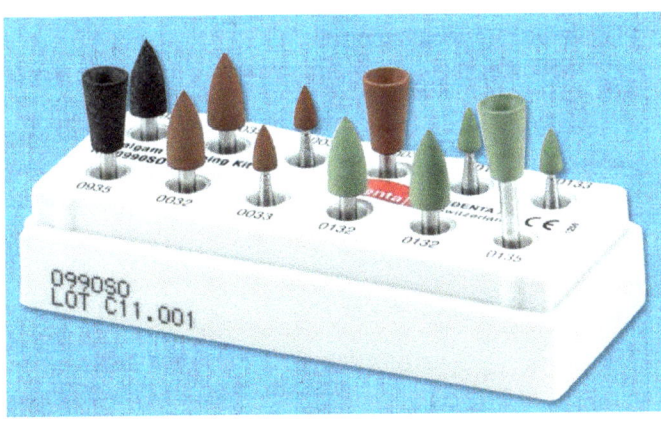

Spotters: 38

Spotter 38: Amalgam Polishing Kit
- Consists of polishing stones of different sizes and grades from fine to coarse
- Used to finish amalgam restoration after 24 hours by attaching it in contra-angle micromotor handpiece.

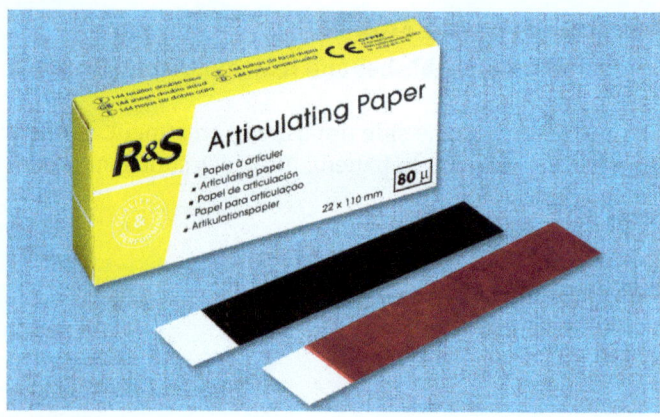

Spotters: 39

Spotter 39: Articulating Paper

Articulating paper is a diagnostic tool used to highlight occlusal contacts and high points. It marks those points on the teeth where the teeth contact during biting and grinding. A strip of articulating paper is placed between the teeth while the desired mandibular movements are performed. It is routinely used to check the occlusal surfaces of recently placed restorations, crowns and bridges and also to highlight occlusal interferences like in persons with bruxism.

MATERIALS

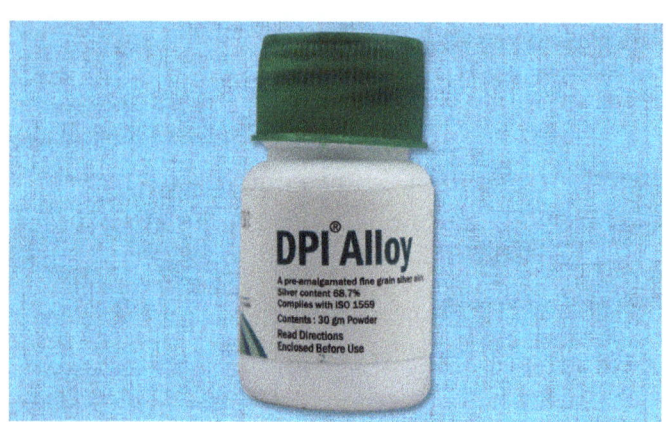

Spotters: 40

Spotter 40: Amalgam Alloy Powder

- Available in form of powder
- Consists of silver, tin, copper, zinc and palladium
- Can be classified as high- and low-copper alloy according to copper content
- Classified as lathe cut and spherical according to shape of alloy
- Mixed with mercury to form dental amalgam.

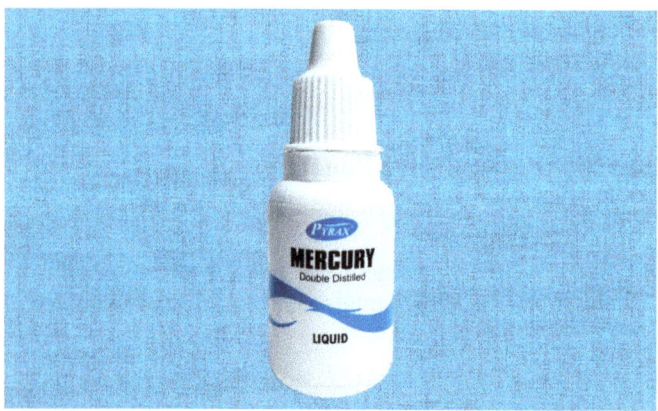

Spotters: 41

Spotter 41: Mercury

- Available in liquid form
- According to Eames technique, it should be mixed in 1:1 ratio with silver alloy powder
- More mercury in alloy results in:
  - More contraction of set amalgam
  - More creep
  - Decrease in strength
  - Should be removed from mixed amalgam by mulling after trituration.

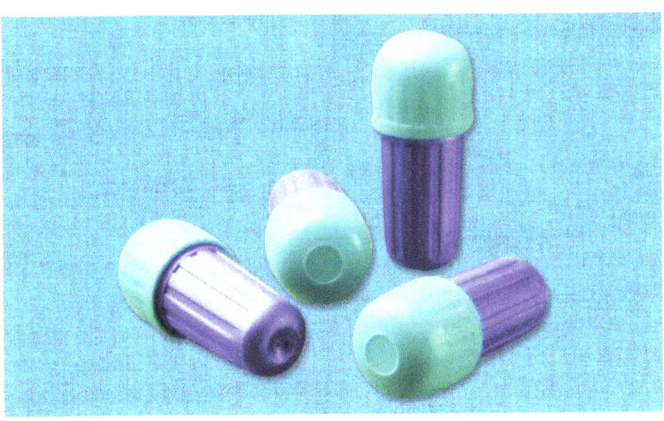
Spotters: 42

Spotter 42: Amalgam Capsule
- It is proportioned capsule containing amalgam alloy and mercury
- To prevent any amalgamation during storage, mercury and alloy are physically separated from each other
- It is triturated mechanically in amalgamator
- Prevents spillage of mercury and provides proper ratio of amalgam alloy and powder.

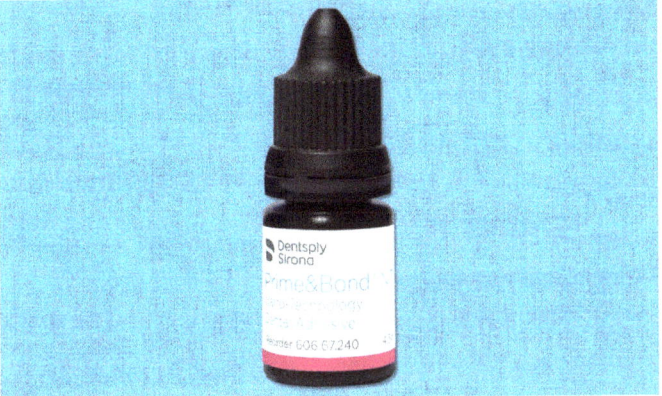
Spotters: 43

Spotter 43: Dentin Bonding Agent
- Available in liquid form
- Mainly consists of HEMA and Bis GMA
- It has a bifunctional structure
- It has both hydrophilic and hydrophobic ends. Hydrophilic end bonds the inorganic part of dentin and hydrophobic end bonds to the composite resin
- It penetrates in etched micropores of tooth surface forming the hybrid layer.

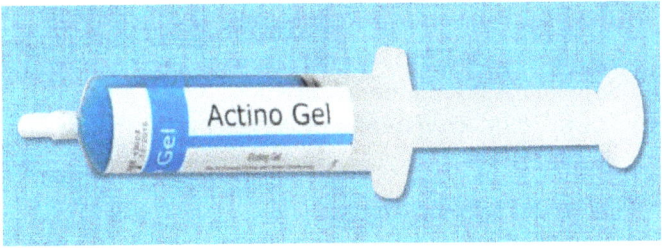
Spotters: 44

Spotter 44: Etchant
- Available as 37% phosphoric acid in form of liquid or gel
- Applied for 10–15 seconds on tooth and then washed off to give a frosty-white appearance it cleanses debris from enamel and produces micropores into which there is mechanical interlocking of the resin
- Increases the enamel surface area available for bonding
- Exposes more reactive surface layer, thus increasing its wettability.

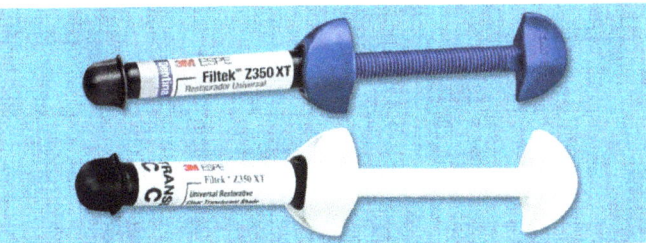
Spotters: 45

Spotter 45: Light-cured Composite Resin
- Restorative resin polymerized by a light source
- Consists of organic part, fillers, coupling agent, activator–initiator system, inhibitors and coloring agents
- Available in different shade for esthetics
- Available as microfilled, hybrid and nanofilled type
- Used for restoration of:
  - Mild to moderate class I and class II tooth preparations
  - Class III, IV and V preparations.

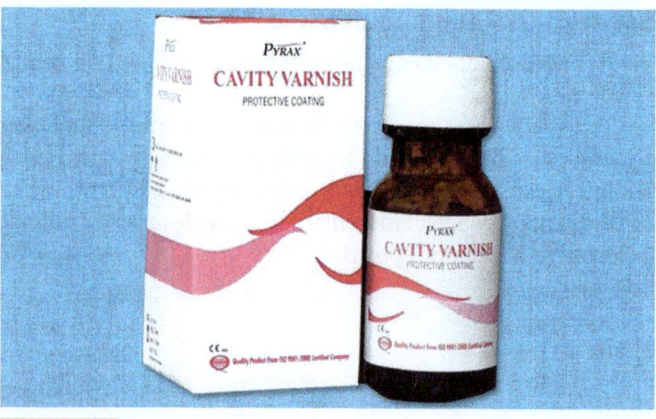

Spotters: 46

Spotter 46: Varnish
- It is an organic copal or resin gum suspended in solutions of ether or chloroform
- Applied on prepared tooth walls and floors in 2-3 coats using a small cotton pledget
- When applied on the tooth surface the organic solvent evaporates leaving behind a protective film
- Used to reduce microleakage, postoperative sensitivity and improve sealing ability of the amalgam
- Prevents discoloration of tooth by checking migration of ions into the dentin
- Not used under glass ionomers because it interferes chemical bonding of tooth and cements.

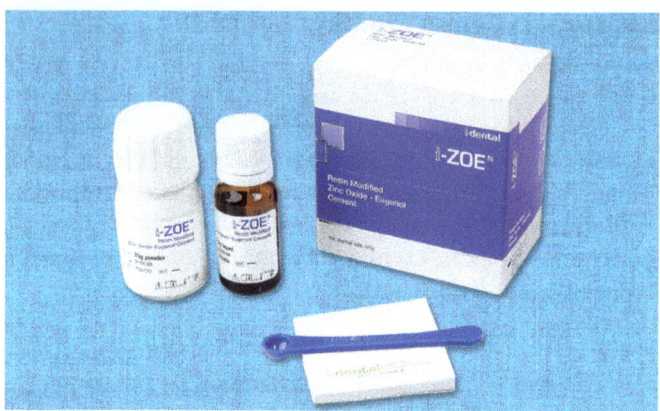

Spotters: 47

Spotter 47: Zinc Oxide Eugenol Cement
- Supplied as powder and liquid
- Powder contains zinc oxide, white rosin, zinc stearate and zinc acetate. Liquid contains eugenol
- Available as Type I (temporary luting), Type II (long-term luting), Type III (temporary restoration) and Type IV (intermediate restoration)
- Used as sedative cement, for temporary luting and restorative purpose.

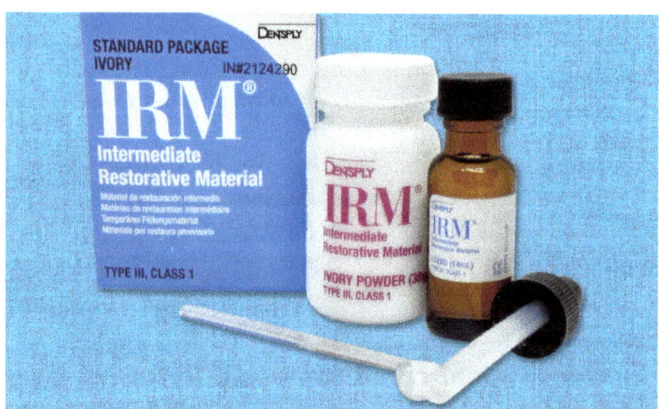

Spotters: 48

Spotter 48: Intermediate Restorative Material (IRM)
- Reinforced zinc oxide eugenol cement
- Supplied as powder and liquid
- Powder reinforced by adding polymethyl methacrylate
- Resin helps in:
  - Improving strength and smoothness of the mix
  - Decreasing flow, solubility and brittleness of the cement
  - Used as temporary restoration.

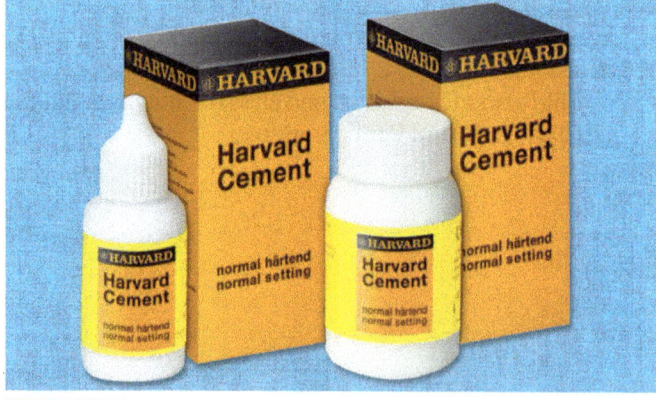

Spotters: 49

Spotter 49: Zinc Phosphate Cement
- Supplied as powder and liquid
- Powder contains zinc oxide, magnesium oxide and bismuth oxide. Liquid contains phosphoric acid, water and alumina
- Available as two types:
  - Type I: used for luting purpose
  - Type II: used as base
- Has high compressive strength and thin film thickness
- Used for luting crowns, inlays and orthodontics bands
- Used as intermediate base and temporary restoration material.

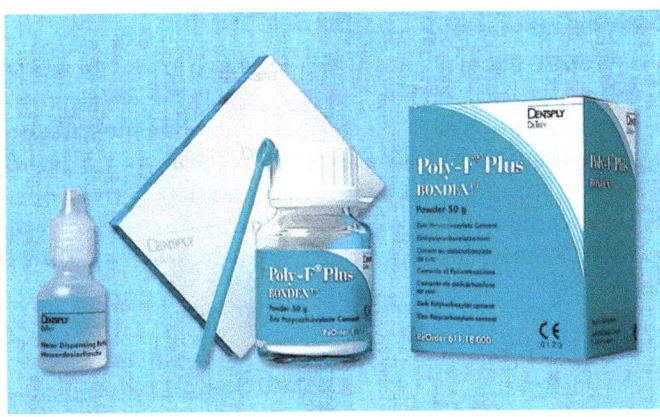

Spotters: 50

Spotter 50: Zinc Polycarboxylate Cement

- Supplied as powder and liquid
- Powder contains zinc oxide and magnesium oxide
- Liquid contains polyacrylic acid
- Bonds chemically to the tooth structure. Polyacrylic acid reacts with calcium ion of teeth via carboxyl group and form chemical bond
- Biocompatibility because of bigger size of polyacrylic acid molecule (unable to penetrate into dentinal tubules) and rise of pH of the cement on mixing
- Used to cement inlays or crowns
- Used as base and temporary restoration.

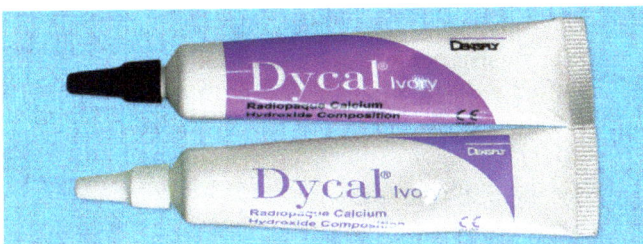

Spotters: 51

Spotter 51: Calcium Hydroxide

- Supplied as base and catalyst
- Its high alkaline pH (12.5) helps in neutralization of acids produced by the microorganisms
- Provides antibacterial properties
- Promotes reparative dentin formation
- Used as sub-base and liner
- Used in pulpotomy and pulp capping procedures.

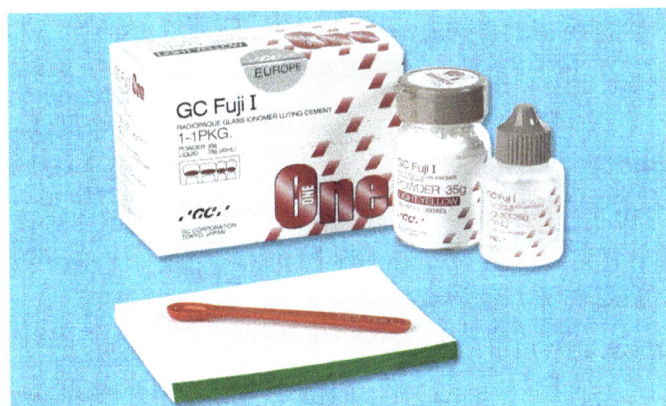

Spotters: 52

Spotter 52: Type 1 Glass Ionomer Cement

- Used for luting purpose
- Supplied as powder and liquid
- Powder contains calcium fluoroaluminosilicate glass and liquid contains polyacrylic acid, itaconic and tartaric acid
- Bonds chemically to tooth structure
- Biocompatible
- Low solubility.

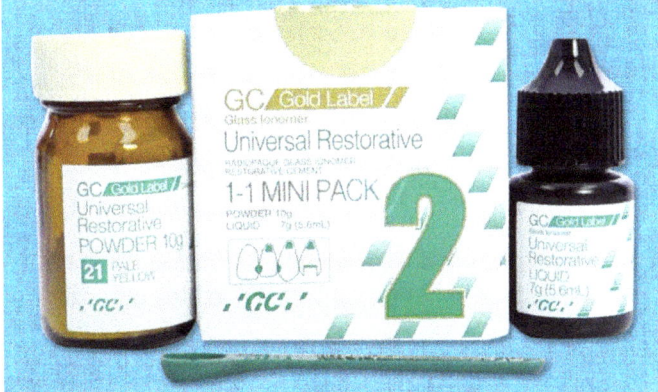

Spotters: 53

Spotter 53: Type 2 Glass Ionomer Cement

- Used as restorative cement
- Supplied as powder and liquid
- Powder contains calcium fluoroaluminosilicate glass and liquid contains polyacrylic acid, itaconic and tartaric acid
- Bonds chemically to tooth structure
- Anticariogenic cement due to release of fluorides
- Biocompatible, esthetic in nature and has low solubility
- Sensitive to both moisture contamination and desiccation during setting phase
- Indicated for class V, III and small class I tooth preparations.

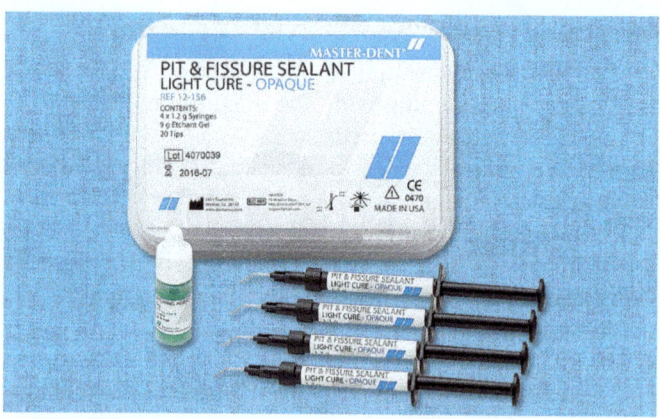

Spotters: 54

Spotter 54: Pit and Fissure Sealant

- Pit and fissure sealant is used as a primary prevention tool when the tooth is at high-risk of caries
- It provides a physical barrier that inhibits microorganisms and food particles accumulation, preventing caries initiation, and arresting caries progression
- It is indicated for pits and fissures of deciduous or permanent teeth in children with high caries risk.

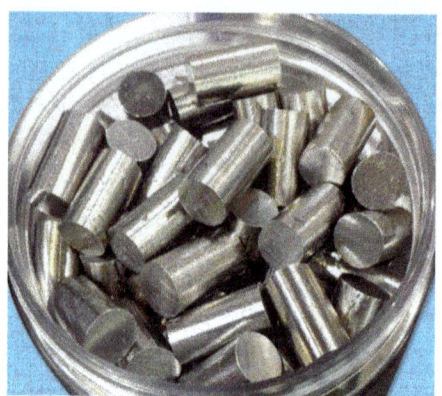

Spotters: 55

Spotter 55: Base-metal Alloy Pellets

- Mainly consists of nickel, chromium and cobalt
- Classified as Type I (soft), Type II (medium), Type III (hard) and Type IV (extra hard) according to their use
- Used for fabrication of inlays, onlays, crowns, bridges and partial dentures.

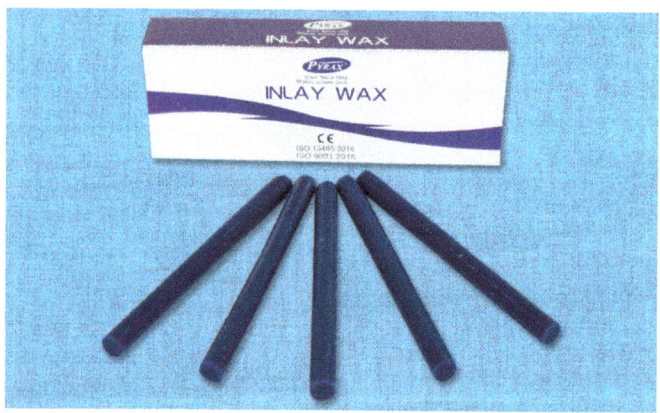

Spotters: 56

Spotter 56: Inlay Wax

- Used for making patterns for inlays, onlays and crowns
- Contains paraffin wax, Carnauba wax, ceresin and gum dammer
- Available as:
  - Type I: Medium wax for direct technique
  - Type II: Soft wax for indirect technique.
- Available in different colors to contrast with die for better demarcation and finishing of margins.

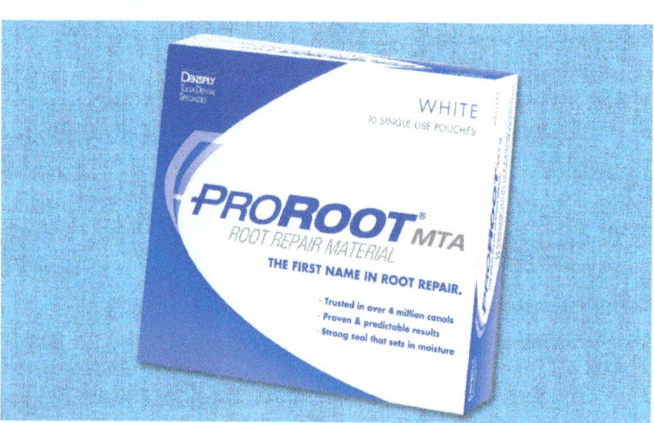

Spotters: 57

Spotter 57: MTA

- Biomaterial used in pulp capping, pulpotomy and apexification
- Mainly consists of tricalcium silicate, dicalcium silicate, tricalcium aluminate, bismuth oxide, tetracalcium aluminoferrite
- Sets in presence of moisture. Mixed with saline and carried with amalgam carrier.

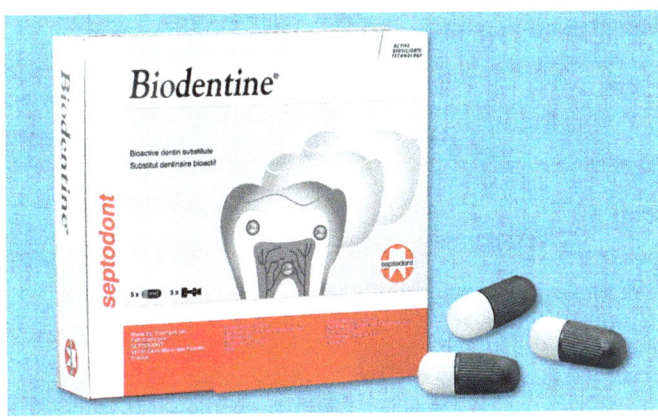

Spotters: 58

Spotter 58: Biodentin

Biodentine is a calcium-silicate based material, known as 'bioactive dentine substitute'. It is which is used for management of root perforations, apexification, resorptions, pulp capping procedures, and dentine replacement.

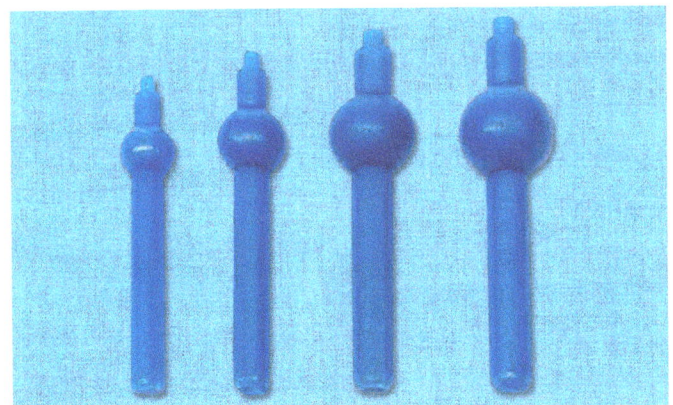

Spotters: 59

Spotter 59: GC Tooth Mousse

- Tooth mousse is derived from the milk protein, casein. It causes remineralization activity due part of casein protein called casein Phosphopeptide (or CPP), which carries calcium and phosphate ions in the form of amorphous calcium phosphate (or ACP).
- Tooth mousse, contain this complex of CPP-ACP, therefore act as delivery system for bio-available calcium and phosphate ions.

Spotters: 60

Spotter 60: Sprue Former

- It is a sprue former which provides channel through which molten metal or ceramic flows into the mold cavity.
- It is attached at 45° to the wax pattern during investment.

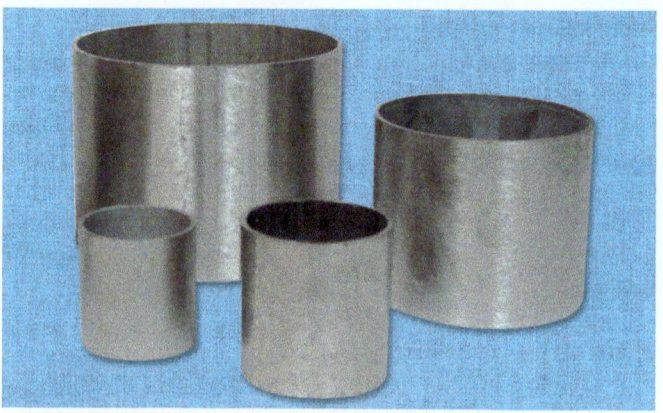

Spotters: 61

Spotter 61: Casting Ring
- It is a metallic ring that holds the wax pattern, sprue former and investment together
- It is available in various sizes for investments of different sized units.

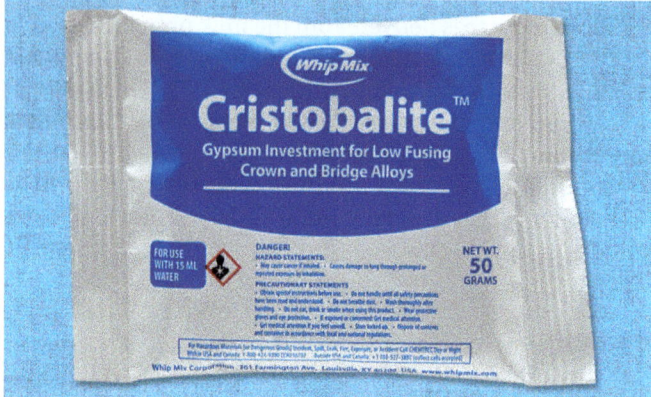

Spotters: 62

Spotter 62: Gypsum Bonded Investment Material
- It contains silica: 60–65%, alpha hemihydrate: 30–35%, chemical modifier 5% and water
- It can withstand temperature of 700°
- It is used in casting for inlays, bridges, removable partial denture frameworks using gold alloys and low fusing alloys.

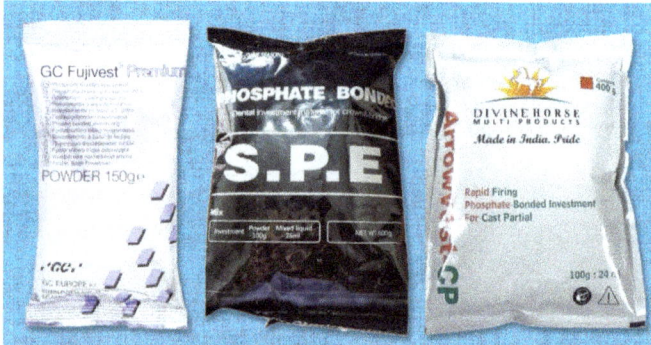

Spotters: 63

Spotter 63: Phosphate Bonded Investment Material
- It is available as powder and liquid. The powder contains ammonium diphosphate, silica, magnesium oxide and liquid is silica solution in water
- It can withstand higher temperatures
- It is used in casting of high fusing alloys, for example, noble metals, metal ceramic and base metal alloys.

Glossary

ABFRACTION: The pathologic loss of hard tooth substance caused by biomechanical loading forces; such loss is thought to be the result of flexure and chemical fatigue degradation of enamel and/or dentin at some location distant from the actual point of loading.

ABRASION: Abrasion is abnormal tooth surface loss resulting from direct friction forces between the teeth and external objects or from frictional forces between contacting teeth components in the presence of an abrasive medium.

ABRASIVE: A substance used for abrading, smoothing, or polishing.

ACCESS CAVITY: It is defined as endodontic coronal preparation which enables unobstructed access to the canal orifices, a straight line access to apical foramen, complete control over instrumentation and to accommodate obturation technique.

ACID-ETCHING: Process of roughening a solid surface by exposing it to an acid and thoroughly rinsing the residue to promote micromechanical bonding of an adhesive to the surface.

ACUTE (RAMPANT) CARIES: Acute caries, often termed rampant caries, is when the disease is rapid in damaging the tooth. It is suddenly appearing, widespread and rapidly burrowing type of caries resulting in early involvement of the pulp and affecting those teeth that are usually regarded as immune to caries.

ADHEREND: A material substrate that is bonded to another material by means of an adhesive.

ADHESION: A molecular or atomic attraction between two contacting surfaces promoted by the interfacial force of attraction between the molecules or atoms of two different species; adhesion may occur as physical adhesion, chemical adhesion, mechanical adhesion (structural interlocking) or a combination of all types.

ADHESIVE BONDING: Process of joining two materials by means of an adhesive agent that solidifies during the bonding process.

ADHESIVE: Substance that promotes adhesion of one substance or material to another. Any substance that join or create close adherence of two or more surfaces.

AFFECTED DENTIN: Softened demineralized dentin not yet invaded by bacteria.

AMALGAM: Technically means an alloy of mercury (Hg) with any other metal.

AMELOGENESIS IMPERFECTA: In amelogenesis imperfecta, the enamel is defective either in form or calcification as a result of heredity and has an appearance ranging from essentially normal to extremely unsightly. It is entirely an ectodermal disturbance since the mesodermal components of teeth are normal.

ANATOMIC TOOTH CROWN: It is the portion of the tooth covered with enamel.

APEX: Refers to tip or most superior point of the structure. Tip of root of the tooth is also known as apex.

APICAL DENTAL FORAMEN: It is the main apical opening on the surface of root canal through which blood vessels enter the canal.

ATTRITION: Attrition is mechanical wear of the incisal or occlusal surface as a result of functional or parafunctional movements of the mandible (tooth-to-tooth contacts).

AXIAL WALL: An axial wall is an internal wall parallel with the long axis of the tooth.

BACKWARD CARIES: When spread of caries along DEJ exceeds the caries in surface enamel, it is termed as backward caries.

BACK PRESSURE POROSITY: Porosity produced in dental castings thought to be the result of the inability of gases in the mold to escape during the casting procedure; synonyms ENTRAPPED AIR / RESIDUAL AIR / SUCK BACK POROSITY.

BALANCE: It is achieved by designing the angles of the shank so that the cutting edge of the blade lies within the projected diameter of the handle and nearly coincides with the projected axis of the handle.

BASES: Bases (cement bases, typically 1–2 mm) are used to provide thermal protection for the pulp and to supplement mechanical support for the restoration by distributing local stresses from the restoration across the underlying dentinal surface.

BEVELS: Bevel are "flexible extensions" of a cavity preparation, allowing the inclusion of surface defects, supplementary grooves, or other areas on the tooth surface. Bevels require minimum tooth involvement, and do not sacrifice the resistance and retention for the restoration.

BLADE ANGLE: It is the angle between the rake face and the clearance face.

BLADE: It is the working end of the instrument.

BUR BLADE: Blade is a projection on the bur head which forms a cutting edge. Blade has two surfaces:
1. *Blade face/Rake Face:* It is the surface of bur blade on the leading edge.
2. *Clearance face:* It is the surface of bur Blade on the trailing edge.

BUTT JOINT: When cavosurface margin is 90 degree, it is a butt joint. It is generally given for amalgam restorations.

CAVITATED CARIES (NONREVERSIBLE): In cavitated caries, the enamel surface is broken (not intact), and usually the lesion has advanced into dentin.

CAVOSURFACE ANGLE AND CAVOSURFACE MARGIN: Cavosurface angle is angle formed by junction of a prepared wall and the external surface of the tooth. Actual junction is referred to as the cavosurface margin.

CEMENT LINERS: Thicker liners that are selected primarily for pulpal medication and thermal protection.

CEMENTOENAMEL JUNCTION: It is the junction of enamel of crown and cementum of the root.

CHRONIC (SLOW OR ARRESTED) CARIES: Chronic caries is slow, or it may be arrested following several active phases. Dentin shows marked brown pigmentation and induration of lesion so called eburnation of dentin.

CINGULUM: It is the lingual lobe of an anterior tooth making bulk of the cervical third of palatal surface.

CLASS I RESTORATION: All pit and fissure restorations are Class I. Assigned to three groups:
1. Restorations on lingual surface of maxillary incisors
2. Restorations on occlusal surface of premolars and molars
3. Restorations on occlusal two thirds of the facial and lingual surfaces of molars.

CLASS II INLAY: It is an intracoronal cast metal restoration that involves the occlusal and proximal surface of a posterior tooth.

CLASS II ONLAY: It is a cast metal restoration that involves the occlusal and proximal surface of a posterior tooth and caps all of the cusps.

CLASS II RESTORATIONS: Restorations on the proximal surfaces of posterior teeth.

CLASS III RESOTRATIONS: Restorations on the proximal surfaces of anterior teeth that do not involve the incisal angle are Class III.

CLASS IV RESTORATIONS: Restorations on the proximal surfaces of anterior teeth that do involve the incisal edge are Class IV.

CLASS V RESTORATIONS: Restorations on the gingival third of the facial or lingual surfaces of all teeth (except pit and fissure lesions) are Class V.

CLEANING AND SHAPING: Use of rotary and /or hand instruments to expose, clean, enlarge and shape the pulp canal space, usually in conjunction with irrigant. To prepare root canal not only for disinfection but also to develop a shape that permits a three-dimensional sealing of canal.

CLINICAL TOOTH CROWN: It is the visible part of a tooth above the gum line.

COLLAR PREPARATION: To increase the retention and resistance forms when preparing a weakened tooth for a mesioocclusodistal onlay to cap all cusps, a facial or lingual "collar" or both may be provided.

CONCENTRICITY: Direct measurement of the symmetry of the bur head itself.

CONDENSATION: Process of packing the triturated mass into the cavity.

CONTACT AREA: Area of mesial or distal surface of a tooth that touches to its adjacent tooth in the arch is called contact area.

CONVENIENCE FORM. Convenience form is that shape or form of the preparation that provides for adequate observation, accessibility, and ease of operation in preparing and restoring the tooth.

CREEP: Amalgam creep is defined as the time dependent plastic deformation of zinc containing amalgam alloys principally resulting from slow metallurgic phase transformation that involve diffusion controlled reactions and produces volume increase.

CUSP: A cusp is an elevation on the crown of a tooth making up a divisional part on the occlusal surface.

DELAYED EXPANSION: Zinc containing low copper or high copper amalgam alloys which get contaminated by moisture during manipulation results in delayed expansion or secondary expansion. This occur 3–5 days after insertion and continues for months. This type of expansion can reach values greater than 400 mm (4%).

DENTAL AMALGAM: Is a metallic restorative material composed of a mixture of silver-tin-copper alloy and mercury.

DENTAL BUR: Bur is a rotary cutting instrument which has bladed cutting head.

DENTIN BONDING AGENT: A thin layer of resin between conditioned dentin and the resin matrix of a composite.

DENTIN BONDING: The process of bonding a resin to conditioned dentin.

DENTAL CASTING INVESTMENT: A material consisting principally of an allotrope of silica and a bonding agent; the bonding substance may be gypsum (for use in lower casting temperatures) or phosphates and silica (for use in higher casting temperatures).

DENTIN CONDITIONER: An acidic agent that dissolves the inorganic structure in dentin, resulting in a collagen mesh that allows infiltration of an adhesive resin.

DENTINAL WALL: The dentinal wall is that portion of a prepared external wall consisting of dentin, in which mechanical retention features may be located.

DENTINOENAMEL JUNCTION (DEJ): It is the interface of enamel and dentin of a tooth crown.

Glossary

DENTINOGENESIS IMPERFECTA: Dentinogenesis imperfecta is a hereditary condition in which only the dentin is defective. Normal enamel is weakly attached and lost early.

DEVELOPMENTAL GROOVE: It is a shallow groove between primary parts of crown or the root.

DOUBLE WEDGING: Here two wedges are used—one is inserted from buccal embrasure and another is inserted from lingual embrasure.

DOVETAIL: A widened portion of a prepared cavity used to increase retention and/or resistance.

EMBRASURES (SPILLWAYS): When two teeth of same arch contact, their curvatures adjacent to the contact areas are called embrasures. Spaces which widen out buccally, lingually, occlusally or gingivally are called buccal, lingual, occlusal or gingival embrasures respectively.

ENAMEL WALL: The enamel wall is that portion of a prepared external wall consisting of enamel.

ENAMELOPLASTY: Enameloplasty is removal of a shallow enamel developmental pit or fissure to create a smooth, saucer-shaped self-cleansing area.

ENDODONTICS: Branch of clinical dentistry associated with the prevention, diagnosis and treatment of the pathosis of the dental pulp and their sequelae.

EROSION: The progressive loss of tooth substance by chemical processes that do not involve bacterial action, producing defects that are wedge-shaped depressions often in occlusal, facial and cervical areas.

EXTERNAL LINE ANGLE: It is a line angle whose apex points away from the tooth.

EXTERNAL WALL: An external wall is a prepared (cut) surface that extends to the external tooth surface, and such a wall takes the name of the tooth surface (or aspect) that the wall is toward.

FACE: The end of the nib or working surface is known as face.

FLOOR (OR SEAT): A floor (or seat) is a prepared (cut) wall that is reasonably flat and perpendicular to those occlusal forces that are directed occlusogingivally (generally parallel to the long axis of the tooth).

FORWARD CARIES: Forward caries is wherever the caries cone in enamel is larger or at least the same size as that in dentin.

FOSSA: It denotes an irregular depression or concavity on the tooth.

HYBRID LAYER: An intermediate layer of resin, collagen, and dentin produced by acid, etching of dentin and resin infiltration into the conditioned dentin.

INCIPIENT CARIES (REVERSIBLE): Incipient caries is the first evidence of caries activity in the enamel, visible as white spot. The lesion can be mineralized by proper preventive procedures, hence called reversible caries.

INFECTED DENTIN: It is softened demineralized dentin containing bacteria.

INITIAL TOOTH PREPARATION: Initial tooth preparation is the extension and initial design of the external walls of the preparation at a specified, limited depth so as to provide access to the caries or defect, reach sound tooth structure (except for later removal of infected dentin on the pulpal or axial walls), resist fracture of the tooth or restorative material from masticatory forces, principally directed with the long axis of the tooth, and retain the restorative material in the tooth (except for the Class V preparation).

INTERNAL LINE ANGLE: It is a line angle whose apex points into the tooth.

INTERNAL WALL: An internal wall is a prepared (cut) surface that does not extend to the external tooth surface.

IRREVERSIBLE PULPITIS: It is the persistent inflammatory condition of the pulp, symptomatic or asymptomatic, caused by a noxious stimulus.

ISTHMUS: The part of class II cavity preparation that connects the occlusal preparation to the proximal box.

LINE ANGLE: A line angle is the junction of two planal surfaces of different orientation along a line.

LINERS: Are relatively thin layers of material used primarily to provide a barrier to protect dentin from residual reactants diffusing out of a restoration or from oral fluids (or both) that may penetrate leaky tooth restoration interfaces.

MAJOR APICAL DIAMETER: It is the apical part of root canal having the narrowest diameter short of the apical foramen or radiographic apex. It may or may not coincide with cemento-dentinal junction (CDJ).

MARGINAL RIDGES: These are the rounded borders of enamel that form mesial and distal margins of posterior teeth and mesial and distal margins of lingual surfaces of anterior teeth.

MATRICING: It is the procedure by which a temporary wall is built opposite to the axial wall, surrounding the tooth structure which has been lost during the tooth preparation.

MATRIX: It is an instrument which is used to hold the restoration within the tooth while it is setting.

MATRIX BAND: It is a piece of metal or polymeric material, intended to give support and form to the restoration during its insertion and setting.

MERCUROSCOPIC EXPANSION: Mercury from Sn-Hg of set amalgam re-reacts with Ag-Sn particles and produce further expansion during new reaction. This mechanism is called as mercuroscopic expansion.

MICROLEAKAGE: Flow of oral fluid and bacteria into the microscopic gap between a prepared tooth surface and a restorative material.

MULLING: It is a continuation of trituration, to increase the homogeneity of the amalgam mass.

NIB: For noncutting instruments, part corresponding to the blade is termed as nib.

NONHEREDITARY ENAMEL HYPOPLASIA: Nonhereditary enamel hypoplasia occurs when the ameloblasts are injured during enamel formation, resulting in defective enamel (diminished form and/or calcification).

OBLIQUE RIDGE: It is a ridge obliquely crossing the occlusal surface of maxillary first molar and is formed by union of triangular ridges of distobuccal cusp and distal cusp ridge of mesiopalatal cusp.

OBTURATION: To fill the shaped and debrided root canal space with a temporary or permanent filling material.

OPERATIVE DENTISTRY: Operative dentistry is the art and science of the diagnosis, treatment, and prognosis of defects of teeth that do not require full coverage restorations for correction. Such treatment should result in the restoration of proper tooth form, function, and esthetics while maintaining the physiologic integrity of the teeth in harmonious relationship with the adjacent hard and soft tissues, all of which should enhance the general health and welfare of the patient.

OUTLINE FORM: Establishing the outline form means:
- Placing the preparation margins in the positions they will occupy in the final preparation, except for finishing enamel walls and margins, and
- Preparing an initial depth of 0.2–0.8 mm pulpally of the DEJ position or normal root-surface position (no deeper initially whether in tooth structure, air, old restorative material, or caries unless the occlusal enamel thickness is minimal and greater dimension is necessary for strength of the restorative material).

PARTIAL ONLAY: Is cast metal restoration that involves the occlusal and proximal surface of a posterior and covers and restores at least one but not all of the cusp tips of posterior tooth.

PERIAPICAL ABSCESS (PERIRADICULAR ABSCESS): A localized collection of pus within the periradicular tissues. It is an inflammatory reaction to pulp infection and necrosis characterized by rapid onset, pus formation, spontaneous pain, tenderness on percussion, and eventually swelling to associated tissues.

PERIODONTITIS (PERICEMENTITIS): Inflammation of periodontium.

PIGGYBACK WEDGING: In this technique, one (larger) wedge is inserted as used normally, while the other smaller wedge (piggyback) is inserted above the larger one.

PITS: These are small pinpoint depressions located at the junction of developmental grooves.

POINT ANGLE: A point angle is the junction of three planal surfaces of different orientation.

POST: A post usually made of metal or fiber-reinforced composite resin that is fitted into a prepared root canal of a natural tooth; yttria-stabilized zirconia is also used as a post material; when combined with a core, it provides retention and resistance for an artificial crown; it is also used as a platform for retentive attachment systems and for a non-retentive overdenture post-coping.

POST-AND-CORE: A post with incorporated core; it provides retention and resistance for an artificial crown; it is also used as a platform for retentive attachment systems and non-retentive overdenture abutments.

PRIMARY CARIES: Primary caries is the original carious lesion of the tooth.

PRIMARY FLARE: First flare that brings proximal preparation out of contact area.

PRIMARY RESISTANCE FORM: Primary resistance form may be defined as that shape and placement of the preparation walls that best enable both the restoration and the tooth to withstand, without fracture, masticatory forces delivered principally in the long axis of the tooth.

PRIMARY RETENTION FORM: Primary retention form is that shape or form of the conventional preparation that resists displacement or removal of the restoration from tipping or lifting forces.

PRIMER: A hydrophilic, low viscosity resin that promotes bonding to a substrate, such as dentin. Resin tag-extension of resin that has penetrated into etched enamel or dentin.

PROPHYLACTIC ODONTOTOMY: Prophylactic odontotomy is presented only as a historical concept characterized by minimally preparing and filling with amalgam, developmental, structural imperfections of the enamel, such as pits and fissures, to prevent caries originating in these sites.

PULP CAPPING: Application of a material to protect the pulp from external influences and promote healing, done either directly or indirectly.

PULP CAVITY: The pulp cavity lies within the tooth and is enclosed by dentin all around, except at the apical foramen.

PULPAL WALL: A pulpal wall is an internal wall that is both perpendicular to the long axis of the tooth and occlusal of the pulp.

RESIDUAL CARIES: Residual caries is caries that remains in a completed tooth preparation, whether by operator intention or by accident.

RETAINER: It holds a band in desired position and shape. Retainers can be a mechanical device, floss, metal ring or impression compound.

REVERSE BEVEL OR COUNTER BEVEL: It is a bevel of which is prepared on the facial (lingual) margin of a reduced cusp with a flame-shaped, fine-grit diamond instrument.

REVERSIBLE PULPITIS: Is the general category which histologically may represent a range of responses varying from dentin hypersensitivity without concomitant inflammatory response to an early phase of inflammation.

RIDGE: It is any linear elevation on the surface of a tooth and is named according to its location. For example buccal or marginal ridge.

ROOT CANAL SYSTEM: The entire space in the dentin where the pulp is housed is called the root canal system.

ROOT SURFACE CARIES: Root surface caries may occur on the tooth root that has been both exposed to the oral environment and habitually covered with plaque.

RUNOUT: Dynamic test measuring the accuracy with which all blade tips pass a single point when the instrumented is rotated.

SCLEROTIC/EBURNATED DENTIN: An arrested, dentinal lesion typically is "open" (allowing debridement from tooth brushing), dark and hard, and this dentin is termed sclerotic or eburnated dentin.

SECONDARY (RECURRENT) CARIES: Secondary caries occurs at the junction of a restoration and the tooth and may progress under the restoration. It is often termed recurrent caries.

SECONDARY FLARE: Is given to provide marginal metal angle of 40 degree.

SHANK: Shank connects handle to working end of the instrument. It tapers from the handle down to the blade and is normally smooth, round or tapered.

SKIRT PREPARATION: Skirts are thin extension of facial or lingual proximal margins of the cast metal onlay that extend from primary flare to a termination just past the transition line angle of the tooth.

SMEAR LAYER: Poorly adherent layer of ground dentin produced by cutting a dentin surface.

SOLUTION LINERS: Any liner based on nonaqueous solvents that rely on evaporation for hardening is designated as a solution liner (or varnish).

STRONGEST ENAMEL MARGIN: The strongest enamel margin is one that is composed of full-length enamel rods supported on the preparation side by shorter enamel rods, all of which extend to sound dentin.

SUSPENSION LINER: Liners based on water have many of the constituents suspended instead of dissolved and are called suspension liners.

TOOTH PREPARATION is defined as the mechanical alteration of a defective, injured, or diseased tooth to best receive a restorative material that will re-establish a healthy state for the tooth, including esthetic corrections where indicated, along with normal form and function.

TRIANGULAR RIDGE: It descends from tip of cusp of molar and premolar towards central part of occlusal surface.

TRITURATION: Process to bring the particles of the alloy in contact with mercury.

UNSUPPORTED ENAMEL MARGIN: An enamel margin composed of rods which do not run uninterrupted from the surface to the sound dentin is termed as unsupported enamel margin.

WEDGE WEDGING: In this technique, two wedges are used, one wedge is inserted from lingual embrasure area while another is inserted between the wedge and matrix band at right angle to first wedge.

WORKING LENGTH: Defined as distance from a coronal reference point to a point at which canal preparation and obturation should terminate.

Index

Page numbers followed by *f* refer to figure and *t* refer to table.

A

Abfraction 26, 32, 33*f*
   clinical features 32
   etiology of 32
Abrasion 1, 26, 31
   cavities 32*f*
   etiology of 31
Abrasive
   classification of 70
   particle size 70
Acellular cementum 15
Acetylene 131
Acidulated phosphate fluoride gel 31
Acrylic teeth, artificial 1
Additives 129
Adhesion 48
   factors affecting 48
Adhesive 48
   cement, role of 48*f*
   dentistry 48
Adjacent tooth 67*f*
Admixed alloy 45
Agents
   activator-initiator 52
   coloring 52
Air pressure casting machine 131
Air-rotor contra-angle handpiece 68, 68*f*
Alloy 44
   melting of 131, 132*f*
   metals 44
   preamalgamated 44
Alumina 40
Aluminum polysalts 42
Alveolar bone 15
Amalgam 44, 94, 112
   capsule 155
   carrier 65, 65*f*, 146
   cusp capping for 112*f*
   insertion of 46
   mulling of 46
   pins 97
   polishing kit 153
   preparation 108*f*
   properties of 45*t*
   retention
      form for 94*f*
      retention to 95*f*
Amalgam alloy
   composition of 44*t*
   powder 154
      types of 45

Amalgam restoration
   cavity preparation for 109, 110*f*, 112
   manipulation of 46
   tooth preparation for 106
Amalgamation reaction 45
Amalgamator pestle 46*f*
Amelogenesis imperfecta 33*f*
Anatomic apex 140
Angle former excavator 63*f*
Anterior teeth, composite restoration in 118*f*
Antibacterial properties 27
Antisepsis 82
Apical constriction 141
Apical foramen 141
Apical root anatomy 141*f*
Arch, opposite 68
Argon laser curing unit 121
Armamentarium 3, 84
Articulating paper 154
Aseptic technique 82
Attrition 26, 31
   etiology of 31
Autocure glass ionomer cement, setting reaction of 42
Axial wall 90, 90*f*
Axiopulpal line angle, rounding of 111

B

Bacteria 26
Ball burnisher 3, 66*f*
Barbed broach 137, 139*f*
Base-metal alloy pellets 158
Bevel instruments, distal 61
Beveled conventional tooth preparation 118, 118*f*, 119*f*
Bibeveled instruments 61
Binangle chisel 63, 63*f*
Binary alloys 44
Biodentin 159
Birth injuries 33
Blue inlay wax 54*f*
Bonding 48
   agent, eighth generation 50, 50*f*
Buccal extension 108*f*
Buccolingual direction 140*f*
Bur
   classifications of 68
   design 70, 70*f*
   end-cutting 70
   entry of 119, 140*f*
   heads, designs of 70*f*
   inverted cone 70, 114*f*
   number, dimensions of 106*f*

parts of 69
pear-shaped 70
round 69
straight 69*f*
types of 69, 69*f*
Burnisher 65, 146

C

Calcium hydroxide 39, 40*f*, 157
   uses of 40
Calcium polyacrylate, formation of 42
Canal instrumentation, principles of 142
Candelilla wax 54
Canine 15, 19, 21
Carbohydrate intake, frequency of 26
Caries
   acute 28
   arrested 28
   complex 28
   compound 28
   detection, methods of 30
   primary 27, 27*f*
   progression, speed of 28
   recurrent 27*f*
   risk assessment 30
   risk, high 30
   secondary 27, 27*f*
   simple 28
   smooth surface 27, 27*f*
Carnauba wax 54
Carry amalgam alloy 47*f*
Carvers 3, 64, 65
Cast gold alloys
   classification of 53
   components of 53
Cast metal 94
   alloys 53
Cast metal restoration 126, 134*f*
   advantages of 126*t*
   cavity preparation for 126
   contraindications for 126*t*
   disadvantages of 126*t*
   indications for 126*t*
Casting
   cementation of 133
   cleaning of 132
   ring 160
   trying in 133
Casting machines 131
   types of 131
Cavitation 29
Cavity liners 96
Cavity preparation 108, 113, 123, 126, 134*f*
   final 108, 111, 114
   stages of 92
Cavosurface angle margin 90
Cellular cementum 15

Cement
   manipulation of 38, 42, 124
   spatulas 64, 64*f*
Cemento-dentinal junction 141
Cemento-enamel junction 6
Cementum 15
Central fossae 8
Central incisor
   distal of 9
   fractured 2*f*
Centres for disease control 82
Centrifugal casting machine 131, 131*f*
Ceresin 54
Cermet cement 41
Cheek retractor 152
Chisel 63, 146
   straight 63, 63*f*
Chlorhexidine gluconate 30
Chronic caries 28
Cingulum 7, 7*f*
Circumferential bevel 61
Cleaning 82
   and shaping 142
Clear plastic matrix strips 73
Cleoid discoid carver 64*f*, 65*f*
Collagen fibers 49
Complex tooth preparation 89, 90*f*, 96*f*
Composite gun 120*f*
Composite placement instruments 119
Composite polishing kit 153
Composite resin
   direct 117
   flowable 53
   instruments 66
   light-cured 155
   newer 53
Composite restorations 117, 123*f*
   advantages of 117*t*
   contraindications for 117*t*
   disadvantages of 117*t*
   fractured 3*f*
   indications for 117*t*
   instruments for 66*f*
   on teeth, steps of 117
   repair of 121
Composite tooth preparation 121
Condensers 3, 65
   types of 65*f*
Conservative tooth preparation 119
   modified 119*f*
Constituent metals, effects of 45*t*
Copper alloy
   admixed high 45
   high 44, 44*t*
   low 44, 44*t*
   unicompositional high 45
Copper content, based on 44

Coves 96
COVID-19 82
    and dentistry 82
Cowhorn 62f
CPITN probe 145
Cross-arch intraoral finger rest 67f
Crown 6
    and root 6
        division of 6f
Crown down 143f
    technique 143
Curing lamps, polymerization using 120
Cusp 7, 7f
    capping 94, 112

D

Dental amalgam 44, 106
    alloys 44
    classification of 44
    composition of 44
Dental bur 68
    parts of 68f
    slow-speed 147
    sterilization of 82
Dental caries 1, 26, 28f
    classification of 27
    diagnosis of 30
    etiology of 26
    histopathology of 29
    prevention of 30
Dental cements 36
    classification of 37
    uses of 36
Dental chair positions 81
Dental composites
    agents in 52f
    composition of 51
Dental handpiece, sterilization of 82
Dental history 30
Dental materials 36
    classification of 36
    properties of 36
Dental operatory 80
    guidelines for preparation of 83
Dental pulp 14, 15f
Dentifrices 31
Dentin 13, 14t
    adhesive systems consist 49
    affected 95t
    bonding 49
    bonding agent 49, 155
        generations of 50
    color 13
    composition 13
    functions of 14
    hardness 13
    hypocalcification, localized nonhereditary 34
    hypoplasia, localized nonhereditary 33
    infected 29, 95t
    intertubular 49
    normal 29
    primary 14t
    secondary 14, 14f, 14t
    structure 14
    subtransparent 29
    supported by 97f
    tertiary 14, 14f, 14t
    thickness 13
    transparent 29
Dentinal caries 29
    zones of 29, 29f
Dentinal tubules 14, 14f
Dentin-bonding agent
    evolution of 49
    generation
        fifth 49
        first 49
        fourth 49
        second 49
        seventh 50
        sixth 50, 50f
        third 49
Dentition, permanent 10f, 11f
Depressions, types of 8f
Diamond abrasive instruments 70
Diamond carver 65f
Diet
    chemical nature of 26
    nature of 26
Digital dental radiography 30
Direct wax pattern 128, 128f
Disinfection 82
Double wedging 75
    technique 76f
Dovetail in maxillary incisor, cavity preparation with 104

E

Egg shaped burnisher 66f
Electric melting units 132
Enamel 12, 14t
    bonding 48
    caries 29
    color 13
    composition 12
    formation, defective 33
    functions of 13
    hardness 13
    hatchet 63, 64f
    hypocalcification, localized nonhereditary 33
    hypoplasia, localized nonhereditary 33
    rods 12f
        direction of 13f
    structure 12
    thickness 13
    translucent
        bluish color of 13f
        gray color of 13f
    walls and margins, finishing of 108, 111

Enameloplasty 93, 94*f*
Endodontic
　basics of 136
　explorer 140*f*
　instruments 137, 137*t*
　　color for 138*f*
Equipment, disinfection of 88
Erosion 1, 32
　clinical picture of 32*f*
　etiology of 32
　intrinsic 32
Esthetic 16
　considerations 112
　improvement 1
　restorations 3*f*
　treatment 2*f*
Etchant 155
Etching and bonding 119
Ethoxybenzoic acid reinforced cement 37
　composition of 37
Ethyl silica bonded investment 129
Eugenol cement 37
Explorer, types of 61, 62*f*
Extrinsic erosion 32

F

Face mask 82
Face shield 82
　and goggles 84
Ferrier double bow separator 76*f*
Fiberoptic transillumination, digital imaging 30
Files 64*f*, 137
Fillers 51
Filling gold, direct 94
Finger rests 67
Finishing and polishing 47, 124, 133
Fissure bur, straight 70
Fissure caries 27
Flat pulpal 94*f*
Floor 90
Fluoride 30
　effects of 30
　products 30
　varnish 31
Fogger machine 84, 84*f*
Foramen, transportation of 143
Fossa 8
Four-number formula 60*f*
Friction-grip angle handpiece shank 69

G

Galvanic corrosion 47
Gingival bevels 128
Gingival floor 90*f*, 93, 94*f*
Gingival margin 93*f*
　trimmer 13, 60, 64 146
　　mesial and distal 64*f*
　　uses of 64

Gingival tissue 17
Gingival wall, preparation of 114*f*
Glass ionomer 41
　powder, composition of 41
　restoration, tooth preparation for 121
Glass ionomer cement 41, 96, 117, 121
　reaction of 44*f*
　resin-modified 42*f*, 96
　setting reaction of 42
　silver alloy admix 41
　steps for placement of 123
　type 1 157
　type 2 157
Gloves 82, 84
Gold inlays 126
Groove 8
Grossman's classification 137*t*
Gum dammer 54
Gypsum bonded investment 129, 131
　material 160
Gypsum investment material 130*f*

H

Hand cutting instrument 62
　parts of 59, 59*f*
Hand hygiene 82
Hand instruments 120*f*
Hand investing 130
Handpiece, types of 68
Hard surfaces, disinfection of 86
Head cap 82
Head covers 85
Hedstrom file 137
HEPA filter 84, 84*f*
Hoe excavator 62, 63*f*
Hollenback's carver 3, 65*f*
Hybrid composites 52
Hybrid technique 143*f*
Hydroxyapatite crystals 14
Hypocalcification 34*f*

I

Immunization 82
Incisal surfaces 9*f*
Incisors 15
　central 18, 20
　lateral 18, 20
　mesial of lateral 9
Incremental layering technique 120*f*
Indirect wax pattern 129*f*
　method 128
Infection, localized 33
Initial cavity preparation 106, 109, 112, 113
　stage 92
Inlay 126
　casting wax 54
　preparation, steps of 126
　wax 158

Instrument 3, 126, 145
   advantages of balancing of 59
   balancing of 59f
   bevels in cutting 60
   cutting 3, 59, 64
   description of 61
   designs, different 60
   excavating 3
   exploring 3
   formula 59
   grasps 66
   handle of 59f
   methods of use of 68
   mixing 3
   noncutting 59
   restoring 3
   triple-beveled 61
   with four-number formula 60f
Interproximal finishing strips 153
Interproximal space 17, 17f, 18f
Inverted pen grasp 66, 66f
Ion leachable glass 41
Irrigants, functions of 142
Irrigating solutions 142
Itaconic acid 40, 41
Ivory matrix
   band retainer 72
   holder 71

J

Juxtapose 1

K

K-file 137

L

Lathe-cut low copper alloys 45
Layering technique, horizontal 120f
Lesion
   body of 29
   smooth surface 92
Light cure unit 149
Light-emitting diode unit 121
Lingual cusps 21
Lingual extension 108f
Lingual portion, axial wall of 108f
Lingual surface 9f
Liquid, composition of 37, 38, 40, 41
Lobe 7, 7f
Loss of gloss 42

M

Magnesium oxide 40
Maleic acid 40, 41
Mamelons 7, 7f
Mandibular first molar 96f, 103
   cavity preparation in 104
   preparation of 93f, 103

Mandibular first premolar 112
Mandibular premolar, cavity preparation in 103
Marginal ditching 48f
Marginal ridge 7, 16
Masks 84
Mastication 15
Materials 154
Matricing 71
Matrix 71
   application 119
   parts of 71
Maxillary anterior teeth, erosion of 2f
Maxillary canine 32f
Maxillary central incisor, restoration of 122f
Maxillary first molar 104, 112
   cavity preparation in 103, 104
   preparation in 103
Maxillary incisor, cavity preparation in 104, 105
Maxillary molars, cavity preparation for 141f
Maxillary premolar, cavity preparation in 103
Maxillary second premolar 134f
Mechanical vacuum investing 130
Mercury 154
Mercury-alloy ratio 46
Mesial
   bevel instruments 61
   pit preparation 104
   wall, dentin from 143f
Mesiolingual cusp 7
Metal reinforced glass ionomer cements 41
Microfilled composites 52
Micromotor 68
   contra-angle handpiece 68f
Miracle mix 42f
Mixing calcium hydroxide cement 40
Molars 15
   and premolar, marginal ridge in 17f
   cavity preparation for 141f
   first 20, 22
   second 20, 22
Mortar and pestle 46f
Mosby's dental dictionary 1
Mouth mirror 61, 145
   sizes of 61, 61f
Mouthrinses 31
Mylar strips 75f, 148

N

Natural gas 131
NiTi instruments
   advantages of 139
   disadvantages of 139
NiTi rotary instruments 139

O

Oblique layering technique 120f
Oblique ridge 7
Occlusal aspect, attrition of 31f

Occlusal bevels 128
Occlusal step
   establishing 109
   proximally, extending 109
Occlusal surface 9*f*, 108, 123*f*
Occlusal thickness, minimum 94
Operating stool 80, 80*f*
Operative dentistry 1, 5, 58, 69*t*
   objectives of 1
   scope of 4
Oral habits, abnormal 31
Oral hygiene 30
   practice, faulty 31
   status of 30
Oral prophylaxis 117
Ordinary hatchet 62
Oxygen 131

P

Palatal and lingual embrasures 17*f*
Palatal extension 108*f*
Palatal surface 9*f*
Palm and thumb grasp 67, 67*f*
   modified 67, 67*f*
Paraffin wax 54
Paste-paste system 38
Pen grasp
   modified 66, 66*f*
   normal 66*f*
Periodontal ligament 15
Periodontium 15*f*
   significance of 15
Periradicular tissue 15
Personal hygiene 82
Personal protective equipment 84, 85*f*
Phosphate bonded investment 129, 131
   material 160
Pickling 133
Piggyback wedging 76
   technique 76*f*
Pigtail 62*f*
Pins 97
Pit 8, 27
Pit and fissure
   caries 27*f*
      in premolar 1*f*
   lesions 92*f*
   sealant 158
Plasma
   air sterilizer 84, 84*f*
   arc curing unit 120
Plaster model 3, 4*f*
Plastic consistency 46*f*
Plastic deformation 47
Plastic filling instrument 65, 65*f*, 146
Plastic wedges 75, 75*f*, 147
Polyacrylic acid 40, 41
Polycarboxylate cement 96

Polymer reinforced zinc oxide-eugenol cement 37
   composition of 37
Polymerization shrinkage 52
Post carve burnishing 47
Post-COVID dentistry 83
Powder 42
   diamond abrasive 70*f*
Precarve burnishing 46
Preclinical conservative dentistry 1, 3
Preclinical operative dentistry 1, 5
Preclinical tooth preparations 3
Premolars 15
   first 19, 21
   second 19, 21
Primary dentition 11*f*
Primary resistance form 93, 107, 111
Primary retention form 94
Primer 49
Probe 63*f*
Protective eyewear 82
Protective gown 82
Proximal box preparation 128
Proximal tooth preparation 93*f*
Pulp
   cavity 136, 136*f*
   chamber 14, 136, 136*f*
   features of 136
   protection 95, 96*t*, 108, 111, 119, 124, 128
Pulpal diseases, etiology of 137
Pulpal floor 90*f*
   rounded 94*f*
   two-level 111
Pulpal pathologies, progression of 137
Pulpal wall 90

Q

Quaternary alloys 44
Quenching 132

R

Rampant caries 28, 28*f*
Reamer 137
Refractory material 129
Remaining caries
   dentin, removal of 108, 128
   removal of 111
Remineralizing agents, application of 31
Reservoir 129
Resin matrix 51
Restoration 48
   design 28
   failure of 94*f*
   fracture of 48*f*
   repair of 1
   retention of 97*f*
   rocking motion of 94*f*
   type of 94, 96
Restorative instruments 64

Restorative material, thickness of 94
Restorative procedures 2*f*, 4*f*
Retention form, secondary 96*f*, 113
Retention grooves 96
Ridge 7
Root 6
Root canal 15, 136*f*, 137
    preparation 143
        techniques of 143
    system, irrigation of 142, 142*f*
Root caries 27, 27*f*
Rotary cutting
    instruments 68
    types of 68
Rubber dam
    clamp 150
    forceps 150
    frame 150
    napkin 151
    punch 150
    sheet 149
    template 151

S

Saliva 27
    composition of 27
    control 4
    pH of 27
    viscosity of 27
Sanitizer dispenser, sensor based 83*f*
SARS-CoV-2, transmission of 83*f*
Sclerotic dentin 14
Scrap amalgam 48
Self-etch
    adhesive 50
    primer 50
Shepherd's crook 62*f*
Silane coupling agents 52
Silica 40
Silver amalgam
    cavity preparation for 106
    phases of 45*t*
Simple box preparation 112
Simple tooth preparation 89, 89*f*
Single-beveled instruments 60, 60*f*
Skinner 52
Slump test 42
Smear layer, removal of 50
Speech 15
Spherical alloy 45
Spoon excavator 61, 61*f*, 63*f*, 146
Sprue diameter 128
Sprue former 159
    angulation of 129
    attachment of 128
    purpose of 128
    types of 128
Sprue length 128

Spruing wax pattern 128
Stannous fluoride 40
Step back technique 143
Straight handpiece 68
    shank 69
Streptococcus mutans 26
Sturdevant's classification 58
Sulcus 8
Synthetic waxes 54
Systemic disorders 33

T

Tapering-fissure bur 70
Ternary alloys 44
Thermal conductivity 47
Three-number formula 60*f*
Three-site technique 120*f*
Tissues, protection of supporting 16
Tofflemire
    band and retainer 75*f*
    matrix, indications of 72
    universal matrix band retainer 72
Tofflemire retainer 74*f*, 147
    and band, placement of 72
    parts of 72, 72*f*, 73*f*
    placement of 74*f*
Tooth 6, 26
    abrasion of 2*f*
    access cavity of anterior 139
    and restoration 48*f*
    anterior 16*f*, 140*f*
    biochemical structures of 26
    buccal surfaces of 9*f*
    carious lesions of 26
    connective tissue of 13
    contour of 16
    deciduous 11
    depressions present on 8
    discoloration of 3*f*
    distal surfaces of 9*f*
    enamel 12
    extracted 4
        natural 1
    fracture of 1, 33*f*, 48
    functions of 15
    inlay on posterior 126*f*
    labial surfaces of 9*f*
    mandibular 20
        anterior 2*f*
    maxillary 18
    mesial surfaces of 9*f*
    morphology of individual 18
    nomenclature of 9
    non-carious lesions of 26, 31
    occlusal surfaces of different 108
    onlay on posterior 126*f*
    overcontouring of 16
    permanent 10, 11, 13*f*

physiology form of 16
position of 26
posterior 16f, 31f
primary 10, 13f
requires, proper alignment of 93f
rotated 112
separation of 73
substance, causes of loss of 1
susceptible areas on 26
tetracyclin stains of 13f
translucency of 12
types of 15t, 16f
typodont 1
undercontouring of 16
Tooth preparation 1, 3, 4, 4f, 71, 91f, 92f, 103, 117, 118, 121f, 123, 124
   classification of 91
   compound 89, 89f
   designs 91t
   different 90
   extend 127f
   external walls of 90f
   final 113
      stages of 95
   finishing external walls of 97
   for composites, designs of 118
   internal walls of 90f
   principles of 89, 117
   steps of 92
   type of 71t, 91
Tooth structure
   causes of loss of 5
   in abfraction, loss of 33
   less 111f
   noncarious loss of 1
   weakened 94
Tooth surfaces 26
   based on 28
   buccal 28
   distal 28
   facial 28
   integrity of 26
   lingual 28
   mesial 28
   number of 28
   occlusal 28
   only one 89f
Total etch technique, mechanism of bonding in 49
Traction principle 76
Transparent crown forms matrices 73
Transverse ridge 7
Trituration 46
T-shaped matrix band 73, 75f
Tungsten-quartz halogen curing unit 120
Turbid dentin 29
Tweezer 61, 62f, 145
Typhodonts 3

U

Under-triturated mix 46
Universal tooth notation system 11f

V

Varnish 95, 96f, 156
Vertical layering technique 120f
Vision using mirror, indirect 61f

W

Wax elimination and heating 130
Wax pattern
   burnout of 130, 131f
   fabrication 128
   investing 129
   washing of 129
Wedelstaedt chisel 63, 63f
Wedge
   types of 73
   wedging 76
      technique 76f
Wedging techniques 75
   modified 75
Wooden wedges 73, 75f, 147

Z

Zinc
   containing alloys 44
   content, based on 44
   free alloys 44
   oxide 40
   oxide-eugenol powder, composition of 37
   polyacrylate cement 40
Zinc oxide eugenol cement 37, 37f, 156
   manipulation of 38
   setting reaction of 37
Zinc phosphate cement 38, 96, 156
   composition of 38
   hydrated 38
   types of 38
Zinc polycarboxylate cement 40, 40f, 157
   composition of 40
   manipulation of 40
Zinc silicophosphate cements 39
   properties of 39
Zoe cement
   manipulation of 38f
   setting reaction of 39f
Zsigmondy-palmer system 9
   tooth notation 10f

EU GSPR Authorised Reprsentative
Logos Europe, 9 rue Nicolas Poussin
1700, La Rochelle, France
Phone: +33 (0) 6 67 93 73 78
E-mail: contact@logoseurope.eu

www.ingramcontent.com/pod-product-compliance
Ingram Content Group UK Ltd.
Pitfield, Milton Keynes, MK11 3LW, UK
UKHW050431150426
5217IPUK00019B/1336